EVERYTHING
You Need to Know about
MENOPAUSE

A Comprehensive Guide

to Surviving—and Thriving—

During This Turbulent

Life Stage

Edited by **Ellen Phillips**
and the Editors of
PREVENTION
Health Books®
for Women

RODALE

© 2003 by Rodale Inc.

Photographs © 2003 by Rodale Inc.

Editorial and Writing Team for *Everything You Need to Know about Menopause*: Ellen Phillips, Shea Zukowski, Karen Neely, Gale Maleskey, Sandi Lloyd, Julia Van Tine, Karen Bolesta, Anne Winthrop Esposito, Lois Hazel

Library of Congress Cataloging-in-Publication Data

    Everything you need to know about menopause : a comprehensive guide to
surviving—and thriving—during this turbulent life stage / edited by
Ellen Phillips and the editors of Prevention health books for women.
        p.   cm.
    Includes index.
    ISBN 1–57954–788–5 hardcover
    1. Menopause—Popular works.   I. Phillips, Ellen.   II. Prevention
health books for women.
RG186.C6246   2003
618.1'75—dc21   2003009702

    4 6 8 10 9 7 5 3   hardcover

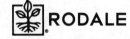

RODALE

CONTENTS

MENOPAUSE: NEW DIRECTIONS

No two women go through menopause in exactly the same way. One experiences hot flashes that will melt steel; others suffer chills—or one of 50 other possible mental or physical changes. In the past, most women confronted by menopause had two choices: Suffer the symptoms (usually in silence), or take a hormone pill. But thanks to the startling findings of the Women's Health Initiative Study, which concluded that the potential health hazards of using Prempro, an estrogen-progesterone combination, outweighed its benefits, and the subsequent National Toxicology Program's classification of estrogen as a carcinogen, women—and their doctors—have been thrown into turmoil. Women who are nearing menopause or are in the midst of it are asking themselves, What do I do now? And they're realizing that there are no easy answers.

In some ways, the flurry of publicity surrounding the study results and the FDA ruling has been a good thing. For one, it's brought menopause out of the closet and into the open. When *Time* magazine runs a cover story on menopause, women find it easier to talk about it—with one another, with their families, with their doctors—rather than suffering in silence, wondering what on earth is happening or is going to happen to them, and fearing the future. For another, it's forced the medical profession to take alternative therapies seriously. Doctors are telling their patients about soy for hormonal imbalances, black cohosh for relief of menopausal symptoms, yoga for stress relief, and a host of other options, as well as discussing all the conventional treatments. Finally, menopause's unlikely entry into the spotlight has given women the opportunity to look at it in new ways. Rather than viewing menopause as a disease to be "cured"—or at least postponed—by medical treatment, or as the gateway to old age, women are starting to see it as an empowering life stage. Bestsellers like Dr. Christiane Northrup's *The Wisdom of Menopause* and Dr. Mary Jane Minkin's pioneering *What Every Woman Needs to Know about Menopause* have paved the way for this very positive change.

But one thing is certain: More than ever, perimenopausal, menopausal, and postmenopausal women have to take their lives and their treatment into their own hands, because virtually every lifestyle change you make today will affect your health and vitality for the rest of your life. These critical changes can make the difference between a slow decline into helplessness and the best years of your life. And that's why we've written this book—to give you the guidance you need to make the best choices for you. We've consulted the top experts in the field, drawn from the latest research, and sifted through all the conflicting data to bring you the definitive guide for what could be the beginning of the most exciting, fulfilling time of your life. Whether you're 35 and just experiencing a few odd symptoms, facing menopause and wondering about your options, or on the other side and looking ahead, this book will give you a wealth of doctor-approved ways to manage your symptoms, your diet, your moods, your stress levels, your looks—even your sex life!

Turn to our extensive "Menopause Symptom Solver" to look up symptoms as you experience them—and for every menopausal woman, the range and severity of symptoms will vary—and find out all the recommended conventional and alternative treatments and preventives for each symptom. Chapters on conventional and alternative treatment options allow you to read in-depth about each treatment, its advantages and drawbacks, when and how it works best, and what can enhance its performance, as well as which remedies should never be combined. Other helpful features are "Straight Talk about Menopause," answering women's most frequently asked questions, and the "Top 10 Menopause Must-Dos," essential for every menopausal or perimenopausal woman.

Menopause confronts women with unique challenges: Our bodies present us with a wide range of often debilitating symptoms, our moods and emotions seem out of our control, we begin gaining midbody weight for no reason, we may lose interest in sex, and new sags and wrinkles mysteriously pop up on our faces and bodies every day, adding the specter of old age to all the other changes. *Everything You Need to Know about Menopause* presents a comprehensive program to help women triumph over each of these challenges, conquer the stress that menopause often piles onto an already hectic lifestyle, and emerge attractive, centered, and vibrantly healthy. Please join us for the journey!

—*Ellen Phillips, Editor*

PART

1

What's Going On?

Your body's changing, medical recommendations are changing, your moods and emotions are changing—suddenly, it seems like *everything's* changing! In this section, we'll tell you what to expect before, during, and after menopause, so none of the possible symptoms will take you by surprise. And we'll give you our top 10 recommendations for getting a fast grip on the situation, minimizing discomfort, and laying the foundation for vibrant good health, good looks, and good times for the rest of your life.

Chapter

1

WHAT TO EXPECT: A MENOPAUSE TIMELINE

IF YOU'RE GEARING UP TO GO THROUGH MENOPAUSE, OR HAVE already done so, you must know you're not alone. Menopause has come out of the closet in a big way, as the huge wave of Baby Boomer females who took control of our reproductive health during the 1970s and beyond are now taking control of our postreproductive years.

Unlike our mothers, most of us never have defined ourselves solely as mothers or wives. So it's only natural that we take that expansive sense of self with us into our later years. We are not buying the traditional role of "little old lady." In fact, we may be the first generation of grandmas who pump iron to prevent osteoporosis and use testosterone to boost sex drive. (A testosterone patch for women is currently in clinical trials.)

In the past, menopause and the years beyond were often painted as a bleak picture—a time of depression, low energy, and terminal crabbiness—mostly because women didn't see their doctors about it unless they had serious symptoms. But more recently, women's experience shows that menopause is *not* all negative for most women. If it seems to be really bad for you, you'd be wise to discuss it with your doctor. A good doctor can

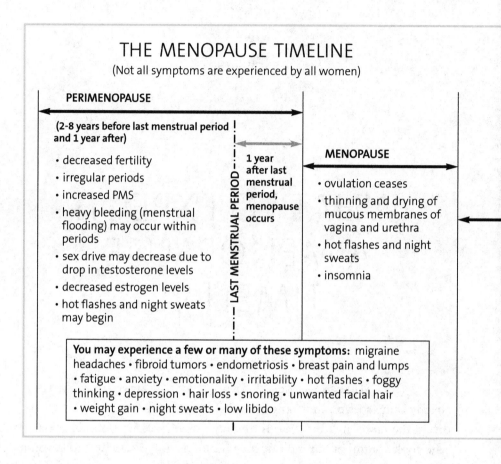

THE MENOPAUSE TIMELINE
(Not all symptoms are experienced by all women)

PERIMENOPAUSE

(2-8 years before last menstrual period and 1 year after)

- decreased fertility
- irregular periods
- increased PMS
- heavy bleeding (menstrual flooding) may occur within periods
- sex drive may decrease due to drop in testosterone levels
- decreased estrogen levels
- hot flashes and night sweats may begin

LAST MENSTRUAL PERIOD

1 year after last menstrual period, menopause occurs

MENOPAUSE

- ovulation ceases
- thinning and drying of mucous membranes of vagina and urethra
- hot flashes and night sweats
- insomnia

You may experience a few or many of these symptoms: migraine headaches • fibroid tumors • endometriosis • breast pain and lumps • fatigue • anxiety • emotionality • irritability • hot flashes • foggy thinking • depression • hair loss • snoring • unwanted facial hair • weight gain • night sweats • low libido

figure out which of your problems are related to menopause and which aren't, and provide help in both cases.

More recently, menopause has also been romanticized as a time of new wisdom, freedom, and inner strength, and that's certainly possible for those who use this time of transition for self-growth. (It doesn't happen automatically!) The groundbreaking book on postmenopausal empowerment is Dr. Christiane Northrup's *The Wisdom of Menopause*. We strongly recommend it.

But even as menopause has finally come out of the closet and started to take on positive overtones, it has become more challenging, too. In the past, women were encouraged by their doctors to normalize their hormone levels and ward off menopausal symptoms by taking estrogen

POSTMENOPAUSE

- skin becomes thin
- cholesterol levels increase
- good cholesterol (HDL) decreases
- bones become more brittle; risk of osteoporosis and fractures increases
- muscles lose tone
- increased risk of heart disease
- hot flashes may continue
- increased risk of cancer

The symptoms in this timeline may look intimidating—even scary. It's important to remember that some women go through menopause without experiencing any symptoms, and most symptoms can be prevented or treated. (We'll show you how in the rest of this book!) The purpose of this timeline is to act as a checkpoint for you, so if you experience symptoms, you'll be able to identify them instantly and then take the appropriate action.

or estrogen/progesterone in pill form, a treatment called hormone therapy (HT, formerly called hormone replacement therapy, HRT). Most doctors are now reluctant to prescribe HT in light of the recent study by the National Institutes of Health that linked hormone therapy to cancer, as well as the inclusion of estrogen replacement therapy on the U.S government list of cancer-causing agents. (See "New Directions" on page v for more about these findings.)

Because of the potential dangers of hormone therapy, all women need to take a more active role in managing their menopause, both to prevent future problems like osteoporosis and weight gain and to minimize or eliminate unpleasant symptoms like hot flashes. And that's what this book is about.

In this chapter, we'll present a timeline of facts about menopause and the years before and after. Menopause is inevitable, and, as with everything else that happens in life, it's up to you to make the best of it, with both good self-care and good medical care. Every woman is different, but most can fit themselves somewhere into this time frame. Keep in mind that while medicine creates premenopausal, perimenopausal, and postmenopausal categories, women's symptoms don't always fit so neatly into that scheme. So read through this short chapter and see the whole range of symptoms and experiences that can occur during these transitional years. Then, whatever you're experiencing, you'll know where it fits in the overall menopause picture.

What Is Menopause, Anyway?

Even the word "menopause" is used loosely. The term actually refers to only *one day* in your life—the 365th day from the date of your last period. (The time after that is called postmenopause.) It's only in retrospect that you know you have reached menopause, and plenty—in fact, most—women have lots of "false starts." They may go for months without a period, and then get one—usually while on vacation.

This demarcation is medically important because menopause means your body no longer produces enough estrogen to support a menstrual cycle. Doctors are much more suspicious of irregular uterine bleeding after menopause—during perimenopause (2 to 8 years before your last menstrual period and 1 year after), it's a given.

The average age of "natural" menopause (that is, not induced by surgery, chemotherapy, or radiation) in this country is 51, and that figure hasn't changed much over the past few centuries. The normal range is ages 46 to 54. But some women reach menopause in their thirties, and a few in their sixties. Women who smoke tend to reach menopause a year or two earlier than nonsmokers. Overweight women tend to have a later menopause since body fat can convert some hormone precursors into estrogen. (This higher estrogen level also puts overweight women at increased risk for breast cancer.) Thin women tend to have a harder time of it at menopause, and are at higher risk for osteoporosis, than women with some extra body fat.

IS IT REALLY MENOPAUSE?

The only way to know for sure if you're in the perimenopause transition, or if you have reached menopause itself, is through a visit to your doctor. He or she will rule out pregnancy or serious health problems like uterine cancer and will take a blood test to assess your estrogen levels.

The most reliable test measures the level of follicle-stimulating hormone (FSH), a hormone secreted by the pituitary gland to stimulate estrogen production. As the ovaries' estrogen production decreases, the pituitary gland increases production of FSH. Levels of 30 to 40 mIU/mL (milli international units per milliliter) or above mean you've reached menopause. Levels from 10 to near 30 mean there's still partial ovarian function.

Even FSH levels, however, can sometimes be misleading. They tend to fluctuate from month to month during perimenopause. To confirm whether you're in perimenopause, your doctor should review not only your FSH results but also your medical history and the physical and emotional changes you're experiencing (irregular periods, hot flashes, and so forth).

Some doctors won't do the FSH test unless you seem too young to be entering menopause. They'll simply assume on the basis of your symptoms that you're menopausal. If you believe yourself to have reached menopause and want to make sure, ask your doctor to check your FSH levels if he or she doesn't volunteer to do so.

What Causes Menopause?

The answer to this question is a simple one: our ovaries. Women depend on their ovaries to produce most of the estrogen in their bodies. Ovaries also produce progesterone, a hormone that is less understood than estrogen but that also has whole-body effects. (A recent study shows that just like estrogen, progesterone can help reduce the incidence of hot flashes and help you sleep better.) Ovaries even produce small amounts of androgen hormones—the male stuff that fuels sex drive in both men and women. Unfortunately, our ovaries have a lifespan that's shorter than our current lifespan of about 75 years. They tend to conk out about 25 years before the rest of our bodies.

The ovaries' manufacture of estrogen and progesterone is dependent on a complex network of other hormones, including follicle-stimulating hormone (FSH) and luteinizing hormone (LH), both secreted by the brain's pituitary gland. Hormone production also depends on the ability of the ovaries to mature and release a ripe egg. The maturing egg "sac," called the follicle, secretes estrogen. After the egg is released, the empty egg sac, called the corpus luteum, secretes progesterone.

Lots of things start working against our ovaries as we age. First, an accelerated depletion of eggs from the ovaries begins somewhere between ages 35 and 40. Many eggs die off during a cycle, and sometimes more than one ripens during a cycle—hence the higher incidence of twins for women in their thirties than in their twenties. The ovaries also become less responsive to the stimulating effects of FSH and LH, so levels of these hormones start to rise. You have fewer cycles in which you ovulate, and because progesterone is produced in the corpus luteum, after ovulation you might see a drop-off of progesterone first, while estrogen levels remain closer to normal. This condition, called estrogen dominance, is the reason some alternative doctors have recommended supplemental progesterone to women during the perimenopausal years.

Finally, there are no more eggs to be released, so there is no egg follicle to secrete estrogen or, after an egg is released, to switch over and secrete progesterone. Progesterone drops to very low levels, but the ovaries continue to make declining amounts of estrogen for a few years after menopause. Eventually, however, they become nonfunctioning as endocrine glands. The adrenal glands, however, continue to make small amounts of sex hormone precursors, such as DHEA (dehydroepiandrosterone). These can be converted to estrogen (or testosterone) in the fat tissues of the body.

In addition to estrogen, your blood levels of testosterone, the "hormone of desire," drop by about 50 percent between ages 20 and 40, and then more slowly trail the decline of estrogen after menopause.

Perimenopause: The Start of It All

The term perimenopause was coined only recently, in the 1990s. *Peri-*, by the way, means "near" or "around," so perimenopause simply means "around the time of menopause." It now officially refers to the 2 to 8 years preceding menopause and the year after menopause. So, for most women, perimenopause begins sometime in the mid-forties, but it can begin as early as the mid- to late thirties. (See "Too Young for Menopause?" below.)

Perimenopause is a time of hormone fluctuations that may begin fairly subtly, then slowly become more exaggerated as a woman approaches menopause. Estrogen levels may go as high as those seen during early pregnancy, only to drop and stay low for some time. Health conditions influenced by unstable hormone levels are likely to worsen during this time. These include migraine headaches, fibroid tumors, endometriosis, PMS, irregular menstrual cycles, and fibrocystic breast disorder.

Women also usually have their first hot flashes and night sweats during this time—and may at first wonder, "What the heck is this?!" Some women complain of fatigue; of emotionality, anxiety, or irritability; of foggy thinking; or of just plain not feeling right. We all need to realize that the feelings we're having at this time aren't simply emotional—they're the result of actual hormonal changes in our bodies. Even the brain has receptor sites for estrogen—and feels deprived when it doesn't get the hormone in the amounts it expects.

For many women, perimenopause is a rougher ride than post-menopause. Luckily, many of the lifestyle changes we suggest in this book are helpful for these symptoms. Natural alternatives—such as black cohosh, soy foods, and progesterone cream—can also make a big difference

TOO YOUNG FOR MENOPAUSE?

Menopause before age 40, technically called premature ovarian failure, is rare. Only about 1 percent of women go through menopause before age 40. It tends to run in families, and tests often show that these women have developed an immune response to their bodies' own ovarian tissue. There also seems to be an association between premature ovarian failure and other autoimmune diseases, such as type 1 diabetes, thyroiditis, and rheumatoid arthritis. Bottom line: If you're in your thirties and experiencing signs of menopause, get your estrogen and follicle-stimulating hormone measured. And get a thyroid-stimulating hormone (TSH) test as part of your workup.

to women during this time. Some doctors will also give women low-dose birth control pills to help control erratic hormone levels. And also, luckily, over time our bodies adjust to lower hormone levels so that by the time we're postmenopausal, some symptoms will have started to subside. But meanwhile, if you're experiencing unpleasant symptoms, check them out in chapter 10, look up the recommended conventional and alternative treatments we recommend, and discuss with your doctor those that make sense to you.

Postmenopause: When It's Finally Over

Once you've gone a full year without periods, you are considered to be in the postmenopausal phase of your life. Your ovaries no longer produce enough estrogen and progesterone to support an ovulation cycle.

But far from its being the beginning of the end, many women see the time after menopause as a new beginning. In survey after survey sponsored by the North American Menopause Society, women consistently report that their postmenopausal years are the most fulfilling and happiest of their lives. Close to 80 percent of women say that cessation of menstruation came as a relief. More than half say that reaching menopause was a positive turning point in their lives. They report having more time and energy to focus on hobbies, relationships, and other interests. And three out of four made some type of health-related improvement, such as finally quitting smoking. And that's all for the best since most women are postmenopausal for about one-third of their lives.

Symptoms linked to hormonal instability tend to diminish as we reach menopause, so migraines, PMS, and endometriosis will tend to improve. Hot flashes will usually continue for a few years after menopause, but they will gradually fade away.

Still, even if you have no immediate obvious symptoms as a result of your having reached menopause, over time you most definitely will have physical changes, as a result of both diminishing hormone levels and aging. You'll have thinning and drying of the mucous membranes of the vagina and urethra, which can set the stage for painful intercourse or urinary incontinence. You'll have gradual thinning of the skin, as well as slowly rising total cho-

HORMONE THERAPY FOR YOUR HUSBAND?

Picture the commercial: A bunch of guys are sitting around watching the big game, drinking a few brews, when one of them pipes up: "Guys, I haven't been feeling myself lately. My doctor thinks I might need to go on HT. I'm not sure what to do."

A big, burly man named Bud comes back with: "I know how you feel, Al. But since I've been on testosterone, I feel great! I'm vibrant, and my sex life has never been better!" The guys raise their beer steins in raucous approval while the name of a prescription flashes on the screen.

This scene might not be so far-fetched. Male hormone therapy is available now and is expected to grow in popularity in the coming years.

The main hormone in male HT is testosterone, says Keith Gordon, Ph.D., associate director for reproductive medicine at Organon in West Orange, New Jersey.

As with estrogen in women, testosterone starts to decline during a man's forties. Early on, testosterone deficiency presents itself as general malaise, depression, and perhaps muscle weakness, Dr. Gordon says. As the decline progresses, it can affect sexual function and, in the long-term, speed up osteoporosis. To ward off all these troubles, a man can take supplemental testosterone.

But just as with our hormone therapy, he'll have to weigh the benefits against the risks. In a man's case, supplemental testosterone could bring on benign prostatic hyperplasia, a condition in which the prostate grows larger and pushes against the urethra or bladder, blocking the normal flow of urine. If a man has the early stages of prostate cancer, testosterone could also speed the cancer's growth, Dr. Gordon says.

lesterol levels and a drop in the "good" stuff—HDL cholesterol. You're likely to lose bone mass and muscle tone, especially if you don't exercise.

Some of these effects take decades to show up, but they do show up sooner or later in most women. These things are also very treatable, both with lifestyle changes and, if necessary, with drugs. Women who choose not to use hormone therapy (HT) to keep their bones strong, for instance, can do resistance training or take a bone-saving drug—a number of them are now on the market. Even some forms of HT can be used selectively to reduce symptoms without much risk. (Case in point: Estring, a vaginal ring that delivers a tiny amount of estrogen to prevent vaginal dryness and atrophy and that also can help maintain the urethra. Its systemic effects are minimal.) Women whose main complaint is loss of sex drive may find that a little testosterone cream applied to the clitoris provides the boost they need. (For details, see chapter 9.)

Fewer than half of postmenopausal women took estrogen before the recent studies implicating it in heart disease and cancer, and these days, with the bad press hormone therapy is receiving, even fewer are likely to take it, or at least to take it in its most commonly prescribed forms—Premarin and Prempro. Using no hormone therapy does make things harder for a woman. There's no easy way to make up for the fact that our bodies have run out of estrogen. But there are ways to compensate—they include alternative therapies like soy foods and phytoestrogen-containing herbs, exercise, and other lifestyle changes. We have literally hundreds of suggestions to help you in the rest of this book. So please join us as we look at the next chapter, "Top 10 Menopause Must-Dos," which includes such tactics as eating and exercising to boost health and beat menopausal weight gain, dealing with stress, managing your moods, and making sex great again, plus a host of suggested supplements and other treatments you can choose from. This book is designed to help you put it all together and have an easy menopause and a vibrant, healthy life once it's over.

Chapter

2

TOP 10 MENOPAUSE MUST-DOs

THE AMOUNT OF INFORMATION THERE IS ABOUT MENOPAUSE MAY seem overwhelming. Where do you start? If you want to make some fast, positive changes that will keep you happy, healthy, and sane throughout the transition into menopause and beyond, start here. These 10 scientifically sound, safe "menopause must-dos" are the best gifts you can give your body—and yourself.

Menopause Must-Do #1: Minimize Weight Gain with Mini-Meals

One annoying, embarrassing, and just plain infuriating thing about menopause is that you'll probably find yourself mysteriously starting to pile on pounds—especially around the middle—even though you're eating as little and exercising as much as ever. What's going on? Aren't hot flashes, irregular periods, menstrual flooding, and crabby moods bad enough?

The good news is: It really *isn't* your fault. When you pass through menopause, at around age 50 or so, your energy requirement drops to about 15 percent less than it was when you were in your twenties. One reason for this is a change in metabolism—the rate at which you burn calories. Basal metabolic rate drops by approximately 5 percent per decade of life. When you hit 40, you are entering your third 5 percent decrease in metabolism. So you need less energy—and that means fewer calories, the body's energy-producing fuel—just to stay in the same place. If you eat the way you always did, it will start to add up—as increased pounds.

At the same time, as you reach middle age—and if you are sedentary—you experience an extreme drop in muscle mass compared with when you were younger. A sedentary person can expect to lose more than 7 pounds of muscle every 10 years! Since muscle mass is your calorie-burning furnace, this loss of muscle results in yet another decreased need for calories—you may need to forgo up to 400 calories a day just to maintain your normal weight.

It's no wonder so many women say they are eating less and still gaining weight during this time. Figuring out how to eat less without feeling deprived and like you're on a permanent diet is a challenge, but there *is* a way—and it's positively ingenious. In fact, you'll probably feel a bit naughty—like you're "cheating"—because this midlife eating plan goes against the "don't eat between meals" rule you've struggled with all your life.

The truth is that you *won't* be eating between meals—you'll actually be eating *more* meals. They'll just be smaller. But because you'll eat every few hours rather than wait until you're ravenous and then wolf down a day's worth of calories at every meal, you'll stay satisfied and maybe even make healthier eating choices since you won't feel like you'll faint from hunger if you don't eat whatever's closest (usually a bag of chips or a chocolate bar) right now or *else*.

A healthy mini-meal consists of 250 to 400 calories and contains a healthy balance of carbohydrates, fats, and protein. This calorie total is important, and here's why: Research shows that the more times you eat each day, the more total calories you tend to consume. You need to be careful that the calories don't creep up—which can happen all too easily if you're eating six times a day!

Ask the Experts:

Mini-Meals

Experts say that if you're trying to lose weight, eating less but more often—the mini-meal concept—may take the edge off your appetite so you don't wind up feeling ravenous and tempted to binge on fast food. But there's more to it than that.

Research suggests that older women burn fat from large meals less effectively than younger women, but they burn fat from smaller meals just as well as younger women. Researchers believe your fat-burning ability drops because of hormonal changes.

In a 1997 study at the Jean Mayer USDA Human Nutrition Research Center on Aging at Tufts University, older women had higher levels of glucagon, a hormone that triggers the release of sugar into the blood—the opposite effect of insulin. With more sugar available to fuel body processes, women burned less fat.

Mini-meals, on the other hand, allow you to burn about 10 percent more calories a day, due to the thermal effect of eating, which keeps your metabolism running on high. This thermal effect is more active when you eat smaller meals more often, rather than fewer, larger meals. You also put less stress on your heart. Eating a big meal can increase your risk of having a heart attack. A heavy meal makes the heart beat up to 30 percent faster. Smaller meals lessen this effect. Plus, healthy mini-meals help stabilize blood sugar, which will help you stave off cravings and mood swings.

Mini-Meal Basics

You'll find a lot more about mini-meals in chapter 3, but here are four tips to get you started. If you follow them faithfully, you'll be on your way to mini-meal success!

- **Use portion control.** Measure out what you plan to eat beforehand, or buy single-serving packages. Follow the Food Pyramid guidelines for serving sizes (and remember, alas, they're a lot smaller than the portions we're used to eating).

- **Eat real foods, not fast food.** Don't get your mini-meals from the snack aisle, snack machines, or McDonald's, or you'll end up eating empty calories—and far too many of them! If you plan ahead, it takes but a minute to pack apples, cheese, almonds, yogurt, skim milk, or whatever you fancy, so you'll have wholesome food at hand when hunger hits.

- **Eat a variety of foods.** We know it's tempting to just grab the yogurt and banana every day, but remember: You may be eating little meals, but you still need to get the full spectrum of nourishment from what you're eating. Meat, poultry, fish, beans, eggs, nuts, and dairy products; grains; fruits and vegetables—choose some from each group (like your mother told you) to get protein, carbohydrates, and a little fat. One trick to make this easier is to fix a bigger meal and break it into two portions, one to eat now, one later.

- **When you eat out, eat for one, not two.** Always get a doggie bag or order an appetizer-size meal. Most restaurant meals these days are at least two servings big—and they will sabotage your mini-meal program.

Mini-meals aren't the only option, but they're one option that definitely works. For more options and more on mini-meals, menopause-savvy eating, and maintaining your figure, see chapter 3.

Menopause Must-Do #2: Take Your Calcium and Vitamin D

Unless you're taking estrogen, you will experience some bone loss at menopause, which sets the stage for osteoporosis. That's because estrogen is involved in maintaining bone mass, and estrogen production drops as menopause progresses. A drop in estrogen levels causes more bone breakdown and less bone building to occur, and the result is bone loss. The total bone loss in the spine, for instance, is about 15 percent over the 5-year period just after menopause. (The bone loss then continues at a much slower pace.) Getting enough calcium can slow bone loss and reduce your risk of fractures.

To reduce your risk of fractures, you need to get 1,200 to 1,500 milligrams a day of calcium once you're over 50. (Most women get about 500 milligrams a day from food.) You can slow bone loss even more by also making sure you get enough vitamin D—400 IU a day up to age 70, and

ASK THE EXPERTS:

Calcium

Make sure you're getting the calcium and vitamin D you need. Experts say it will help protect you from broken bones. Recent clinical trials have suggested that supplementation with calcium, or calcium plus vitamin D, can reduce fracture incidence by about 30 to 50 percent in people with low calcium intakes.

But just as bone loss occurs over time, it takes a while to get maximum protection from calcium supplements. In one large study done in France, it took 18 months for older women getting calcium and vitamin D supplements to show a 40 percent reduction in hip fractures. In another study, at the end of 3 years, calcium and vitamin D supplementation had reduced fracture rates at all sites by 55 percent.

The people in most of these studies were women age 65 or older, when bone loss starts showing up as fractures. But don't wait until then to start taking calcium and vitamin D. The goal is to prevent bone loss as well as bone breaks!

600 IU a day after that. (Take 800 IU if you are housebound since vitamin D is naturally produced by your body when you're outdoors and exposed to sunlight.)

We recommend that you get at least some of your daily calcium from dairy products because dairy products provide a ratio of calcium, protein, and phosphorus that is ideal for bone health. (Milk is also fortified with vitamin D.) And if you drink fat-free milk and eat fat-free yogurt and cheese, you won't need to worry about piling on calories while you're taking in calcium. (For more tips on calcium-rich foods, see chapter 3.)

Calcium Basics

If you take calcium supplements to make up for what your diet doesn't provide, keep these tips in mind.

- **Don't take more than you need.** Take no more than 500 milligrams at one time. Your body can't absorb more than that.
- **Save by taking calcium with food.** If you take your calcium with meals, just take the cheapest form, calcium carbonate.

- **If absorption could be a problem . . .** If you need to take calcium between meals or have low stomach acid, take calcium citrate or calcium aspartate, the most absorbable forms.

- **Give your bones a phosphorus boost.** If you rely on calcium supplements *alone* (because you eat no dairy foods), consider taking a calcium–phosphorus combination, tricalcium phosphorus.

- **Give calcium time to work.** Remember, it takes time for calcium to stop bone loss. (See "Ask the Experts: Calcium" on page 17.) That's why starting a calcium supplement regimen early on is such a smart move—you'll prevent problems rather than having to try to reverse them. But the good news is that the effects are cumulative, so as long as you continue supplementation, you'll continue building protection right into your bones!

There are other options for keeping your bones healthy, including exercise and bone-building drugs like Fosamax. (We'll discuss those exercises next here and in chapter 4. You can read more about Fosamax, estrogen replacement, and other options in chapter 11.) But no matter what else you do, you should still supplement your diet with calcium because your body requires optimal calcium intake for maximum bone density. To find out more about the kinds of calcium supplements that are available and what each one does, see chapter 5.

Menopause Must-Do #3: Try These Three Easy Exercises

There's more to protecting your bones than getting enough calcium every day. Weight-bearing exercises keep your bones strong (and your muscles toned, and your skin taut and youthful . . . but we're getting ahead of ourselves). We're not talking about lifting huge barbells or anything, either. Putting weight on a bone or joint is what matters. The goal is to target the three areas most likely to break if you have weak bones: spine, hips, and wrists.

Keeping your spine strong is important because fractures of the spinal vertebrae are painful and crippling. Remember that good posture helps.

ASK THE EXPERTS:

Exercise

New research shows that you can actually make bones stronger with resistance training exercises that build up the muscles around the bones. Here's what researchers at the Department of Physical Medicine and Rehabilitation at the Mayo Clinic found: Women ages 58 through 75 who were assigned to routinely do an exercise that strengthened their back extensor muscles were only about one-third as likely to go on to have compression fractures of the spinal vertebrae, compared with women who did nothing to strengthen these muscles. This was a long-term effect—the women were still protected from fractures 10 years after they had completed the study.

In another study of postmenopausal women, done at Oregon State University, a control group that didn't exercise lost 3.8 percent of total hip bone mass during the 5 years of the study, while the exercise group lost less than 1 percent. On average, the control group lost 4.3 percent of the bone mass in the upper part of the femur, the big bone in your thigh, compared with a 0.2 percent loss for the exercise group. At the femoral neck of the hip, where most hip fractures occur, the control group lost 4.4 percent of its bone mass, while the exercisers *gained* more than 1.5 percent.

Standing, walking, and sitting with your head held high and your back straight, shoulders back, will not only benefit your bones; it also will make you look years younger. And it's a lot cheaper than plastic surgery!

Exercises that target the hips, such as squats, can strengthen the femoral neck of the hip. (The femoral neck is the site of more than 50 percent of all hip fractures in the United States.) You can enhance bone density in your wrists and forearms with weight resistance, and for that, forearm curls are best. Pushups are also great.

Exercise Basics

Okay, let's not waste another second. You can start strengthening your bones while you're reading this chapter! Here's how to do the exercises:

- **Forearm curls.** Sit or stand at a table or bench with your arm bent at 90 degrees, supported along its entire length, with only your wrist and hand protruding over the edge of the surface. Hold a dumbbell with your fingers underneath so that the palm of your hand is facing forward and up. Close your hand by rolling the dumbbell upward in a continuous motion. Bend your hand toward your forearm at the wrist, hold, and then, in an even motion, return to the starting position. Use a weight heavy enough so that each arm is fatigued after eight repetitions—but remember, that can be a 2-, 3-, 5-, 8-, or 10-pound weight. Try several at the store or gym, and see what works for you.

- **Squats.** Stand in front of a chair, your feet about shoulder-width apart. Bending at the knees and hips, slowly lower yourself as though you're going to sit down on the chair. Raise your arms in front of you for better balance. Keep your back straight, and make sure you can always see your toes. Stop just shy of touching the chair. Hold for a second, then stand up. Do three sets of 10 repetitions two to three times a week.

- **Back extensors.** Lie on the floor facedown, arms extended forward, legs flat on the floor. (If necessary, put a folded blanket or mat under your hips.) Extend your arms and legs in a stretch. Contract your buttocks, pressing your hips toward the floor. Next, working from your lower back, raise your arms and upper body off the floor a few inches. Hold for a count of 10, then slowly lower your body. Try to do three sets of 10. Then do the same sequence, but this time lift your legs a few inches off the floor.

For other menopause-friendly exercises, see chapter 4. You'll find illustrations showing you step-by-step how to do the exercises correctly, as well as information on how they'll benefit you during menopause and beyond.

Menopause Must-Do #4:
De-Stress with Deep Breathing

During menopause, it's more important than ever to manage stress. That's not just because there's more to feel stressed-out about, either. It's really because when you're feeling the heat of stress, your body responds by pumping out more of the hormone cortisol. Even though your estrogen and progesterone levels are in decline during menopause, you definitely don't want more cortisol as some sort of hormonal consolation prize.

ASK THE EXPERTS:

Breathing

Experts agree that breathing deeply into your belly—also called diaphragmatic breathing—is a simple way to calm down. It has even been used to reduce the incidence of hot flashes. Diaphragmatic breathing, it seems, short-circuits the arousal of the central nervous system that normally occurs in the initial stages of a hot flash.

Cortisol is bad for you, as you're about to see. It raises your blood pressure by constricting blood vessels, so it contributes to the development of heart disease. It dampens your immune response, making you prone to infection, perhaps even cancer. And it prompts your body to store fat around your midsection—the kind of fat that puts you at higher risk for diabetes and heart disease. Is just reading this enough to make you feel stressed? Read on—help is at hand.

One of the quickest, most direct ways to short-circuit your stress response is to alter your breathing. When we are stressed, we often breathe rapidly and shallowly. This is part of the "fight-or-flight" response, which prepares us to handle threatening situations. It's associated with arousal—muscle tension, blood vessel constriction, higher blood pressure, and, alas, more cortisol. When you recognize that you're taking rapid, shallow breaths, you can begin breathing slowly and deeply to interrupt this response.

Deep-Breathing Basics

Breathing to de-stress is as easy as, well, breathing. You can do deep breathing sitting up or, if you need to, lying flat on your back. Here's how it works.

- Prepare for deep breathing by sitting up straight and loosening your belt or waistband if it feels tight.

- Begin by exhaling through your nose slightly longer than you normally would.

- Then inhale through your nose slowly and deeply, filling your lungs from the bottom up while keeping your belly relaxed.
- When your chest is fully expanded, exhale fully and deeply, as if sighing.
- Be aware of your breath without trying to control it too much.
- Continue this pattern of inhaling and exhaling until you feel calm and refreshed.

Deep breathing is a fast, simple, foolproof way to de-stress. You'll find lots of other options in chapter 7.

Menopause Must-Do #5: Slip In Some Soy

Eating more soy foods has become a menopause mainstay. That's because diets that contain one or two soy servings a day reduce hot flashes and vaginal dryness, and may even help maintain bone mass. Studies also suggest that soy foods can protect you from the deadly duo that tops America's mortality list: heart disease and cancer. Soy lowers cholesterol levels and reduces the risk for heart disease—women's number one killer after age 50. And it reduces the risk for women's most common cancers—breast, colon, and lung.

You may be envisioning an endless stream of tofu blocks, but there are lots of other ways to eat your soy—and many of them have higher levels of isoflavones than tofu and its sister food, tempeh. (Isoflavones are chemical compounds that have weak estrogenic properties; they're found in some foods.) Many women get their daily soy quotient by drinking soymilk. Look for a brand fortified with calcium and vitamin D, as some are, or take supplements if your brand isn't fortified. Experiment with different brands and flavors to find the ones you like. (We're partial to chocolate soymilk.) There are also soy flour breads, soy cereals, soy burgers (and all those other soy pseudo-meats), soy butter, roasted soy nuts, soy yogurt, soy cheese. . . . The list is, well, maybe not endless, but certainly extensive. Check it out the next time you're in the health food store or a large supermarket. And almost all groceries now carry soymilk and some soy "meats." For more on soy foods, see chapter 3.

Ask the Experts:

Soy

Studies have shown that women who eat about 4 ounces of soy foods a day—which supplies 30 to 50 milligrams of isoflavones—are less likely to have bothersome menopausal symptoms such as hot flashes and vaginal dryness. (Isoflavones have weakly estrogenic properties.) In one study, women eating about 1½ ounces of soy flour a day reported that the severity or incidence of hot flashes dropped by 40 percent.

For soy's effect on bones, clinical research is scarce, but a population study done of postmenopausal Japanese women found that those who consumed the highest levels of soy had significantly stronger, thicker bones than those who consumed the lowest levels. The women who ate more soy also had the lowest rates of backache and joint stiffness and pain. And researchers in China found that premenopausal women ages 31 through 40 gained bone mass after dietary intake of soy protein. The best mix for bones seems to be a combination of soy protein and isoflavones, found in whole soy foods.

As for heart disease, researchers think that eating soy foods increases the activity of LDL receptors, "traps" on the surfaces of cells that seize harmful LDL molecules from the bloodstream and ship them to the liver, where they're eventually excreted. In one large study that analyzed the results of 38 separate studies, researchers concluded that consuming 1 to 1½ ounces of soy protein (rather than animal protein) a day lowered total cholesterol by 9 percent and harmful LDL cholesterol by 13 percent.

Animal experiments, population studies, and clinical research all point to a role for soy in prevention of and perhaps treatment for cancer. Soybeans contain at least five compounds with anticancer activity. Most research has focused on two soy isoflavones, genistein and daidzein. Research suggests that these and probably other soy isoflavones help protect against prostate, breast, colon, lung, and skin cancers. These isoflavones are "estrogen mimics." They have the ability to modulate estrogen activity in the body. In addition, soy isoflavones are potent antioxidants and are antiangiogenic—that is, they interfere with unwanted blood vessel growth in disease states.

Soy Basics

You're feeling clueless about how to slip some soy into your diet without embracing veganism or macrobiotics? Try these tips.

- **Buy a burger.** Next time you're in the mood for a burger, ask for a soy burger (or veggie burger, as they're often called). You're right; they don't taste like hamburgers, but add lettuce, tomato, ketchup, and mustard, and they do taste good!

- **Eat Chinese.** A block of plain tofu looks about as appetizing as a particularly anemic sponge. But tofu in a Chinese restaurant (where they may call it bean curd) is a totally different vegetable. Ask for a spicy Szechuan tofu dish if you like pepper heat, or, for great chewy texture, check out the dish called bean curd home-style. We've also had phenomenally delicious tofu appetizers in Vietnamese and Thai restaurants.

- **Try flour power.** If you enjoy baking, try substituting soy flour for part of the wheat flour you use in breads and other baked goods. (Because the gluten in wheat holds the dough together, substitute no more than one-third of the flour.)

- **Eat your cereal.** Not only are many cereals now soy-based (look for this when you choose one), but you can serve them with soymilk rather than cow's milk. (The difference is less distracting when you've got the cereal, too.) Two soy boosts for the price of one!

If eating any form of soy still curls your toes (come on, now—we *know* you haven't tried our suggestions!), you can try scrambled egg substitute, lentil soup, a sandwich made with half a banana and 1 tablespoon of peanut butter, or pasta primavera.

Menopause Must-Do #6: Save Your Smile

Nothing says youthful sexiness like a dazzling, for-real smile. You already know that menopause causes bone loss. But did you know it also causes loss of calcium from—you guessed it—your teeth? Estrogen therapy helps preserve teeth, just as it preserves bones. If you're not taking estrogen, you'll want to take extra precautions with your smile.

ASK THE EXPERTS:

Teeth

In one study, healthy people age 65 or older who had taken supplemental calcium and vitamin D were about half as likely to have lost a tooth, compared with people who had not taken the supplements. The people took the supplements for 3 years, and then were examined 2 years later. Only 13 percent of those who had taken the supplements had lost one tooth or more—compared with 24 percent of those who had not taken the supplements.

Osteoporosis can affect your jawbone, allowing your teeth to loosen as you age. Luckily, the same things that keep bones strong also work for teeth. Once teeth loosen, gum disease can set in, and it's possible you'll lose teeth; in fact, gum disease causes more lost teeth in adults than cavities do. Gum disease is also associated with increased risk for heart disease, stroke, and diabetes. (That may be because it can raise levels of C-reactive protein, an inflammatory protein now closely linked with heart disease.) If your gums bleed, see your dentist. Gum disease can be handled with antibiotics and other treatments—the sooner, the better.

Tooth Care Basics

If you're like us, keeping your own teeth for your whole life is a major priority. Try these tips to make sure yours stay with you.

- **Use a soft-bristle brush.** We promise; it really will clean your teeth. And brush carefully along the gum line. Be thorough, but be gentle.

- **Use dental floss daily.** Ask your dental hygienist for a brushup lesson if you need it. And ask what type of floss she recommends— there are flat flosses, like Glide, as well as the threadlike types, and of course some are waxed and some aren't. You may find one more comfortable or easier to use than others.

- **Use a plaque-control toothpaste.** Give yourself a fighting edge with one of the many toothpastes, such as Colgate Total, that contain plaque-fighting ingredients.

- **Keep your mouth moist.** If a drug you take causes dry mouth, drink extra water, and avoid sugary snacks and beverages.

- **Go for the buzz.** If arthritis limits your dexterity, get an electric toothbrush.

Menopause Must-Do #7: Get Your Sleep

Many women complain of poor sleep as they approach menopause and beyond. The immediate culprit might be hot flashes or night sweats, which (as you can imagine) are terribly disruptive to sleep. So anything that relieves these problems—such as black cohosh, deep breathing, or even a chilly bedroom—will help you sleep better. (For more on relief from hot flashes and night sweats, see chapter 10.)

But there's more to it than that. As you age, your sleep patterns change. You still require 7 to 9 hours a night. But you may have more trouble falling asleep, sleep less deeply and tend to wake up during the night, or wake up very early in the morning. As a result, you might be sleepy during the day.

Sleep problems can be brought on by health problems, such as sleep apnea or depression. But even healthy older adults secrete less of two hormones that control the sleep–wake cycle—melatonin and growth hormone.

Getting a good night's sleep is important. Good sleep is as restorative as exercise and a healthy diet. Sleep is a recovery period for the body's stress response system. The loss of REM, or rapid eye movement, sleep is associated with higher levels of the stress hormone cortisol, which—as you recall from Menopause Must-Do #4—adds to the body's wear and tear and may predispose you to a host of diseases. Lack of sleep is also linked to memory problems and to insulin resistance, a risk factor for diabetes.

Sleep Basics

Okay, we hope we've convinced you that getting a good night's sleep is important enough to be a Menopause Must-Do. Get your 7 to 9 hours, and you'll feel better, look younger, and be more alert and less stressed. You'll also be less likely to get some scary diseases. So, here's how to get a good night's sleep despite getting older.

ASK THE EXPERTS:

Sleep

Experts have shown that poor sleeping habits can affect insulin resistance, which can lead to diabetes. In one study, people who were permitted only 4 hours of sleep a night for six nights had much higher blood glucose levels after breakfast. And the rate at which sugar cleared from the blood was nearly 40 percent slower when they hadn't gotten enough sleep than when they had slept for 9 hours.

- **Lighten up.** Get at least 30 minutes of natural light a day. Natural light helps reset your inner clock so you'll fall asleep at the right time.

- **Take a walk.** In one study, people who took a daily brisk walk cut their risk of sleep disturbance by half. If you have trouble falling asleep, walk early in the day. If you fall asleep early but wake up before the birds, walk in the late afternoon.

- **Sleep in the dark.** Darkness helps your body produce melatonin, a hormone that induces sleep. You can also dim the lights a few hours before bed. Too much bright light in the evening causes the body's internal clock to shift to late-night bedtimes and sleepy mornings. If you wake up during the night, resist turning on the lights unless you're sure there's no way you're going to fall back to sleep.

- **Don't drink late.** Drink no alcohol after dinnertime. It might put you to sleep earlier, but it'll leave you wide-awake at 4 in the morning.

- **Watch when you nap.** If you're a napper, follow these rules: Don't nap closer than 4 hours before bedtime, and don't nap longer than 30 minutes to 1 hour.

Menopause Must-Do #8: Stay Sexual and Sensual

Menopause may cause women to question their sexuality and sex appeal for any number of reasons. We may feel like we're starting to look old, losing our sexual attractiveness. Or we may find that we just don't feel like having sex. Or—and this is really cruel—we may feel like having sex but find that it hurts. If you can relate to any of this, you'll find help here.

This book will help you look desirable and feel great—see chapter 3 (page 39); chapter 4 (page 75); and chapter 6 (page 145). And there's a whole chapter especially devoted to menopause and sex, chapter 9 (page 230). But while you're waiting to plunge into the other chapters, here are a couple of things you can do right now.

No matter how "in the mood" you are, once menopause hits—and especially once you're years beyond—without added estrogen, you will experience vaginal dryness, thinning of the vaginal walls, and atrophy. Estrogen helps keep vaginal tissue moist and healthy. So estrogen replacement clears this up nicely, and it is possible to use a form of estrogen replacement that targets only the vagina, without any risk of systemic effects.

One such product is Estring, a soft, flexible silicone ring inserted into the vagina that slowly releases estrogen for a period of 90 days. (You then remove and replace it.) A prescription product, Estring provides the least bodywide exposure to estrogen of any hormonal treatment available for vaginal dryness. It can even be used by some women who've had breast or endometrial cancer.

If your problem is a lack of desire for sex, you may benefit from using a touch of testosterone, the hormone that promotes sex drive in both men and women. (Are you surprised? We're conditioned to think of testosterone as a male hormone, but all women have it, too.)

Some doctors prescribe a cream made with methyltestosterone or micronized testosterone that is applied, initially, directly to the vulva. Then, after a week or two, when this tissue has been resensitized, the cream is applied to the inside of the thighs or the wrist. (This treatment is less likely to have systemic effects than oral testosterone, most commonly prescribed as Estratest, an estrogen–testosterone combination.)

Soy, black cohosh, and a vaginal moisturizer can also help. (And so can a candlelit bedroom and a light supper!) Read more about them, and about lots of other ideas for rejuvenating your sex life and sensuality, in chapter 9.

Ask the Experts:

Sex

If you haven't felt like having sex for a while now, but you'd like to start enjoying sex again, the experts recommend a little testosterone boost. But short of a sex change, how do you go about getting some? You might want to talk to your doctor about trying testosterone cream. Ask your OB/GYN about it—if you need to, search for a gynecologist who specializes in menopause. A compounding pharmacist—one who makes up drugs for doctors—may know if there is a doctor in your area who prescribes this cream.

Sexy Basics

There's more to feeling sexy than sex itself. You may find yourself in the mood a lot more often if you try these tactics for increasing your sensual pleasure and "sensualizing" your environment.

- **Dress for success.** Lose the sweatpants, the work clothes, the granny gowns (you'll have a different way to stay warm), and the industrial-strength undies. (You can put them back on afterward; we promise.) We're not telling you to cram yourself into a thong, or anything else that makes you feel uncomfortable or ridiculous. But putting on pretty underwear or slipping into a slinky dress or nightgown can make *you* feel pretty, and trust us, he'll see the difference—and get the point.

- **Revisit dating.** Okay, we know you're married. But that doesn't mean you can't date. The hottest couples we know—the ones who seem to have defied time and kept the bounce in their relationships—set aside one night a week (often Friday) for "date night." They get a sitter or leave the older kids in charge and head out the door. You'd be surprised at what this regular "adults only" time together can do for your relationship.

- **Talk about it.** Maybe you want sex when he wants to watch pro football, or he wants sex when you're falling asleep on your feet. Instead of getting mad—or, worse, getting hurt and giving up—try talking about your mutual needs. Thinking back, you may realize that it's been years since you've even talked about sex; it's become so mechanical and unfulfilling. You may be amazed at what you discover about yourselves once you sit down and open up to each other.

- **Try something new.** Maybe your bedroom just isn't that exciting anymore—it's turned into a catchall for everybody's old stuff, the bedspread is 1,000 years old, and you think of the bed as a place to watch TV until you fall asleep. A makeover could be just what it needs— from old mess to love nest. Think about how you could transform the bedroom into a romantic hideaway (keeping in mind that no matter what you do, it still needs to be comfortable for the two of you, both physically and emotionally). Or try having sex in the *other* rooms, the way you did when you were first married. And don't forget—darkness may be a girl's best friend, but there are 24 hours in every day, and all of them are great for sex, cuddling, and romance.

That's a start. Now it's your turn. Think about what you'd really enjoy, turn to chapter 9 for more great ideas, and then try something new tonight. And tomorrow night. And . . . okay, we'll stop. But trust us; you (and your spouse) will be really glad you did. After all, feeling sexy is part of feeling alive. And it's another good way to stay close and connected to your partner.

Menopause Must-Do #9: Look Good to Feel Great

It's important to look good whatever your age. But you *really* want to look good when you're trying to cope with menopausal symptoms—and the idea of growing older—in a society where youth is idealized. If your coworkers are starting to look like toddlers, you need to look vital and vibrant, not tired and stressed. And it's nice to think that your spouse or partner still finds you a little too hot to handle! How you pull your look together can make a huge difference in how attractive you appear. Turn to chapter 6 for tons of great tips on making the most of your looks. But first, try these ideas out and see what they can do for you.

ASK THE EXPERTS:

Beauty

Your makeup might have looked great on you when you were 30, but at 50-plus most women need to seriously revamp their routine, says New York City makeup artist Deborah Grayson.

"The biggest mistake older women make is to continue to use matte products, such as lipstick and foundation, which are designed for oily skin," Deborah says. "These products look pasty and masklike on older skin."

Instead, use moisture-based lipstick and foundation formulas. Use foundation sparingly, just where you need it, such as the sides of the nose or on red spots. Apply it with a damp makeup sponge to blend edges. Then use a subtly toned moisturizing lipstick or neutral-colored gloss. If you must use lip liner, make sure it's a neutral tone and applied on the lips, not beyond them.

"Don't look to makeup as a cover-up," Deborah says. "Instead, use it with finesse to enhance your features, to reflect the woman you've become."

Beauty Basics

Here are five can't-fail makeup tips that will take years off your face and make you look radiant. Try them and see for yourself!

- **Cover up.** Under eyes, use a lightly textured concealer, and blend with moisturizer before applying.

- **Be natural.** Choose colors that are natural against your skin tone. Don't go for vibrant or contrasting tones. They're aging.

- **Don't go for glow.** Steer clear of shimmer or pearl products. These exaggerate the texture of skin, intensifying the appearance of fine lines and wrinkles.

- **Skip the Alice Cooper look.** Use mascara on the upper lashes only. The same goes for eyeliner. Makeup applied to the lower eye area inevitably travels down, causing what looks like two black eyes.

- **Blush like an apple.** For a fuller look, instead of applying blush to your cheekbones, smile and apply it to the "apples" of the cheeks, then blend like there's no tomorrow. Think of looking sun-kissed, not gaunt.

How you dress, eat, exercise, sleep, feel, and handle stress affect how you look. So do how well you stay hydrated, how good your posture is, and how energetically you move. The more vibrant you feel, the more vibrant you'll look. And that's what youth and beauty are *really* all about.

Menopause Must-Do #10: Cultivate a Giving Spirit

Dissatisfaction, whether in your career or in other areas of your life, can happen at any stage of life. But in midlife, it typifies the emotional growing pains that almost everyone feels. The need to find meaning, purpose, and connection in your work and life—to feel like you're making a difference—becomes more of an issue now, even for people who consider themselves happy and successful.

It can take a while—perhaps the rest of your life—to really figure out what your life is all about. In the meantime, there's one sure way to feel like you are really making a difference, and maybe even live longer in the process. It's giving to others.

Giving Basics

You'll find many more ways to revitalize your relationships and enrich your life in chapter 8. But if you want to start right now to become a more giving person, here are four tips to try. And remember, you'll live longer!

- **Do something that makes you feel good.** Make sure it meets your own emotional needs. Don't act out of some puritanical commitment. Give with joy.

- **Get personal.** Find situations that put you into direct contact with others who need the help. You'll get greater satisfaction. Even making phone calls is better than stuffing envelopes.

ASK THE EXPERTS:

Giving

Experts say that being a giver imparts a sense of control, instills a sense of abundance in your life, boosts self-esteem, satisfies emotional needs, and widens your social circles. In doing so, it increases your sense of self-preservation and your chances for survival. (See page 173 for more on giving.)

Researchers at the University of Michigan recently found that older people who were helpful to others reduced their risk of dying by nearly 60 percent, compared with peers who provided neither practical help nor emotional support to relatives, neighbors, or friends.

The study analyzed data on 423 older couples, a random, community-based sample of people who were first interviewed in 1987 and then followed for 5 years to see how they coped with the inevitable changes of later life. During the first set of interviews, the husbands and wives were asked a series of questions about whether they provided any practical support to friends, neighbors, or relatives, including help with housework, child care, errands, or transportation. They were also asked how much they could count on help from friends or family members if they needed it. Finally, they were asked about giving emotional support to and receiving emotional support from their spouses, including their willingness to listen if the spouse needed to talk.

Over the 5-year period of the study, 134 people died. In the analysis of the link between giving and receiving help and mortality, the researchers controlled for a variety of factors, including age, gender, and physical and emotional health. This was to rule out the possibilities that older people gave less and were likelier to die, that females gave more and were less likely to die, and that people who were depressed or in poor health were both less likely to be able to help others and likelier to die.

The researchers found that people who reported having provided no help to others were more than twice as likely to die as people who had given some help to others. Overall, the study found that 75 percent of men and 72 percent of women reported having provided some help without pay to friends, relatives, or neighbors in the year before they were surveyed.

TOP 10 MYTHS OF MENOPAUSE

Well, we hope you've mastered the Top 10 Menopause Must-Dos (or at least read them!). Now, in case you're wondering, here are the Top 10 Myths of Menopause. See how many of these you've heard — and what the truth really is.

1. **Menopause makes you crazy.** Perhaps the most pervasive myth associated with menopause is that mental health problems result from decreased hormone production. No scientific research shows that natural menopause is responsible for true clinical depression, anxiety, severe memory lapses, or erratic behavior.

2. **Your age when you first started menstruating determines your age when menopause begins.** Contrary to folklore, age at onset of menstruation plays no part. Nor does your contraceptive or sexual history.

3. **Menopause can be cured.** Many doctors have approached menopause as if it were an estrogen deficiency disease. It's not. This is a natural transition, and while hormone therapy (HT) can ease unpleasant side effects, it can't turn back the hands of time.

4. **All the physical changes associated with menopause are bad.** Just consider: No more estrogen-stoked migraines. No more PMS. No more debilitating cramps. No more bleeding! Lots of women who've suffered these ailments agree "menopause is probably the best thing that ever happened to me." P.S. No more concerns about pregnancy and birth control, either.

5. **Menopause makes you irritable.** Night sweats and hot flashes may disrupt healthy sleep patterns, as can falling estrogen levels. Without enough deep sleep, anyone can feel tired and cranky, but it's a myth that menopause itself makes you irritable.

- **Don't overcommit yourself.** The last thing you need is another source of stress. It's better to start small and add on.

- **Give thanks.** If life finds you on the receiving end, give what you can in return: Gratitude. Love. Thanks. Let people know how much you appreciate their help.

That's it: Top 10 menopause must-dos. We hope you try them all. They'll help you have an easier menopause, a more positive experience,

6. **You're no longer a "real" woman.** If you feel this way, retool your self-image and realize you're a person whose value has to do with a great deal more than the ability to make babies, says Patricia Love, Ed.D., a marriage and family therapist and relationship consultant in Austin, Texas, and coauthor of *Hot Monogamy*. You are more than a uterus. Act like it.

7. **Menopause makes you lose interest in sex.** Often, previous attitudes dictate a woman's view of her sexuality as she ages. In general, women who enjoyed sex in their younger years will continue to do so during midlife and beyond, says Dr. Love. She notes that many women in their seventies and eighties enjoy satisfying sex lives. With age, there's a gradual decline in sexual drive for both women and men. However, a decline does not mean an abrupt halt.

8. **The best years are over.** Ovarian failure doesn't mean your mind, your humanity, and your spirit stop growing. People don't simply fossilize. A majority of menopausal women today believe these are the best years of their lives.

9. **Menopause makes you unattractive.** Beauty, grace, and allure are not a function of age or fertility. European women are considered attractive well into their sixth and seventh decades, notes Dr. Love. Think of Sophia Loren.

10. **Energy drops after menopause.** Actually, it's the opposite. Hormone cycling is an enormous energy drain. Women exhibit extraordinary stamina after menopause, says Dr. Love, especially if they exercise and eat right.

and a healthier, happier, richer life. And they're just the beginning. In the chapters ahead, we'll give you in-depth information about eating, exercise, supplements, beauty, stress, moods, and sex, all geared specifically to menopause. And we'll discuss menopause symptoms and all the solutions that are available—both conventional and alternative. Dig in!

PART
2

Looking Good, Feeling Great

Menopause is a time of transition, with day-to-day changes and symptoms that can last for years. But life doesn't screech to a halt—and neither should you. In this section, we'll show you how to live life to the fullest, minimizing negative changes (like weight gain and hair loss) while discovering positive changes that will dramatically improve your life.

Chapter
3

THE MENOPAUSE EATING PLAN

THERE ARE PLENTY OF REASONS TO CHANGE THE WAY YOU EAT AS you approach menopause. If you don't, you'll start gaining weight—even if you're eating the way you always did in the past. The foods you eat—or don't eat—can also increase or minimize menopausal symptoms, from hot flashes to bloating and gas. And foods are also key weapons in the fight against the major postmenopausal diseases: cancer, osteoporosis, and heart disease.

With all this in mind, we've developed an eating plan that will help you combat weight gain, menopausal symptoms, and diseases. And it will help you look and feel great. We'll start with our core strategy: eating five or six mini-meals a day, rather than two or three biggies. (Find out why this works in the next section, "Mini-Meals Fight 'Menopause Midriffs.'") Then, in "Eating for an Easier Menopause" on page 51, we'll tell you about the menopause superfoods, the ones that promote overall radiant health and energy while reducing menopausal symptoms. Finally, we'll give you the latest recommendations on foods that fight disease in "Cutting Your Cancer Risk" on page 60, "Give Your Bones a Break from Osteoporosis" on page 62, and "Heading Off Heart Disease" on page 66.

Food is one of the most basic, easiest, and cheapest health care options available. Making smart food choices now can help you breeze through menopause, and keep you looking good and feeling great in your post-menopausal years.

Mini-Meals Fight "Menopause Midriffs"

The heart of our Menopause Eating Plan is mini-meals. There are four great reasons that mini-meals are the right choice for menopausal women. First, they help minimize midlife weight gain. Second, eating small meals at regular intervals helps control the unpleasant digestive symptoms of menopause, including bloating, gas, and diarrhea. Third, eating frequent mini-meals gives you the steady supply of fuel you need to stay calm, focused, and energetic all day, freed at last from the soar-and-crash seesaw caused by large, infrequent meals. And fourth, because you're never ravenous, you can make the smart food choices you'll need to stay healthy and vibrant, rather than panic in your hunger and grab the first high-fat, high-sugar energy booster you can lay your hands on.

Scientific research supports the mini-meal concept. Some studies have suggested that eating five or six smaller meals a day is better for you than eating the traditional three squares, and can make it easier to control your weight, particularly as you age. Menopause specialists also support the idea of mini-meals. Larrian Gillespie, author of *The Menopause Diet*; Debra Waterhouse in *Outsmarting the Midlife Fat Cell*; and Dr. Christiane Northrup in *The Wisdom of Menopause* all recommend mini-meals to combat midlife weight gain.

To show you how it works, here's a tale of two menopause-age dieters on a typical day.

Woman number one is a mini-meal muncher. She breakfasts each morning on some cereal and orange juice, then heads off to work. About midmorning she takes a break and gets a plain bagel to nibble on while she works up proposals. A few hours later she stops for lunch—a sandwich and some veggies. By late afternoon she's at the vending machine, getting some pretzels. After work she heads home and whips up some baked fish and a small potato for dinner. Later, when her chores are done, she sits down to watch TV and snacks on low-fat yogurt and some grapes. Then it's time for bed.

Woman number two is a calorie watcher. She's out the door in the morning without any breakfast, and ignores her hunger pangs until lunch. Finally, it's lunchtime. She picks at a small salad and then ignores her hunger all afternoon. About 5:00 P.M., she heads home, polishes off a nice dinner, watches some TV, and heads for bed.

Who's going to be the winner at losing?

Woman number one.

Why More Is Best

You'd think skipping meals would result in eating fewer calories, which in turn would result in less body fat. But your body doesn't work that way. It actually burns fat more effectively when you eat small amounts of food more often. In fact, scientists have discovered that eating four to six small meals a day actually helps to speed up your fat-burning system. Here's why.

- If you bypass breakfast and skimp on lunch, you're going to overload at dinner. "After an all-day fast, the body is ravenous and you end up doubling the quantity of food you eat," says Diane Grabowski-Nepa, R.D., nutrition educator at the Pritikin Longevity Center in Malibu, California. Too much food at any one time is more than your body can handle, and it encourages fat storage. On top of that, your body is more efficient at storing fat in the evening than earlier in the day, when you're more active. So if you overeat at dinner, more calories get stored as fat than, say, if you overeat at breakfast.

- Skipping meals can slow your metabolism by as much as 5 percent. That's because an empty stomach makes your brain think your body is starving, so it turns down its calorie-burning thermostat in an effort to live longer off its stored fat. On the other hand, when you eat small meals all day long, your stomach never gets a chance to be empty, thus keeping your metabolism purring along.

- When you eat a big meal such as a huge dinner, your body produces insulin, which stimulates an enzyme called lipoprotein lipase, or LPL. LPL opens up the door of fat cells, which can expand quite easily, and lets those lipids settle in. The more insulin you have, the more those

(continued on page 44)

MINI-MEAL MENU SAMPLER

It can be a little daunting to figure out how to eat all day and still lose weight, so we asked Anne Dubner, R.D., a nutritionist in private practice in Houston, to put together a sampling of daily menus to show how satisfying mini-meals can be.

The trick to losing weight on mini-meals, she says, is to listen to your stomach. Eat when you start feeling a little hungry—don't wait until you're famished—and stop as soon as your hunger goes away, not when you're stuffed. That way, you'll stay satisfied all day. Here are 3 days' worth of menus to get you started.

DAY ONE

Breakfast: Half a whole wheat bagel with pureed roasted peppers mixed with reduced-fat or fat-free cream cheese, an 8-ounce glass of fat-free milk, and ½ cup of blueberries

Snack: The other half of the bagel with roasted peppers

Lunch: Half a turkey club sandwich (made with turkey breast, sliced tomato, and lettuce) and a mixed garden salad with 1 tablespoon of reduced-fat Russian dressing

Snack: The other half of the sandwich

Dinner: 2 cups of pasta primavera (made with rotini pasta, frozen mixed vegetables, garlic, Parmesan cheese, and 1 tablespoon of olive oil) and a slice of Italian bread topped with 1 teaspoon of reduced-fat margarine mixed with 1 teaspoon each of crushed fresh garlic and grated Parmesan cheese

Snack: An oatmeal raisin cookie

DAY TWO

Breakfast: One slice of raisin bread with 1 tablespoon of peanut butter and a 4-ounce glass of orange juice

Snack: A reduced-fat fig bar and an 8-ounce glass of fat-free milk

Lunch: Half a chicken salad pita sandwich (made with low-fat, cubed cooked chicken, toasted walnuts, raisins, small grapes, and honey) and 1 cup of raw vegetables such as baby carrots and celery

Snack: The other half of the sandwich

Dinner: Cheese quesadilla (made with a fat-free flour tortilla, 1 tablespoon each of shredded reduced-fat Cheddar and hot-pepper Monterey Jack cheese, $1\frac{1}{2}$ teaspoons of chopped canned green chile peppers, $1\frac{1}{2}$ teaspoons of sliced black olives, and salsa, chili powder, and sliced scallions to taste) with $\frac{1}{2}$ cup of white rice mixed with 2 tablespoons of salsa

Snack: 8 ounces of fat-free flavored yogurt with three graham crackers

DAY THREE

Breakfast: An English muffin with scrambled egg substitute, an orange wedge, and an 8-ounce glass of fat-free milk

Snack: A sandwich made with half a banana and 1 tablespoon of peanut butter

Lunch: A small Greek salad (made with chopped tomatoes, cucumbers, sweet red peppers, and onions, with feta cheese and a dressing of lemon juice and olive oil with oregano and garlic) and a slice of Italian bread

Snack: Six crackers with tuna salad (made with tuna, 1 tablespoon of reduced-fat mayonnaise, and a squirt of lemon juice)

Dinner: Potato skins (made with one quartered baked potato, 1 cup of shredded reduced-fat Cheddar cheese, some scallions or chives, and paprika) with $\frac{1}{2}$ cup of steamed broccoli

Snack: 3 cups of reduced-fat popcorn sprinkled with 2 teaspoons of Parmesan cheese

fat cells can hold. High insulin levels also stimulate appetite, which makes you want to eat more. On the other hand, when you eat small meals all day long, you never experience the insulin surge that larger meals create.

- Spreading your daily calories over four meals or more can help you dampen your appetite by keeping food in your stomach at all times. Instead of always feeling deprived, you always feel full, so you don't binge.

- Your stomach expands and contracts with food load, and apparently it loses its tone when repeatedly pushed to the max. So once your stomach is overstretched, it takes more food to satisfy you, according to studies by scientists at the obesity research center at St. Luke's–Roosevelt Hospital Center in New York City. Eating small amounts of food all day doesn't stretch the stomach, so you feel full more quickly.

Mini-Meal Magic

Ready to give it a try? Think variety. Continue to eat from all the food groups—grains, fruits, vegetables, dairy, and protein—throughout the day. But you don't need to balance your intake of food groups at every meal as you did when you were eating three meals. Instead, you want to achieve balance over the course of an entire day, which means about eight grains, three or four fruits, four vegetables, two or three dairy products, and five lean meats or other protein foods each day.

Here's the best advice from experts for getting into the mini-meal mindset.

Give your regular meals the split. Try dividing what you eat for breakfast, lunch, and dinner in half to create six meals, suggests Anne Dubner, R.D., a nutrition consultant in private practice in Houston. If you usually eat a bagel for breakfast, for example, eat half when you get up and the other half later. If you have a sandwich for lunch, eat the halves at two different times. That way, you won't spend any more time preparing food.

Watch the fat and the portions. In determining your daily intake, it's important to keep your eye on those two waist-expanding monsters, fat and calories. While fat reduction is the most important priority for good health and weight loss, you don't want calories to fall too low or climb too high.

Eat "fight fat" foods. That means foods high in fiber and low in fat and added sugar—things like fruit, vegetables, and whole wheat bread. Avoid empty-calorie snacks, like doughnuts.

Select a serving. Favor foods that are already portioned into individual servings, like a baked potato, a container of yogurt, or a bagel. Eating a set portion ensures that you'll stop when you're full (or nearly

MAKING THE SWITCH TO MINI-MEALS

Because she was overweight and diabetic, Anita Beattie's doctor gave her a harsh ultimatum: "Enter a hospital program to lose weight or don't come back to see me because you are wasting my time and your money." That push was just the encouragement Anita needed to drop the extra 38 pounds that she was lugging around and, with her doctor's guidance, to taper off the insulin that she used to control her diabetes.

"My doctor put me in the hospital for 4 days to teach me enough about diet and exercise so that when I left the hospital, I could carry out these lessons on my own," Anita explains. "The hospital nutritionist put me on an exercise program and a low-calorie diet. I started walking for 20 minutes a few times a week, and I began eating several mini-meals throughout the day, instead of the all-day meal I used to eat. My husband was a great support—he measured all my food and created my menus. He helped me learn about portion sizes. I was surprised to learn, for instance, that a piece of cheese as long as the distance from the tip of your pointer finger to your first knuckle constitutes one serving, and there are 100 calories in that serving.

"After I got out of the hospital, I continued eating four or five mini-meals throughout the day. I have breakfast, lunch, dinner, and a nighttime snack of a rice cake or some sugar-free Jell-O, and occasionally I have a midmorning snack as well.

"I eat smaller portions and make better food choices. I used to eat eggs and bacon for breakfast, but now I eat half a grapefruit, a serving of oatmeal with skim milk, half a bagel, and, of course, coffee. I haven't eliminated any foods from my diet, except sweets because of my diabetes. I've just learned to recognize what serving sizes are, and I apply that knowledge to whatever I eat.

"I have also kept up with my exercise plan, and now I walk $2\frac{1}{2}$ to $3\frac{1}{2}$ miles five times a week. Walking coupled with my new mini-meal habits has helped me maintain my weight at 126 pounds for the past 3 years. And it has done wonders for my diabetes!"

full) because you'll run out of food, says Michele Harvey, R.D., a diabetes educator and private nutrition consultant in Boca Raton and Delray Beach, Florida.

Choose no-risk foods. As you adapt, choose low-calorie foods. Reach for the fat-free milk, apple, and air-popped popcorn, or a sweet potato and a mixed-greens salad dressed with lemon juice or balsamic vinegar. (Say no thanks to the Caesar salad and sweet potato fries.)

Go to pieces. Mini-meals will be more satisfying if you eat them in small bites. So instead of one big rice cake, have a few of the bite-size variety. Instead of eating a big pretzel, have lots of small ones. You can even cut a cookie into pieces and eat the pieces individually.

Don't tempt yourself. If you know that you have no resistance to certain foods—cookies, for instance—stay away from them. If you don't, you'll probably end up eating well beyond fullness. Choose mini-meal foods that you know you can control, says Donna Weihofen, R.D., nutritionist at the University of Wisconsin Hospital and Clinics in Madison.

Watch out for fat-free. Most of the new packaged fat-free foods won't fill you up for long. Also, many fat-free foods have added sugar to make up for the loss of fat. Look at the total calories, not just the fat—many of these foods are only 20 or so calories lower than the full-fat version! (And trust us—if you've ever walked for half an hour on a treadmill, only to discover at the end that you've burned a total of 150 calories, a 20-calorie drop isn't *nearly* low enough!)

Be a Time Machine

You might be afraid that eating six meals a day would really cut into your time. But remember—these are mini-meals, not formal dinners. Eating mini-meals doesn't have to be time-consuming, according to Natalie Payne, R.D., nutritionist at the Washington Cancer Institute and Washington Hospital Center in Washington, D.C. Here are some time-saving strategies.

Take mini-meals on the road. Keep a snack stash in your car, carry snacks in your purse when you go to the mall, and stock your briefcase when you fly. Good portables include small boxes of raisins, mini-boxes of cereal, cans of low-sodium vegetable juice cocktail, and whole wheat hard pretzels. (This practice has another benefit: If you find yourself ravenous on the road or at the mall or airport, you won't be tempted to grab the closest high-calorie fast-food fare!)

Switch meals. Consider some easy-to-prepare, easy-to-eat (but somewhat unusual) choices for your meals. Make a turkey sandwich in the evening, for example, and put it in the fridge. Then grab it on your way out the door in the morning and eat it for breakfast on your way to work.

Keep it cold. If you don't have access to a refrigerator where you work, freeze a juice box overnight and put it in the bottom of your lunch bag the following day. The frozen juice will keep easy-to-eat items such as yogurt and cheese cold.

Stash some safe bets. At work, keep a desk drawer stocked with canned fruit (in water or fruit juice), dried fruit, low-fat crackers, and other nonperishable convenience foods. (And don't forget a can opener.)

Slice at night. When cutting up carrots and other raw vegetables for dinner, don't forget to slice some extras to take along and munch the next day at work.

Dinner—Don't Overdo It

Dinner can be the toughest time to eat a mini-meal. If you go out to eat, you're served too much food. If you eat at home, you might linger at the table with the family and eat more than you planned. Yet calories consumed at night are most likely to pack on the pounds since your metabolism actually slows while you sleep. Here are some of Anne Dubner and Michele Harvey's most effective ideas for downsizing at dinnertime.

Have an appetizer. Have a snack ready in the fridge for when you walk in the door after work. After you've eaten your appetizer, change into comfortable clothes, take a shower, or do whatever else you do to ready yourself for an evening meal with your family. Then you can spend as much time at the dinner table as you like, but you won't overeat because you won't be as hungry.

Don't stay on course. Switch back and forth between courses by alternating bites of your main dish (chicken or pasta, for example) with a

DROP THE DIET AND START LOSING WEIGHT

For 20 years, Ann has been a chronic yo-yo dieter—up 10 pounds, down 5, up 5, down 10. Either she's dieting to starvation by existing on raw vegetables and canned tuna or eating all the wrong things. For Ann, there is no in between. Lately, though, she seems to have more "eating days" than "diet days," and her weight just keeps going up. What's happened to her willpower?

The reality is that Ann's new weight problem may have nothing to do with willpower. As we've seen, as a woman approaches menopause, her metabolism slows and she may gain weight even when eating and exercising the same way she always did. And in Ann's case, her constant dieting may have made her situation even worse. After so many years of dieting, Ann's body is probably tired from all the bouncing up and down on the scale. And like all yo-yo dieters, she has probably set unrealistic goals. When she keeps falling short of meeting them, she loses her desire to even try to fight her weight gain. For women like her, a sensible weight loss of only a pound a week is viewed as failure. Like many yo-yo dieters, she eats out of frustration for failing and promises to start all over again tomorrow.

It's going to be difficult for Ann to reclaim her willpower as it's been years since she's eaten sensibly. But she can do it if she changes her habits. First, she needs to set realistic weight-loss goals. She needs to realize that the only way she'll achieve long-term success is through gradual steps. If she doesn't lose weight right away, she shouldn't consider herself a failure.

Second, she needs to believe that all foods are allowed; otherwise, the foods she deprives herself of on her "diet days" are exactly the foods she'll want on her "eating days." Most important, she needs to get on a regular eating plan with three small meals a day, spaced fairly evenly, and enough snacks in between to keep her from bingeing later on. Once Ann quits playing yo-yo with her eating habits, her weight is bound to settle down, too.

bite of salad. If you do that, you won't finish eating before the rest of your family does.

Fill 'er up. Before ordering dinner at a restaurant, drink a big glass of water to quiet your appetite. Then take a sip of water after every bite so that you'll eat more slowly.

Hold the bread. Ask the server not to serve bread. Or take one roll and send the basket back.

Request less. Ask the server for a smaller portion. You can request a meal that's half the usual size, for instance.

Don't entrée right away. When eating out, have a small bowl of noncreamy soup like minestrone or a small salad before making a decision on your entrée. That way, you won't be as hungry and you'll order a smaller meal.

Or don't order it at all. Instead of ordering an entrée, order an appetizer.

Start low, end high. Eat your vegetables first, then the starches, such as potatoes and bread. Leave the highest-calorie and fattiest items, like meat, for last. That way you'll fill up on the lowest-calorie items and feel too full to finish the high-calorie foods.

Take it home. Before the server brings the meal, ask for a doggie bag. When he brings the dinner, immediately divide your food, putting half in the take-home container and leaving the rest on your plate. Or ask the server to do it for you. Store the take-home container under your chair so you won't be tempted to nibble from it.

Don't worry about detours. Every once in a while—at Thanksgiving, for instance—you'll stuff yourself. Don't feel guilty. "You are not going to get lost when you take a detour, as long as you don't keep slapping yourself across the face," says Michele Harvey. You will get lost, however, if you continually berate yourself, she says, because then you'll feel so bad about yourself that you'll keep eating.

More Tricks for Keeping the "Mini" in Mini-Meals

It's obvious: If you're eating mini-meals but you don't downsize each meal, you won't lose weight. But how can you keep the portions from creeping up on you? Here are some top-notch tips from Edith Howard Hogan, R.D., L.D., a nutrition counselor specializing in women's health and a spokesperson for the American Dietetic Association in Washington, D.C.

- **Choose "one-fisted" snacks.** A piece of fresh fruit, a miniature box of raisins, a cup of yogurt, a little box of cereal, a snack pack of applesauce, or a pop-top can of tuna automatically limits your portions.

BALANCE YOUR PORTIONS

Here's another trick for minimizing menopausal weight gain. Select the right balance of foods on your plate, says Jackie Newgent, R.D., a spa cuisine instructor at Peter Kump's New York Cooking School. Jackie's bottom line: Slice starches, dice fat, value vegetables!

Menopause slows your metabolic rate. To compensate, one of your best moves is to limit fat consumption. "But the downside of cutting too much fat is that it leaves you hungry," says Jackie. Many people then make the mistake of taking gluttonous helpings of carbohydrates instead. Then they find to their horror that their waistlines keep expanding.

The key to success, according to Jackie, is to practice just as much portion control with breads and pastas as with cheese and meat portions. If you're hungry, load up on veggies and legumes.

"It's just a matter of balance," Jackie says. "Remember that less fat, fewer starches, and more vegetables will help you maintain your premenopausal waistline and ease the burden on your postmenopausal heart."

She offers this Confetti Veggie Couscous as a quick and delicious example of a balanced one-dish meal.

- **Shrink your sweets.** Bite-size chocolate bars, presliced brownies, or mini bagels will give you the taste you love with portion control. Just be sure to say no to seconds.

- **Downsize your dishes.** Use a salad plate instead of a dinner plate for meals, a cup instead of a bowl for soup, and a juice glass instead of a tumbler for beverages (unless it's water, which you want to load up on).

- **Take control.** Finally, remember these wise words from Edith: "When your eating is under control, everything else feels more in control, too. Instead of eating for comfort and making everything worse, eat for health and energy to support positive change."

Confetti Veggie Couscous

1 tablespoon extra-virgin olive oil
3 large cloves garlic, minced
6 ounces water
1 can (14½ ounces) vegetable broth
1 cup chopped red bell peppers
1 cup chopped zucchini or yellow squash
½ cup shredded carrot
10 ounces whole wheat couscous
¼ cup chopped fresh oregano, basil, parsley, or a mixture
Salt to taste
Lemon juice

Add the oil to a large saucepan over medium heat. Add the garlic and cook for about 1 minute, being careful not to brown the garlic. Add the water, broth, peppers, zucchini or squash, and carrot. Bring just to a boil over high heat. Stir in the couscous and herbs. Cover and immediately remove from the heat. Let sit for 5 minutes. Fluff with a fork and add salt. Serve immediately or chilled with a squirt of fresh lemon juice.

MAKES 6 SERVINGS

Per serving: 295 calories, 3 g fat

Eating for an Easier Menopause

Mini-meals will help you keep midlife weight gain under control, but they won't do much to minimize menopause's more unpleasant symptoms (hot flashes come to mind). Fortunately, there's plenty you can do to help yourself have an easier menopause just by making the right food choices. We'll give you specific disease-fighting foods in the sections on the big menopausal diseases—cancer (page 60), osteoporosis (page 62), and heart disease (page 66)—that follow. But first, we'd like to present a few foods and beverages that we think *all* menopausal women should include in their diets for reduction of menopausal symptoms, overall well-being, and preventive care. And there are a few foods and beverages that you should avoid. Here are our top recommendations.

Avoid Flash Foods

Tea, coffee, and other hot or spicy foods and drinks can provoke the sweaty spells we all dread. During menopause, your body struggles to control its internal thermostat. All too often, it fails. Toss in caffeine, with its stimulating effects, and things get worse. Serve it up hot, and if you're prone to hot flashes, you'd better head for the deep freeze.

"I tell my patients that hot coffee and hot tea are no-nos if they want to minimize hot flashes," says Mary Jane Minkin, M.D., clinical professor of obstetrics and gynecology at Yale University School of Medicine and coauthor of *What Every Woman Needs to Know about Menopause.* Hot drinks add warmth to your body, and this burst of heat can overload your erratic temperature mechanisms. Caffeine also relaxes your capillaries and allows more blood and heat to reach your skin, creating the unwelcome flush. Alcohol has a similar warming effect.

Spicy foods can also superstimulate more than just your tongue. Limit your intake of whole peppercorns, crushed red pepper, and even freshly ground pepper, says Dr. Minkin. Steer clear of chiles in Southwestern, Mexican, Indian, and Chinese foods. Remember that the smaller the chile, the hotter it usually will be.

Don't Forget Fiber!

In terms of warding off diseases that often strike at midlife, fiber may be the most important dietary supplement ever. There's evidence that a high-fiber diet may help protect against breast cancer. It can also help to lower blood cholesterol, stabilize blood sugar in women with diabetes, and prevent GI tract ills—constipation, diarrhea, hemorrhoids, diverticulosis, even colon cancer.

As the indigestible part of plants, fiber isn't absorbed by the body. It travels pretty much intact from the stomach to the intestines. There it soaks up water like a sponge, softening and bulking up the stool so it moves through the GI tract quickly and efficiently. This not only alleviates many bowel disturbances; it also prevents harmful, cancer-causing substances from camping out and getting a stronghold. Fiber's amazing cholesterol-lowering effect is achieved in the same process. While absorbing water in

HOW TO EAT MORE FIBER

Want to make sure you're getting plenty of lifesaving fiber? Eat your cereal. Not surprisingly, some breakfast cereals top the charts for fiber content. One-third cup of Kellogg's All-Bran Bran Buds packs a whopping 13 grams. One-half cup of Kellogg's All-Bran contains 10 grams. A 1-cup serving of Kellogg's Raisin Bran has 8 grams. A 1¼-cup serving of Post Spoon Size Shredded Wheat'n Bran also has 8 grams. Here are a dozen more sources of fiber that can help you get closer to meeting your daily needs.

- Black beans, ½ cup: 7.5 grams
- Dried figs, three: 6.9 grams
- Dried pears, five halves: 6.5 grams
- Kidney beans, ½ cup: 6.5 grams
- Artichoke, one medium: 6.5 grams
- Lentil soup, 1 cup: 5.6 grams
- Potato with skin, one baked: 4.8 grams
- Raspberries, ½ cup: 4.2 grams
- Split pea soup, 1 cup: 4 grams
- Apple with peel, one medium: 3.7 grams
- Blackberries, ½ cup: 3.8 grams
- Sweet potato, baked, one medium: 3.4 grams

the intestines, fiber also sucks up bile, a fluid secreted by the liver that aids digestion. To make more bile, the liver pilfers cholesterol from the blood-stream, resulting in lower blood cholesterol.

If that's not enough to win you over, consider this: Fiber has been called the most powerful weight-loss aid in the world. That's because high-fiber foods make you feel full on fewer calories. And when you're fighting off "menopause middle," that's really good news.

Getting Enough

In spite of its many benefits, few women get the recommended 20 to 35 grams of fiber per day—the amount studies suggest for blanket health protection. Most of us get half that amount or less. Yet fiber is extremely easy to add to your diet. Just look to fruits, vegetables, legumes (beans and peas), and whole grains like oats and whole wheat. Or, for an extra boost, supplement your meals with a granulated fiber product like wheat bran or psyllium. But don't rely solely on fiber supplements to meet your recommended daily requirements. You'll miss out on a slew of disease-fighting vitamins and minerals that are available only in food.

Don't forget to drink lots of water, at least eight 8-ounce glasses a day, while eating a high-fiber diet and/or taking fiber supplements. If you run dry, you risk becoming constipated or experiencing other unpleasant GI disturbances like gas (already a common problem during menopause) or a more serious complication like a bowel obstruction.

The Menopause Superfood: Soy

Soy's extraordinary potential to relieve hot flashes and other menopausal symptoms and reduce cholesterol has made it *the* superfood for menopausal women. (For more on soy's role in fighting high cholesterol—plus a yummy recipe for Cranberry-Almond Muffins—see "Enjoy Soy's Flour Power" on page 72.) Soy may also fight breast cancer, protect against colon cancer and endometrial cancer, and prevent strokes—among other life-extending benefits.

"There almost isn't a disease that soy can't help in some way," says John Glaspy, M.D., of Jonsson Cancer Center at UCLA, who is studying soy's protective effect against breast cancer.

The "magic" ingredients responsible for soy's healing prowess? Isoflavones—specifically genistein and daidzein—estrogen-like compounds abundant in soybeans. Soy is "the" life extension food. Doctors and scientists add soy to their diets, and advise women to do the same.

One of the richest sources of isoflavones (30 milligrams per ½ cup) is tofu—spongelike blocks of soybean curd sold in supermarkets. But if you're like many women, you know your family will never, ever eat it. (And you're not too fond of it yourself.) It's soft, mushy, and bland.

Chinese, Vietnamese, and Thai cuisines work wonders with tofu, changing the texture so it's chewy or crispy and adding a variety of robust, mouthwatering flavors. We suggest that you try a few tofu (often listed as "bean curd" in Chinese restaurants) dishes when you're eating out and see if your opinion of tofu doesn't improve.

BE SOY SAVVY

Soy is loaded with estrogen-like plant substances, which in moderation may help replace your body's subsiding hormone reserves. Women in Japan and China eat lots of soy foods. These women also don't need hormone therapy (HT) since they have few menopausal symptoms, not to mention low rates of breast cancer. Better yet, research suggests that plant hormones in soy called isoflavones are responsible for building bone, thus lowering the risk for osteoporosis, which normally soars in menopausal years. Studies show that another plant hormone in soy, genistein, shows promise in fighting cancerous tumors.

Can eating soy help you avoid menopausal problems as it does for your sisters living in the Far East? The medical community is not sure. Researchers have a number of misgivings and unanswered questions about this ancient Asian wonder.

"The truth is, the Asian women who avoid symptoms have been eating soy all of their lives and may be benefiting from other factors in their diets or lifestyle," says Walter Willett, M.D., Dr.P.H., professor of epidemiology and nutrition and chairperson of the department of nutrition at the Harvard School of Public Health.

In fact, some studies suggest that adding excessive doses of plant estrogens, like those found in soy products, to your diet later in life may actually *increase* your cancer risk.

So what should you do about this promising but perplexing legume? Dr. Willett recommends incorporating soy into your diet, within limits. One or two servings of soy foods daily may be enough to give your estrogen a little lift, especially if you forgo HT (women on hormone therapy shouldn't need any help). Try a cup of calcium-fortified vanilla soymilk on your cereal. Snack on roasted soy nuts from the health food store. Marinate sliced tofu and portobello mushrooms, then grill and toss the mixture into a pita pocket or into pasta.

Still can't face tofu, or just want to get the benefits of soy more often than the occasional Chinese take-out? No problem: Here's a list of 15 *other* tasty ways to work soy into your diet without eating tofu, starting with those with the highest isoflavone content per serving. (Isoflavone content varies from product to product.) Many are found in supermarkets; others, in health food stores or through mail order.

- Textured vegetable protein—62 milligrams of isoflavones per ¼ cup of dry granules; one brand is Beef (Not) Textured Soy Protein Granules. Use as a meat substitute in chili, barbecue, sloppy joes and the like
- Soy cereal—60 milligrams of isoflavones per ¼ cup (sold under the brand name Nutlettes; mild and slightly nutty, like Grapenuts)
- Soy shakes—52 to 57 milligrams of isoflavones (smooth, creamy drinks from milk and fat-free ice cream)
- Soy protein bars—49 milligrams isoflavones per bar (available in chocolate mint, peanut butter, and mocha)
- Canned soybeans—41 milligrams of isoflavones per ½ cup (chestnutty and creamy; they work well in soups and chili)
- Tempeh—36 milligrams of isoflavones per ½ cup (sold in cakes, then marinated, sliced, and fried)
- Soymilk—30 milligrams of isoflavones per cup (a slightly beany liquid best used in shakes, puddings, and hot cocoa, though vanilla soy milk poured over cereal is tasty)
- Roasted soy nuts—30 milligrams of isoflavones per 3 tablespoons (look like tiny peanuts—delicious as a snack)
- Soy pudding—30 milligrams of isoflavones per ½ cup (chocolate almond is heavenly)
- Miso—29 milligrams of isoflavones per ¼ cup (a flavoring for soups and stews; tastes a little like teriyaki)
- Soy cheese—9 milligrams of isoflavones per ounce (used in cooking as a nondairy stand-in for the real thing). If you don't like one soy cheese, try a different brand. Tastes and textures vary.
- Soy burgers—8 milligrams of isoflavones per patty (an easy-to-digest substitute for beef, it tastes a little like bean dip with vegetables)
- Soy flour—8 milligrams of isoflavones per tablespoon (replace one-quarter to one-third of the flour in recipes for muffins and other baked goods—you'll never taste the difference)

PLEASE READ THE LABELS!

Not every soy product automatically supplies isoflavones. Avoid "soy protein concentrate"—most of the isoflavones may have been processed out. Instead, look for "isolated soy protein," "soy protein isolate," or "textured soy protein" on the label. (If you're unsure, write to or call the manufacturer.) Roasted soy butter has only 1 milligram of isoflavone per serving. And don't count on soy sauce or soybean oil—they contain *no* isoflavones.

- Soy hot dogs—7 milligrams of isoflavones per frank (resembles chicken burgers and works well with relish and other fixings)
- Soy ice cream—5 milligrams of isoflavones per ½ cup (available in chocolate supreme, vanilla almond bark, and butter pecan and tastes like premium ice cream)
- Soy ice milk—3 milligrams isoflavones per ½ cup (sweet, ice milk consistency with a bit of an aftertaste)

Experts recommend that you get 30 to 50 milligrams of isoflavones a day—a cinch with so much variety.

Helpful Hints

Plain soymilk is Band-Aid brown and beany tasting. Look for chocolate, vanilla, mocha, or other flavors. Or stir in some cocoa powder, coffee, almond extract, or whatever strikes your fancy. Example: Heat 1 cup of soymilk in the microwave for 1 minute, add a little instant coffee or chocolate mix, and you have a healthy latte or hot cocoa.

Go against the Grain

Americans are virtually addicted to white flour, white rice, and white sugar. Perhaps refined foods may look and feel lighter. But in reality, it's the darker, whole grains that can keep *you* lighter—and keep you alive longer.

When the diets of 34,000 women ages 55 to 69 were analyzed by researchers at the University of Minnesota, those who had diets high in whole grains were 40 percent more likely to live longer. Women who ate at least one daily serving of whole grains had a substantially lower risk of cancer, cardiovascular disease, diabetes, and other diseases than women who ate almost no whole grains. And there's more good news: The whole grain eaters were significantly slimmer than the fans of refined foods.

"Women who eat more fiber usually weigh less, making it a welcome ally in the battle against menopausal weight gain and heart disease. That may be because high-fiber foods tend to be low in calories, yet bulky and filling, and they take longer to digest than processed foods," says Christine Rosenbloom, R.D., Ph.D., associate professor of nutrition at Georgia State University in Atlanta.

Although the processed food industry so often removes stay-slim fiber from common foods, make the effort to get the right grain. When the germ and hulls are removed to make white flour and white rice, for instance, they lose fiber, along with precious nutrients. Whole grains, on the other hand, tend to be more satisfying because of their fuller, more satisfying flavors as well as the chewier textures that you can really sink your teeth into.

Most women eat 12 to 14 grams of fiber daily. But actually, you need to eat twice that amount, particularly as you go through menopause, says Dr. Rosenbloom. A great habit to increase fiber is to do your own baking with whole flours and oat bran, and base lots of meals around brown rice and wild rice, bulgur wheat, and buckwheat (kasha).

When you do buy processed foods, let the numbers talk. A "high-fiber" food supplies 5 or more grams per serving, while a food labeled as "a good source of fiber" provides 2.5 to 4.9 grams per serving. Look for multigrain or whole grain cereals and crackers, and switch to whole wheat pasta, pita pockets, and tortillas. For a bigger fiber boost, smash up bran cereal and use it as a topping for casseroles, vegetables, fruit, even frozen yogurt. And don't pass by popcorn—it's truly a fiber-friendly snack.

Wheat Germ: Treat This Germ like a Gem

Wheat germ is packed with so many nutrients that many researchers consider it the ultimate health food for menopausal women. It's a concentrated source of vitamin E and folate, both of which have been shown to protect against heart disease, says Densie Webb, R.D., Ph.D., a nutritionist in Austin, Texas, and associate editor of *Environmental Nutrition* newsletter. "It's also packed with manganese, magnesium, phosphorus, and potassium—trace minerals recently shown to be critical for strong bones."

Wheat germ is a part of the wheat kernel, which, along with the fibrous bran coating, gets processed out to make white flour, so most women don't get very much of it. But you can add it back into your diet in a variety of ways. When you're baking muffins or quick breads, replace ½ cup of flour with wheat germ. In cookies, go up to 1 cup. You can also swirl it into smoothies, stir it into yogurt, or sprinkle it on cold cereal and salads.

At room temperature, wheat germ spoils quickly, so refrigerate it in a tightly sealed container. That way, it will stay fresh for up to 9 months, says Dr. Webb.

Water Down Symptoms

Being even a little dehydrated can trigger a range of menopause aggravations. So drink up.

Staying well-hydrated is vital for cooling down those hot flashes and fending off constipation, irritability, insomnia, and other symptoms of menopause, says Felicia Busch, R.D., author of *The New Nutrition: From Antioxidants to Zucchini.*

Getting enough water also can help you feel more energetic and can even diminish skin dryness.

Here are a few solid ways to avoid dehydration and to minimize menopausal symptoms.

- Drink six to eight 8-ounce glasses of water daily. If you're active, especially in hot and humid weather, drink more.

- Cool water is absorbed more quickly into your body than warm water, says Felicia. So chill your water bottle in a freezer for a few minutes before you head out to the golf course or tennis court. Your water is also more apt to stay cold until the end of your game.

- Plain water is fine, but if you prefer the flavor or carbonation of bottled water, that works just as well. Do whatever it takes to keep your tank full.

- Limit your consumption of cola, coffee, and other caffeinated drinks since they are diuretics, which move water out of your body.

- Think you're hungry? Have a glass of water first. Thirst often masquerades as hunger.

Cutting Your Cancer Risk

As if the thought of cancer weren't already frightening enough, the risks of certain kinds of cancer, including breast cancer and endometrial cancer, rise after menopause. (See "Color Your Life with Cancer Protection" below for more on breast cancer risks.) If you choose to combat menopausal symptoms with hormone therapy (HT; formerly called hormone replacement therapy, or HRT), new studies show that your risk of developing breast cancer can rise even higher.

So it's a smart move for all of us, as we enter menopause, to start doing everything we comfortably can to reduce our cancer risks. And one of the easiest things we can do is to modify our diets. Even small changes—like adding more of the fruits and vegetables we all know we *should* be eating anyway—can make a big difference. Read on for tasty ways to add cancer-fighting foods and flavorings to your daily meals.

Color Your Life with Cancer Protection

Many postmenopausal women fear breast cancer—and with good reason. The older you get, the higher your risk of this dreaded diagnosis. One out of eight women experience breast cancer by age 80. But there's something that can protect you, and fortunately, it's right out back in your garden, says Cyndi Thomson, R.D., Ph.D., a diet and breast cancer researcher at the University of Arizona in Tucson.

Eat a minimum of seven servings of fruits and vegetables daily in all hues of the rainbow, she suggests. That's because carotenoids, the plant chemicals that create bright colors in fruits and vegetables, may help prevent cancer. So make it a habit to dine on blueberries, grapes, raisins, plums, dark green lettuce, spinach, kale, collards, carrots, strawberries, tomatoes, beets, and red, green, orange, and yellow peppers.

Try a new fruit or vegetable each week, and learn new ways to prepare old favorites. You don't have to give up meat completely; just shift toward a more colorful, plant-based diet. A good tool for expanding your produce menu is a vegetarian starter cookbook, such as *Vegetarian and More!* by Linda Rosensweig.

HEALTHY, HEARTY PASTA

The next time you think "spaghetti," skip the meatballs and instead, try this Chickpea Pasta Sauce from Jackie Newgent, R.D., a spa cuisine instructor at Peter Kump's New York Cooking School.

Chickpea Pasta Sauce

1	tablespoon extra-virgin olive oil
1	large onion, thinly sliced
2–3	cloves garlic, minced
1	can (20 ounces) chickpeas, with juice
1	can (16 ounces) chopped tomatoes, with juice
1	tablespoon chopped or crushed fresh rosemary
	Salt and freshly ground pepper
	Hot-pepper sauce
2	tablespoons freshly grated Parmesan cheese (optional)

Heat the oil in a large saucepan over medium heat. Cover the pan with a tight-fitting lid and "sweat" the onion and garlic by allowing them to soften and slowly release their own water without browning. If they begin to brown, reduce the heat.

In a blender, puree half the chickpeas and half (or all) of the chickpea juice. Stir the pureed chickpeas, whole chickpeas, tomatoes (with juice), and rosemary into the onion–garlic mixture. Simmer, uncovered, stirring occasionally for about 20 minutes, or until the sauce thickens.

Season with the salt and pepper and the hot-pepper sauce. Stir in the Parmesan, if using. Serve over your favorite pasta or couscous or use as a sauce for baked or grilled chicken.

MAKES 8 SERVINGS

Approximately ½ cup sauce with 1 cup cooked ziti: 275 calories, 4 g fat, 13 percent of calories from fat

Cancer-Fighting Flavorings

Nonfattening flavor enhancers will not only spice up your meals but also help you break away from eating habits that can undermine your postmenopausal health. Old family favorites may suddenly seem bland and joyless when you banish their fat-laden ingredients in order to reduce your cancer risk, lower your cholesterol, and corral your postmenopausal risk of heart disease. But there is life after sour cream and bacon bits. You can avoid dieting doldrums by flavoring food in new ways that will tempt your taste buds, protect your heart, and fight cancer, too.

Here's how:

- Start by replacing butter with extra-virgin olive oil, suggests Jackie Newgent, R.D., a spa cuisine instructor at Peter Kump's New York Cooking School. The flavor is robust, so you don't need much. And for weight control, think teaspoons, not tablespoons. Olive oil supplies a more heart-healthy kind of fat, but it's still high in calories.

- Cook with plenty of onions and fresh garlic, too, says Jackie. They're rich in organosulfides, compounds that create their characteristic "fragrances" and protect against heart disease and cancer. For best flavor and least fat, learn to "sweat" your vegetables (you sweat an onion, for example, by allowing it to soften and slowly release its own water, without browning it).

- Experiment with different herbs. Jackie recommends rosemary in particular. "Its pine fragrance entices you to indulge in dishes even if they lack the familiar smack of saturated fat," she says. Rosemary is also packed with carnosol, an antioxidant that may prevent cancer.

- One last trick: Replacing ground beef with beans will eliminate the saturated fat and load you up on antioxidants that can defend cells against cancer-causing agents, Jackie says.

Give Your Bones a Break from Osteoporosis

We've all got enough to do without worrying about broken bones. But osteoporosis is one of the major diseases women face after menopause, and along with it comes the specter of dowager's humps and broken hips. One out of every two women in the United States has an osteoporosis-induced fracture in her lifetime. Decades of chronic pain and disfigurement can follow all-too-common vertebral compression fractures. If the injury is to the hip, a woman's golden years are likely to be blackened by permanent disability or premature death. One-quarter of the people who survive hip fractures require long-term care.

Needless to say, it's imperative to take this insidious disease seriously, particularly when estrogen decline at menopause increases its likelihood. So start protecting your bones now with weight-bearing exercises (for more on these, see chapter 4, "The Menopause Exercise Plan") and bone-strengthening foods and supplements.

Catch Up with Calcium

Calcium helps slow bone loss after menopause. But to get enough each day, you must think beyond the obvious. When menopause occurs, a woman can begin losing up to 7 percent of her bone mass annually. Over time, that loss can lead to osteoporosis, the bone-thinning disease known as the silent crippler of women.

Doctors recommend that women up to age 50 get 1,000 milligrams of calcium daily and that those over age 50 consume 1,200 milligrams daily. A glass of milk or 1 cup of yogurt is an excellent start. Each contains 300 to 400 milligrams of calcium. But to get a full dose, you're probably going to have to make a few changes in your diet, says Sheah Rarback, R.D., assistant professor at the University of Miami School of Medicine in Florida.

Here are just few ways to enhance your calcium intake.

- Replace the nondairy creamer in your coffee with ¼ cup of fat-free milk to be 75 milligrams of calcium richer.

- Sprinkle an ounce of shredded low-fat cheese on your salad, and you get another 200 milligrams of calcium.

- Top 1 cup of steamed broccoli with a tablespoon of sesame seeds, and get a vegetarian bonanza worth 82 milligrams of calcium.

- Scatter 2 tablespoons of slivered almonds on your green beans and get a 50-milligram calcium bonus.

- Snap up beans. Most contain between 50 and 130 milligrams of calcium per cup.

Get Hip to Vitamin K

If you're trying to avoid fractures caused by menopause-related bone loss, maybe you're eating plenty of dairy foods already. But a lesser-known security for your skeleton is to kick up your vitamin K intake.

Research shows that middle-aged women who get the most vitamin K from food have the lowest rates of hip fractures. The minimum recommended level of vitamin K is 65 micrograms daily, but experts say that to *really* bolster bones, you might need almost twice as much—about 110 micrograms.

"Green vegetables are the best source of vitamin K, which activates osteocalcin, a protein that makes your bones stronger," says Liz Ward, R.D., a nutritionist in Stoneham, Massachusetts, and coauthor of *Super Nutrition after 50*. Just one brussels sprout or ½ cup of broccoli, cabbage, spinach, kale, Swiss chard, or collard greens will do it. For variety, try 1 cup of cooked asparagus, green beans, or turnip greens, or ½ cup of raw cauliflower. Vitamin K is also found in soybean oil and egg yolks.

Yell for Yogurt

Want a supercharged source of calcium to strengthen your menopausal bones? Put yogurt at the top of your shopping list. Yogurt is a plain and simple skeleton helper. Plain yogurt packs a whopping 400 milligrams of calcium per cup, and it's more readily digested than milk, says JoAnn Hattner, R.D., a nutrition counselor in Palo Alto, California.

In fact, as we age and head toward menopause, many of us lose the ability to break down lactose, the sugar in milk, and end up with bloating, cramping, or diarrhea. Many women who can't handle milk, however, do just fine with yogurt. That's because, in the yogurt-making process, friendly bacteria digest a lot of the lactose for us.

Also, with age, many women experience mild gastrointestinal symptoms. "Live and active cultures in yogurt keep your intestinal tract healthier," says JoAnn. And that's in contrast to the problems some women have with calcium supplements. "Among the women I counsel, some become constipated from calcium carbonate supplements, while others develop loose stools from calcium supplements that contain magnesium. I tell them they'll do better with low-fat or fat-free yogurt."

JoAnn shares another bone-friendly tip: "In its natural state, plain yogurt is higher in calcium than sweetened varieties. You can sweeten it yourself with honey and get a bonus because honey seems to fight infection."

You can use yogurt as a condiment by dolloping it atop soups and mixing it with grated lime peel as an accompaniment for fruit. Or try this simple, luscious yogurt-based dip for vegetables.

Creamy Mustard Dip

Use as a dip for fresh vegetables or dried tomatoes.

> 1 **cup calcium-added low-fat cottage cheese**
> ½ **cup fat-free plain yogurt**
> ⅓ **cup brown mustard**
> 1 **teaspoon chopped fresh thyme**
> 2 **teaspoon minced shallots**
> 1 **teaspoon chopped fresh dill or ¼ teaspoon dried**
> ½ **teaspoon lemon juice**

In a food processor or blender, whip the cottage cheese until smooth. Add the yogurt, mustard, thyme, shallots, dill, and lemon juice. Stir until blended.

MAKES ABOUT 2 CUPS

Per 2 tablespoons: 1 g fat, 100 mg calcium

Say "Cheese!" for a Healthy Smile

When we think of postmenopausal bone loss, we tend to think of hip fractures and spinal compression. But there's another set of critical bones that need protection: your skull and jawbone. Calcium loss in the jaws can lead to loose (and ultimately lost) teeth. The teeth themselves can suffer from calcium loss.

After menopause, your gums are also more vulnerable to decay. That's because the loss of estrogen that occurs during menopause affects all the cells in your body, including the gum tissue surrounding your teeth. As your gums recede, tooth roots, which are not protected by hard enamel, become exposed to cavity-causing bacteria. And to make matters worse, baked, starchy foods like pastries, pretzels, crackers, and cookies stick between your teeth, providing the bacteria and the acidic conditions that rot teeth. Dry mouth, another menopause symptom and a side effect of some medications, can also lead to gum disease.

For past generations, the answer to tooth loss was dentures, something that seemed as inevitable as reading glasses. But women today would like to keep their own teeth, thank you. And because of better at-home dental care and routine dental cleanings, we have a better chance of doing so than our mothers and grandmothers.

Our food choices can also help in the fight to keep our teeth. Just chomping on a piece or two of cheese, such as aged Swiss, Cheddar, or Monterey Jack, every day may actually protect against cavities, says Mary P. Faine, R.D., associate professor of nutrition at the University of Washington in Seattle. Dairy products, and cheese in particular, contain a protein that prevents plaque from sticking to teeth, she says.

Here are other tips to smile about:

- Brushing your teeth or drinking water after snacks will help fend off cavities.

- If you experience dry mouth, chew high-fiber foods, such as celery or carrots. They stimulate saliva flow, which protects your teeth.

- A cup of fat-free milk is good saliva substitute because it won't cause cavities and it helps provide the calcium you need to keep your jawbone strong and your teeth sturdy.

Heading Off Heart Disease

It wasn't so long ago that everyone thought of heart disease as a man's problem. What a shock when the news broke that it's also a major killer of women! The risk rises after menopause, so you need to act now to keep your heart healthy and your cholesterol and blood pressure low. Once again, your food choices can help you. From nuts and salmon to psyllium supplements and orange juice, here are some easy ways to pack more heart-healing punch into your meals.

Put the Crunch on Heart Disease

Pecans, almonds, and other nuts can help slash your heart disease risk after menopause. It's an injustice to their other health benefits if you shun them just because they contain fat. Eating just 1 ounce daily, about ¼ cup, can lower "bad," low-density lipoprotein (LDL) cholesterol levels, slightly raise "good," high-density lipoprotein (HDL) cholesterol levels, and lower triglyceride levels—a triple treat that protects against postmenopausal heart disease, says Kenneth I. Burke, R.D., Ph.D., professor and associate chairperson of the department of nutrition and dietetics at Loma Linda University in California.

Walnuts, for instance, are the best land-based source of omega-3 fatty acids, the heart-protective oil found in salmon and other cold-water fish. Pecans, just like olives, are rich in oleic acid, another cardiovascular power broker. And almonds are a bountiful source of heart-healthy natural vitamin E.

Just be sure to crunch with control. Each level measuring tablespoonful of these nuts packs about 50 calories, which can lead to weight gain and, in turn, overtax your heart. So measure your portions. Sprinkle a tablespoon of toasted walnuts on your hot or cold breakfast cereal, stir a tablespoon of sliced almonds into yogurt, or scatter 2 tablespoons of chopped pecans on a dinner salad until you've reached your daily ¼-cup quota.

Befriend Broccoli

Cruciferous (cabbage family) vegetables are well-established cancer fighters. Now comes word that broccoli is also a potent ally in your fight against postmenopausal heart disease.

Like apples and onions, broccoli is a good source of flavonoids, a group of antioxidant compounds that scavenge free radicals before they can oxidize low-density lipoprotein (LDL) cholesterol. If oxidized, this bad cholesterol can glom onto your artery walls, increasing your heart attack risk.

Researchers at the University of Minnesota hailed broccoli after they analyzed the eating habits of 34,000 postmenopausal women. After 10 years, those women who had eaten the most flavonoid-laden foods had a 32 percent lower risk of dying from heart disease than those who had eaten the least of this nutrient. Of all the beneficial foods studied, broccoli demonstrated the most promise.

"This is the only study done exclusively on postmenopausal women that looked at flavonoids," explains Laura Yochum, R.D., a senior health care analyst in Phoenix, who was the study's lead researcher. "It suggests that getting plenty of foods rich in flavonoids, especially broccoli, can lower the heart disease risks that escalate after menopause."

One cup of cooked broccoli is also good source of heart-friendly fiber and folate, as well as vitamins A, C, and E. To get the most nutritional benefit, buy broccoli that is bright emerald green with small, tightly closed flower buds, she says.

TAKE IRON INTAKE TO HEART

After menopause, your body's iron requirements change. You'll need to adjust your intake to protect your heart—and your overall health.

As long as you were having regular menstrual periods, you lost precious iron, critical for carrying oxygen for energy. That's why you always needed more iron than your mate (15 milligrams daily to his 10 milligrams) to avoid iron deficiency anemia. But after menopause, your iron needs drop to about 8 milligrams daily.

You still need this mineral, but you must make your intake more moderate, insists Kathleen Zelman, R.D., an Atlanta-based spokesperson for the American Dietetic Association. Some researchers suspect that excess iron can damage the heart and other cells in the body.

To get the right age-adjusted iron dose, take a senior formula daily multivitamin that contains 4 milligrams of iron, she suggests. Get your remaining daily iron needs from food.

Iron from lean meat, chicken, and fish is absorbed better than the iron from plant sources, like beans, bread, fruit, and vegetables. Animal protein also increases the absorption of iron from those plant sources. So add an ounce or two of chicken to your beans, have a dab of lean meat with your potatoes, or have a bit of fish with your pasta. "You'll get all the iron you need without overdoing it," says Kathleen.

Get Hooked on Deep-Sea Fish

Eating certain fish can help keep your arteries clear and lower your risk of heart problems as you go through menopause. As menopause kicks in and your estrogen levels tumble, your risk of heart disease shoots up. But adding fish such as salmon, turbot, haddock, and cod to your menu two or three times a week can help keep your cardiovascular system healthy, says Clare M. Hasler, Ph.D., the executive director of the Functional Foods for Health program at the University of Illinois at Urbana–Champaign and Chicago.

That's because these deep-water ocean fish have developed a kind of body fat—called omega-3—that stays pliable no matter how low the temperature goes. When you eat these omega-3s, they become part of your own cell membranes, which in turn become more supple, says Dr. Hasler. That means the walls of your arteries are more flexible and the platelets in your blood are more slippery, a combination that can lower your risk of blood clots. (A blood clot that gets stuck in the artery that supplies blood to your heart is what typically causes a heart attack.)

Eat your fish baked, broiled, steamed, poached, grilled, or even canned. But don't fry it—that only adds heart-clogging saturated fat to your meal. When you're eating out, order grilled salmon, have anchovies on your Caesar salad, or go for a tuna sandwich.

Take Psyllium with Supper

Throughout your childbearing years, estrogen keeps cholesterol under control, providing natural protection against heart disease. But with menopause, estrogen dwindles, which allows cholesterol levels—and your risk of heart disease—to soar.

Psyllium, the ground husk of the plantain plant and a well-known ingredient in laxatives, may be one of your best weapons in the battle against postmenopausal heart disease, says Gail Frank, R.D., Dr.P.H., professor of nutrition at California State University at Long Beach. Psyllium is loaded with soluble fiber, a gummy substance that clings to digestive secretions called bile. As this fiber passes through your digestive tract, it traps bile, which normally helps your body absorb fat and cholesterol from food. Without bile, more cholesterol is excreted from your body.

Just a little psyllium is mighty potent: 1 tablespoon contains as much soluble fiber as *14 tablespoons* of oat bran, which is better known for its soluble fiber content. So even if you're already eating a diet low in saturated fat and cholesterol, adding 4 level teaspoons daily of ground psyllium seed husk to drinks and foods may further reduce your cholesterol load.

But beware: You can't eat psyllium by itself. It soaks up water in your digestive tract, which could cause constipation. Instead, stir it into at least 8 ounces of juice or milk, or add it to cookies or muffins in place of a few teaspoons of flour. Psyllium also works well in meat loaf because it helps soak up the juices.

Add psyllium to your diet gradually. Start with 1 teaspoon a day for about a week. Add another teaspoon each week until you reach 4 teaspoons a day. If you develop gas or bloating at some point, cut back to your previous amount. If even 1 teaspoon triggers these symptoms, stick it out for a week—your body may adjust. If it doesn't, cut back to ½ teaspoon for a week, then gradually increase the amount as previously described.

Make sure you drink your daily requirement of at least eight 8-ounce glasses of water. Getting plenty of water helps psyllium do its job. In addition, fluids will cut down on gas, bloating, and other side effects, says Dr. Frank. (For more good reasons to drink lots of water, see "Water Down Symptoms" on page 59.)

Psyllium is available at most health food stores. Check with your physician before using the supplement because it may alter the absorption of any medications you are taking. And don't take psyllium if you have a bowel obstruction.

Sweeten Your Cholesterol Numbers with Oranges

Help yourself to a little citrus sunshine. It's a surprising weapon in the fight against postmenopausal heart disease.

Researchers have long known that eating less saturated fat will lower levels of low-density lipoprotein (LDL), the so-called bad cholesterol. But food wasn't thought to have any effect on "good," high-density lipoprotein (HDL) cholesterol. So Elzbieta Kurowska, Ph.D., a nutrition researcher in the department of biochemistry at the University of Western

SPREAD ON BENECOL'S BENEFITS

If you're tired of the battle of butter versus margarine in your low-cholesterol campaign, try Benecol on your bread. Benecol, a margarine-like spread available in most dairy cases, can help keep menopausal estrogen loss from pushing your cholesterol sky high. More than 20 clinical studies have shown that as little as three Benecol servings daily can drop total cholesterol by 10 percent and the "bad," low-density lipoprotein (LDL) cholesterol by 14 percent.

Benecol is a combination of canola oil and a powerful plant compound that helps block the absorption of cholesterol in your digestive tract. Unlike some margarines, regular Benecol spread—but not the "light" version—can be used to bake or sauté.

"It tastes good, and it actually melts," says Nadine Pazder, R.D., the outpatient dietitian at Morton Plant Hospital in Clearwater, Florida. Try it on air-popped popcorn, baked potatoes, bagels, toast, and cooked veggies, pasta, or rice. You can even use it when you scramble up your egg substitute.

Benecol's convenient premeasured packets make it easy to get the dose just right. "It is more expensive than butter or margarine, but I tell my patients it costs less than open-heart surgery," says Nadine.

Although Benecol is not a drug, be sure to check with your physician before using this product if you are taking cholesterol-lowering medication or if you are allergic to soy products.

Ontario in London, Canada, was surprised when a group of individuals she studied, including postmenopausal women (none on hormone therapy), had a 20 percent increase in HDL after drinking three 8-ounce glasses of orange juice daily.

Oranges are packed with vitamin C, folate, and other nutrients that could have a positive impact on cholesterol. But further studies will be needed to confirm Dr. Kurowska's results and to pinpoint the precise mechanism.

Dr. Kurowska is not advocating that you drink three glasses of orange juice a day. That's simply far too many calories for just one food, she says. Not to mention that some women in this small preliminary study developed high triglycerides, another risk factor for heart disease. Instead, she suggests that you drink one glass of orange juice daily if you are menopausal. That way, you'll still probably increase your good cholesterol without causing your triglycerides to sneak upward.

Enjoy Soy's Flour Power

While all of soy's benefits to the postmenopausal woman are not completely understood, it is clear that enjoying soy foods daily can lower your total cholesterol level by about 10 percent. After the onset of menopause, a woman's total and "bad," low-density lipoprotein (LDL) cholesterol levels are likely to rise, while her "good," high-density lipoprotein (HDL) cholesterol levels wane, probably because of a dwindling supply of estrogen. Soy, because of its estrogen-like properties, may help halt that trend.

Soy flour is a concentrated source of protein, with about 20 grams per one-half cup. It takes about 25 grams per day to get soy's cholesterol-lowering effect, says Barbara Gollman, R.D., coauthor of *The Phytopia Cookbook* and a Dallas-based consulting dietitian, nutrition educator, and culinary arts expert. This is an amount considered safe even if you're at risk for breast cancer (in some studies, excessive soy consumption is associated with cancer risk).

Since soy flour lacks gluten—the elastic component in wheat flour that allows bread or muffins to capture air so they're light and fluffy—you can't completely replace white flour with soy flour in recipes. "Try replacing about one-fourth of the wheat flour with soy flour, and watch the cooking time," says Barbara. "The soy will make muffins moist and tender, but they will brown a little more quickly." As a general rule, nip 5 to 10 minutes off the baking time suggested in a regular recipe.

To get you started on your soy adventure, try a Chef Gollman favorite.

Cranberry-Almond Muffins

½ cup light and firm silken tofu
    Peel of 1 orange, grated
½ cup sugar
2 eggs, lightly beaten
2 tablespoons canola oil
¼ cup soy flour

    1¼ cups unbleached all-purpose flour
      1 teaspoon baking powder
     ¼ teaspoon baking soda
     ¼ teaspoon salt
     ⅓ cup unblanched almonds, finely chopped
     ½ cup dried cranberries, coarsely chopped

Blend the tofu in a small food processor or blender, or whip with a hand-held blender, until it reaches the consistency of mayonnaise. (Do not use an electric handheld mixer.) Be patient as this takes several minutes.

Preheat the oven to 375°F. Coat a muffin tin with cooking spray. Set aside.

In a small bowl, mix the orange peel with the sugar until the sugar is orange-colored. In a medium bowl, combine the egg, oil, and tofu. Turn the sugar into the egg mixture. Beat with a wire whisk until smooth.

In a large mixing bowl, combine the soy flour, all-purpose flour, baking powder, baking soda, and salt. Stir well. Add the nuts and cranberries. Add the tofu mixture and stir quickly, until just blended. The batter will be lumpy.

Fill the muffin cups about three-quarters full. Bake for 15 minutes, or until golden and springy to the touch.

MAKES 12 MUFFINS
Per muffin: 166 calories, 6 g fat, 1 g saturated fat, 35 mg cholesterol

We've given you a lot to digest in this chapter (pardon the pun), but eating right is a key to your menopausal and postmenopausal health. Here, we've focused on eating to maintain your youthful figure, enhance your overall health and well-being, and ward off serious bodily illness. But diet can do more than nourish your body—it can also help you manage your moods. If menopause is making you moody, turn to "Calming Cuisine: A Week of Relaxing Foods" on page 192.

But there's more to making menopause an easy transition than good eating. Exercise is equally essential in midlife and beyond. In fact, it's probably even more important during the second half of life than it was in your early years.

If you exercise regularly, turn to chapter 4, "The Menopause Exercise Plan," to find a program of exercises that are especially suited for menopause and beyond. They'll strengthen your bones, improve your overall health, and help minimize menopausal symptoms. (They'll also make you look younger!) And if you're an exercise avoider, chapter 4 presents a host of easy options that will let you slide into exercising without breaking a sweat, joining a gym, or springing for costly, space-eating equipment.

DASH AWAY FROM HIGH BLOOD PRESSURE

More than half of all women over age 55 have high blood pressure. But dietary changes can begin to tame this "silent killer" in as little as 14 days.

When women reach menopause, usually in their late forties or early fifties, they are likelier than men of the same age to develop hypertension, also known as high blood pressure. Untreated, high blood pressure can lead to heart disease or stroke. But there's plenty that you can do to slash your risk of hypertension at menopause. For starters, eat less salt, lose weight, and cut down on alcohol. But to really take a load off your cardiovascular system, consider adding a powerful new weapon to your hypertension-busting plan—the DASH diet.

When people tried the Dietary Approaches to Stop Hypertension (DASH) program in research centers around the country, the results were remarkable. Research shows that shifting from a typical American high-fat diet to an eating plan that's low in fat, high in fruits and vegetables, and rich in low-fat dairy products can lower blood pressure as much as medication can, and in just 2 weeks, says Lawrence J. Appel, M.D., associate professor of medicine, epidemiology, and international health at the Johns Hopkins Medical Institutions in Baltimore.

The diet is pretty un-American since it includes about double the national average consumption of fruits, vegetables, and low-fat dairy products. But it's well worth the effort if you can get your blood pressure down without drugs, Dr. Appel says.

For best results, try to stay as close as possible to the following food proportions used in the DASH diet. If you're taking medication for high blood pressure, don't stop without your doctor's permission.

- Grains and grain products: 7 to 8 servings daily
- Low-fat or fat-free dairy foods: 2 to 3 servings daily
- Fruits and vegetables: 8 to 10 servings daily
- Meat, poultry, or fish: 2 or fewer 3-ounce portions daily
- Nuts, seeds, and legumes: 4 to 5 servings per week
- Fats and oils: 2.5 teaspoons a day

Chapter

4

THE MENOPAUSE EXERCISE PLAN

WHEN IT COMES TO MENOPAUSE AND EXERCISE, IT'S TIME TO use it or lose it, where muscles are concerned. "Most women lose about one-third to one-half pound of muscle a year after age 35. By the time they're 80, some can't perform routine tasks, like getting up out of a chair or climbing stairs," says Miriam Nelson, Ph.D., director of the Center for Physical Fitness at Tufts University School of Nutrition Science and Policy in Boston and author of *Strong Women Stay Young* and *Strong Women Stay Slim.*

Part of this loss of strength is from aging, "but it's also from inactivity, and *that* you can do something about," Dr. Nelson says. Research shows that people who strength train seem to preserve their youthful body compositions very well.

Dr. Nelson's own studies show that women in their fifties and sixties who do high-intensity strength training can develop strength scores more typical of women in their late thirties or forties. "We have seen an increase in muscle mass in people even in their nineties," she says. "I'm not saying we are going to make a 90-year-old look like a 20-year-old, but we can see the body shape change and take on a more youthful appearance."

If you already know that you should be exercising and are looking for a quick and easy plan, turn to "The Menopause Exercise Program" on page 89. But if you need further convincing, read on.

What Can Exercise Do for Me?

In addition to helping you look younger, exercise of any type can make you feel really good physically and psychologically after a stressful day. And the effects of exercise may go even deeper than that. Some researchers have shown that it can actually relieve depression and anxiety.

However, unless you're a police officer, construction worker, gym teacher, or carpenter, your normal daily activities are not likely to make a big impact on your cardiovascular health, muscle strength and endurance, or flexibility, all of which are important for general health and fitness and for disease prevention, says Maggie Greenwood-Robinson, Ph.D., a certified nutrition consultant in Newburgh, Indiana, and author of Natural Weight Loss Miracles.

So if you're like most people, you need a plan for exercise. Setting time aside in your day allows you to take care of yourself and anticipate a chance to relax and unwind. "And it's a time to socialize if you participate in an exercise class," adds Tia Willows, assistant vice president of group exercise at Bally Total Fitness in Chicago.

Does It Really Matter What Type of Exercise I Choose?

Aerobic exercise, such as jogging or brisk walking for 30 minutes or more, increases your body's ability to process and utilize oxygen. It keeps your heart and lungs healthy, and it can help prevent diabetes, high blood pressure, and certain types of cancers, says Janet P. Wallace, Ph.D., professor of kinesiology and associate professor and director of adult fitness at Indiana University in Bloomington.

Weight training, on the other hand, is an anaerobic workout. Your body doesn't have the same oxygen needs as it does when performing an aerobic exercise. Lifting weights builds lean muscle tissue, keeps you

ENOUGH EXCUSES!

In high school, we pleaded cramps or "forgot" our ugly gym suits at home to get out of phys ed class. Now, as grown women, we have more sophisticated excuses for weaseling out of working out. Below are the top 10 excuses for not exercising, according to Judith Young, Ph.D., executive director of the National Association for Sport and Physical Education in Reston, Virginia.

1. "I'm too tired."
2. "I have a bad back/knee/ankle."
3. "I can't stick to a routine."
4. "It's so boring."
5. "My job/kids/home obligations eat up my time."
6. "I never see results."
7. "I'm too embarrassed by my body to join a gym or walk in the park."
8. "I get winded easily and can't keep up."
9. "I don't know where to start."
10. "I'm too old."

You can probably make up a great list of your own. But when you're finished, take it out to the backyard and bury it. Then start working on your list of the 10 best reasons to exercise!

strong, gives you more energy, and prevents bone loss—a major concern for women in their postmenopausal years.

Then there are flexibility exercises, such as yoga and stretching, to keep your muscles, ligaments, and tendons limber and less susceptible to injury, says Tia Willows.

But do you really need to incorporate these different types of exercise into your daily routine? The answer is most likely *yes* if you want to accomplish most or all of these seven goals.

Lose body fat. Aerobic exercise is one of the best ways to do it, along with diet adjustments, of course. Resistance training (also called weight training) can help, too, because building muscle mass through resistance training will bump up your resting metabolic rate. And that means you'll burn more calories throughout the day even when you're not exercising. But that works only to support or help maintain your weight-loss efforts. "You're not going to see a big difference, either way, in the scales from weight training alone," says Lisa Womack, associate director of the Cardiac Health and Fitness Memorial Gym at the University of Virginia in Charlottesville.

Get toned. Here's where resistance training does the job and where aerobic training doesn't. "Regular resistance training will make your muscles denser so that you look better," says Priscilla Clarkson, Ph.D., professor and associate dean of the department of exercise science at the University of Massachusetts School of Public Health and Health Sciences in Amherst. "They'll become firm rather than flabby, which is often a concern in areas like the backs of your arms and your stomach."

Get stronger. Appearance aside, strength training will make you stronger. Aerobics, on the other hand, won't do much to help you lift your daughter's 3-year-old or carry heavy stuff without asking for help.

Build endurance. Aerobic work recruits the muscle fibers that specialize in endurance much more than resistance training does. So it makes perfect sense that aerobic exercise is the one that will help you enjoy those long hikes or bike rides.

Get a strong heart. This is a job for aerobics. It's your heart that has to pump all that oxygen to your muscles via your bloodstream when you're doing aerobic work. That's why your heart rate goes up. And that's why aerobic exercise is a proven strengthener of your cardiovascular system and a risk reducer for heart disease.

Spot train. It bears repeating: Neither aerobic exercise nor diets can target fat in any one body part for elimination. For that matter, neither

HOW MUCH EXERCISE DO I NEED?

On average, 2 hours of aerobic activity will burn about 1,000 calories. If your goal is weight loss, you need to burn 3,500 calories to lose 1 pound of fat. So, if you spend 30 minutes jogging four times a week, you can knock off 1 pound of fat in 3½ weeks through exercise alone.

can resistance training. "If you could spot reduce, everyone who chewed gum would have a skinny face," Lisa says. But what resistance training can do—and aerobics can't—is target body parts for muscle toning. When you do toning exercises, you can say, "I'm going to work on my thighs today." Not so with aerobics.

The Health Connection

The immediate reward of any exercise program is the deep satisfaction of looking good on the outside and feeling great on the inside. But if you step back and look at the big picture, exercise can help prevent heart disease, osteoporosis, and other high-risk health problems of the postmenopausal years—as doctors have been telling us for years. Here is a brief summary of those benefits.

Lower Your Risk of Breast Cancer

Being overweight is linked to a higher risk of breast cancer, especially for women after menopause if they gained weight during adulthood. With that in mind, it seems like a no-brainer to assume that exercise will lower your risk of breast cancer. But in reality, the link between exercise and cancer risk is a fairly new area of research, and the results are hardly conclusive.

What we do know so far is that some studies seem to indicate that women who don't exercise and are overweight appear to have a higher risk of breast cancer than leaner women who exercise. Case in point: A Norwegian study found that compared with women who didn't exercise at all, women who exercised at least 4 hours a week had a 37 percent lower breast cancer risk. In other research, postmenopausal women who were moderately active (walking, gardening, or doing housework several times a week) had a 50 percent reduced risk of breast cancer compared with sedentary women. However, more research is being done to confirm similar findings.

Until then, make sure to include moderate exercise in your strategy to lower your risk of breast cancer. The American Cancer Society recommends that women try to stay at a healthy weight to help lower their risk—and exercise is a definite means to that goal.

Lift Yourself from Depression

Exercise can blast away fat, shave years off your figure, boost your energy, and fight disease, but to say that it can prevent stress and depression altogether is a bit of a stretch. Nonetheless, research shows that regular aerobic activity can relieve symptoms of depression and significantly reduce stress—to the point where it's barely noticeable.

Experts theorize that's because regular exercise helps enhance your sense of mastery so you feel more mentally and physically in control. Also, when you're stressed-out, your body releases large amounts of cortisol and adrenaline, hormones that tense your muscles and speed your heart rate, blood pressure, and breathing. Exercise keeps these hormone levels down and protects you from irritability, panic attacks, throbbing headaches, stomachaches, ulcers, and heart disease.

Research shows that regular aerobic exercise produces mood-enhancing chemicals called endorphins that keep us cheerful, bolster self-esteem, and restore feelings of hopefulness in depressed women. So moving your body definitely helps. There's even evidence that exercise can reduce the amount of antidepressant medication you take, depending on the severity of your depression. In one 4-month study, for example, researchers found that depressed men and women who walked or jogged three times a week for 45 minutes improved as much as a control group taking antidepressants.

Enjoy Heart Health

Researchers have found that exercise can give your body's systems the capacity to work as well as those of someone 20 years younger. So it's not surprising that physically active people—regardless of their biological ages—have lower rates of heart disease and are less vulnerable to strokes.

If you haven't exercised for years, don't be put off: "As soon as you start to exercise, your risk of cardiovascular problems drops by 25 percent," says Gerald Fletcher, M.D., professor of medicine at the Mayo Clinic in Jacksonville, Florida.

"Studies show that even if you start a regular exercise program in your sixties, you lower your risk of heart disease for the rest of your life," says James M. Rippe, M.D., director of the Center for Clinical and Lifestyle Research at Tufts University School of Medicine in Boston and author of *Fit after Forty*. "If you're 60 years old, you may have another 25 years left, so the quality of life during those years is something to think about."

Don't let a heart attack hold you back. "Exercise has been proven to be a great therapy," says Kenneth H. Cooper, M.D., president and founder of the Cooper Clinic and the Cooper Institute for Aerobics in Dallas, who is also known as the father of aerobics. Studies have shown that people who became involved in an exercise program after their first heart attacks were 20 to 40 percent more likely to be alive 7 years later than those who had survived heart attacks and then remained totally sedentary.

Exercise is so important that cardiologists often prescribe (not just recommend or suggest) exercise for patients with heart disease. In one study, researchers followed 68 patients who were on a waiting list for heart transplants and who also participated in a walking program. After 3 to 6 months, the hearts of 30 patients had improved to the point that they no longer needed new hearts. Two years later, their hearts were still going strong.

How does aerobic exercise perform these miracles? It makes your heart pump more vigorously to carry extra blood and oxygen to hardworking muscles. Over time, the demands of exercise make your heart physically fit—stronger and more efficient. The heart becomes a bigger, stronger pump that pumps more blood with each beat.

You get practical payoffs as well: The well-exercised heart doesn't have to beat as fast when you do something demanding. Even though your body is stressed, your heart isn't. When nonexercisers shovel the sidewalk after a snowstorm, for instance, their likelihood of a heart attack jumps to 107 times their normal risk! But someone who exercises five times a week has only 2.4 times the normal risk.

Bone Up on Exercise

What's true for muscle is also true for bones, Dr. Nelson says: Use 'em or lose 'em. If women decide to sit back at menopause and allow nature to take its course, they can count on losing up to 20 percent of bone mass in the first 5 to 7 years, followed by a continuous slower loss. But exercise that stresses the bone, such as high-intensity strength training, can change that. It can actually preserve bone mass, and in some cases it even leads to a slight increase, says Dr. Nelson.

"Even that slight increase, or just maintaining bone mass, is important," Dr. Nelson says. "The alternative is allowing your bones to become so brittle and weak over time that you can begin to have fractures."

So no matter what your age, today is the day to start exercising. Even women who already have osteoporosis can strength train, as long as they start out very slowly. While they probably won't regain enough bone mass to stop potential fractures, they can regain muscle strength, which will help them maintain balance and prevent falls, Dr. Nelson says. But she cautions, "Women who have osteoporosis need to work with their doctors to develop a total program, which includes exercise, nutritional support, and perhaps drugs."

FORGET TOE TOUCHING! TRY THIS

Have you ever bent over to touch your toes and wanted to convince yourself later that the reason they seem so hard to reach is because your legs must be growing longer?

Well, take heart. According to many experts, you shouldn't feel bad if you can't touch your toes. The talent of toe touchers—who are actually in the minority—is due to bone structure and joint alignment, not just flexible muscles. Some people really can't touch their toes, period, and if they try too hard, they're likely to strain their lower-back muscles.

It's true that you should stretch your hamstrings and gluteals, the muscles on the backs of your upper thighs and buttocks. Keeping these muscles flexible helps you avoid back and knee injuries. But you don't have to touch your toes to stretch them. You can safely do a forward bend with your knees bent a bit—that takes the strain off your lower back. Ease gently into the stretch.

Or, if you find it comfortable, you can safely stretch these muscles by lying with your torso and buttocks flat on the floor and your legs straight up a wall at a 90-degree angle.

Avoid Exercise Injuries

Given all the health benefits to gain from exercising, the last thing you want to do is backslide with exercise-related injuries. And while injuries can happen anytime, the first few weeks on any exercise program tend to be particularly risky, says Jean Reeve, Ph.D., a triathelete and associate professor of physical education at Southern Utah University in Cedar City. "Mentally, you may be raring to go; but at the same time, your body is just getting used to the idea of regular workouts," she says. "You need to slowly build up strength, especially around vulnerable knee and shoulder joints."

If you're overweight, you need to be especially careful about high-impact activities, like running or jumping. They could hurt your joints. And if you're out of shape overall, Dr. Reeve suggests that you may do better by initially steering clear of activities that require good balance and coordination, such as step aerobics. "You're better off building up some muscle first with light resistance training and stair climbing," she says.

If you're already suffering from an injury, take heart. You don't have to mothball your entire workout. "You probably can continue to do certain exercises," Dr. Reeve says. "But you may need to avoid using your injured area, or use it less strenuously. A physical therapist can help you figure out what moves to avoid until you're healed, and what exercises may actually help your injury heal faster."

Here are five things to do as you begin your exercise program.

Get your doctor to sign off. If you are age 45 or older, or if you have back or joint problems, osteoarthritis, osteoporosis, high blood pressure, or any other kind of chronic medical problem that makes you wonder if it's safe to exercise, Dr. Reeve suggests that you clear your plans with your doctor first. The evaluation should include a treadmill stress test, which can detect serious coronary artery blockage, and blood pressure and cholesterol measurements. If necessary, your doctor can suggest activities that you need to avoid.

Start like a tortoise, not a hare. Begin with a routine that is suited to your level of fitness. "For people who haven't exercised in a long time, start slow and easy," says Michelle F. Mottola, Ph.D., associate professor of anatomy and kinesiology and director of the exercise and pregnancy lab at the University of Western Ontario in London, Ontario. You'll beef things up as you progress. If you're lifting weights, for example, you may find that 2-pound weights are all you can handle when you start. Eventually, you'll get the weights up to the point where doing 16 reps leaves your muscles pretty much pooped out.

Warm up and cool down. Older bodies take time to get in the mood for exercise, get more blood flowing into muscles, and limber up, Dr. Nelson says. Conversely, they also need more time to slow heart rate and cool off after a workout. A proper warmup helps reduce your risk for injuries because it helps your muscles work at their optimal level. And, along with cooldown, it's mandatory if you have heart disease. You can get light-headed or have chest pains from angina if you start or stop too quickly. And some medications for high blood pressure or heart disease make your body warm up and cool down more slowly than normal, she

MOVING TOO MUCH

There *is* such a thing as exercising too much, says certified personal trainer Jana Angelakis, owner of PEx Personalized Exercise in New York City. If you're so sore the next day that you can hardly move, you're working too hard. Getting sick is another sign that you should cut back on your workouts. Knowing when to stop means you're listening to your body so you won't hurt yourself, and you'll stay healthy and energized. Here are a few more red flags.

- Your performance has decreased.
- Your form and technique have deteriorated.
- You need more recovery time than usual.
- You experience a loss of appetite.
- You feel fatigued or nauseated during workouts.
- You get headaches during workouts.

If you experience such symptoms as undue breathlessness, light-headedness, chest pains, and an irregular heartbeat, you could just be overdoing it with exercise, but you should consult a physician to be sure.

adds. A 5- to 10-minute warmup is adequate for most people, on or off medication. However, if you're feeling particularly stiff or sluggish, give yourself a few more minutes.

Don't be a heartbreaker. If you're afraid to exercise because you have heart disease, your doctor can write you a prescription for cardiac rehabilitation, which allows you to learn to exercise in a safe, monitored environment. The best place for such exercise is in a cardiac rehabilitation program in a hospital or other health facility, where medical personnel can monitor you.

Rest up. Give your muscles 48 hours between sessions to recover. Strength training two or three times a week is great for women of all ages, Dr. Nelson says. "Even older women can recover within 48 hours," she says. If you don't recover within this period of time, you are doing too much during your sessions. You'll know that you overdid it if you are still very stiff and it's painful to move your muscles through their full range of motion.

Adjust Your Exercise Attitude

"Basically, at the turn of the 20th century, something like 85 percent of our workforce worked in agricultural-related jobs," says Barbara Moore, Ph.D., president of Shape Up America! in Washington, D.C., a nonprofit organization that helps people lose weight for life. "Their lives were very physically demanding. In today's information-based society, so much of the work we do requires sitting and only sitting."

According to a study from the United Kingdom, people there burn about 800 fewer calories per day than they did in 1970, mostly because of automation and laborsaving devices. It's the same story on this side of the Atlantic.

"Physical activity has been pushed out of our lives," says Dr. Nelson of the Center for Physical Fitness at Tufts University. "This means we have to choose ways to work activity back into our lives. We have to consciously get up more, walk more, take the stairs more. Whenever possible, we need to seek out activity."

WHY DO I HATE TO EXERCISE?

No woman "hates" to exercise. What she hates are her preconceived notions about exercise—that it's painful and inconvenient, that she doesn't do it correctly, that it's a chore rather than an activity that can be both fun and beneficial to her physical and emotional well-being, that she looks ridiculous in exercise clothes.

When women associate exercise with physical pain, it's often because they lifted more weight than they should have or did too many repetitions during their first visits to the gym. When they couldn't move the next day, they blamed the exercise itself, rather than an overambitious workout.

Other women think they dislike exercise because they feel foolish doing it. They think that it requires physical skill or feel pressured to exercise flawlessly, much in the way they feel pressured to be perfect mothers or perfect workers. But doing an arm curl or leg extension doesn't require any unique skills whatsoever.

Women may also hate working out because they believe it should be unpleasant or boring—that if it feels good, it can't possibly have any serious benefits. But, as many women who have "hated" exercise have learned, exercise comes in many different forms. You just have to find the form that works for you, whether it's Pilates or power yoga, kickboxing or bicycling in the park.

If you "hate" to exercise, challenge your assumptions about it. Then try to reframe your idea of exercise in a positive light. Think of it as a gift from you to yourself, as a time-out from the hustle and bustle of your daily life.

Remember, too, that it takes some time to make exercise a habit—at least 6 weeks. If you can stick to an exercise program for that long, you may find that far from "hating" exercise, you actually look forward to your workouts.

Find the Time

Most moderate-intensity activities—walking briskly, raking leaves, mowing the lawn with a push mower, vacuuming—will burn 150 calories in about 30 minutes. So in addition to just counting calories, add up your minutes of activity each day. To lose weight and keep it off, you actually need about 60 minutes of activity a day, according to the latest research.

It doesn't make any difference if you do it all at once or break it up into smaller chunks of time. "Everything counts," says Dr. Moore.

Here are a few ways to motivate yourself to get those 60 minutes in each day.

Step up the intensity. Michelle Edwards, a health educator and certified personal trainer at the Cooper Institute for Aerobics in Dallas, advises her clients to start by simply increasing the intensity of any physical activity that they're already doing. That can mean taking the stairs a little faster, choosing parking spots at the far end of the lot, or making wider arm circles when wiping off the kitchen counter. The idea is to put a little more effort into every activity in order to burn more calories.

Keep a diary. For the next few days, clock yourself every time you walk, clean, garden, climb a flight of stairs, or perform any other activity that involves moving the muscles in your arms and legs. At the end of the day, add up your active time. This helps create a vivid picture of how the minutes add up, explains Michelle. Once you do this, you'll probably find yourself thinking of all kinds of ways to add a few more minutes here and there throughout the day.

One of the keys to becoming more active is learning to identify opportunities in your day and taking advantage of them. "Five minutes here; 10 minutes there. It all adds up," she says.

It also helps to record how much time you spend sitting each day, and to do the reverse. Figure out ways to gradually replace the sitting with activity.

Get a pedometer. If you want to get a clearer picture of the amount of physical activity you are doing in a day, record how many steps you take on an average day and then find ways to add more. Studies show that people who are active for 30 minutes each day accumulate about 10,000 steps, while the average person who works in an office typically takes about 2,000 to 4,000 steps a day. "A pedometer can be a very motivational tool, a way to self-monitor," says Michelle. "And we know from experience that people who self-monitor are more likely to reach their activity goals than people who do not."

Be prepared. Keep walking shoes in your car or desk so that you can walk whenever you have a few minutes.

Schedule it. We tend to keep our appointments, so make an appointment to exercise. You can start by scheduling exercise in the morning

BURNING CALORIES

If you are a 150-pound woman, how long does it take to burn 150 calories? That depends on what you do. (If you weigh more, it may take less intensity to burn the same number of calories.)

Ironing	59 minutes
Cooking	48 minutes
Washing and waxing a car	45 to 60 minutes
Playing volleyball	45 minutes
Strolling through the mall	44 minutes
Grocery shopping	36 minutes
Doing yoga	36 minutes
Vacuuming	34 minutes
Playing horseshoes	33 minutes
Gardening	30 to 45 minutes
Bicycling leisurely	30 minutes (at 10 mph)
Brisk walking	30 minutes
Dancing fast	30 minutes
Pushing a stroller	30 minutes
Raking leaves	30 minutes
Mowing the lawn with a push mower	29 minutes
Inline skating leisurely	26 minutes
Stacking firewood	25 minutes
Bowling	23 minutes
Housecleaning	21 minutes
Scrubbing floors	20 minutes
Swimming	19 minutes
Climbing stairs	15 minutes
Shoveling snow	15 minutes

instead of later in the day, suggests Denise Bruner, M.D., president of the American Society of Bariatric Physicians (a group of doctors who specialize in weight-loss treatments) and a physician practicing in Arlington, Virginia. "Women seem to be more successful in general if they put activity on the front end of the day, versus the end of the day, when either work-related issues or home issues can end up taking precedence over exercise time," she says.

The Menopause Exercise Program

As we've already said, all forms of exercise give you more energy. And for optimal energy, you need a program that combines cardiovascular activity, strength and toning exercises, and stretching. So wouldn't it be great to have one workout that does all those things and lasts no longer than an episode of your favorite sitcom? Well, here it is!

Our Menopause Exercise Program for total body toning is a muscle-toning, strength-training program specially designed by *Prevention* magazine to raise your heart rate and increase your flexibility. So you get all your fitness benefits rolled into one fat-blasting 25-minute routine.

The concept behind this plan is circuit training, and it works like this: You have a series of strength-training exercises, which you perform back-to-back with little rest in between. Like traditional strength training, circuit training builds muscle, which helps you burn more calories when you're not exercising.

(continued on page 98)

LIFTING WEIGHTS VERSUS JOGGING

Research has shown that when volunteers performed just 20 minutes of circuit training 3 days a week, they improved their fitness levels by up to 11 percent. That's about the same cardiovascular boost a similar group got when they jogged for 30 minutes, 3 days a week.

More recently, researchers found that when previously sedentary adults did 40 minutes of either circuit training or endurance exercise, such as cycling or cross-country skiing, 3 days a week, both groups had similar aerobic benefits, with the circuit trainers reaping the added benefit of increased muscle strength.

Another advantage of circuit training is that it's fun. That's because you're constantly moving to a new exercise, which keeps it interesting, says *Prevention* magazine fitness advisor Wayne Westcott, Ph.D.

Circuit 1

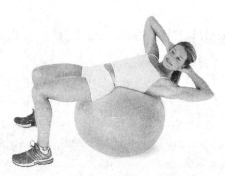

1. Twisting crunch on a ball: Sit on an exercise ball with your feet on the floor, shoulder-width apart. Place your fingertips lightly behind your head. Lean back (the ball will roll slightly forward) so your rear and the small of your back are pressing against the ball. Use your abs to lift your shoulders up and forward, twisting your right shoulder toward your left side as you lift. Pause, then lower. Repeat, alternating sides, for a total of 60 seconds. Rest 15 seconds before moving on to the next exercise.

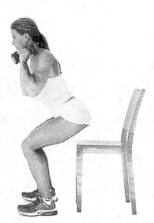

2. Dumbbell squat: Stand with your back to a chair, your feet about shoulder-width apart. Hold the dumbbells at your shoulders, palms facing in. Keeping your back straight, bend at the knees and hips as though you were sitting down. Don't let your knees move forward beyond your toes. Stop just shy of touching the chair, then stand up. Repeat for 60 seconds. Rest 15 seconds before moving on to the next exercise.

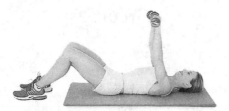

3. Chest press: Lying on the floor (or a bench), hold the dumbbells end to end just above chest height; your elbows should be pointing out. Press the dumbbells straight up, extending your arms. Hold, then lower. Repeat for 60 seconds. Rest 15 seconds before moving on to the next stretch.

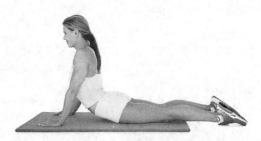

4. Cobra stretch: Lie facedown with your feet together, your toes pointed, and your hands on the floor, palms down just in front of your shoulders. Press your hands into the floor and gently extend your arms, lifting your upper body as far as is comfortably possible. If you feel any strain in your back, alter the pose so that you keep your elbows bent and your forearms on the floor. Hold for 15 seconds.

Circuit 2

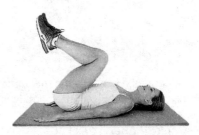

1. Reverse curl: Lie on your back with your arms at your sides, palms down. Bend your hips and knees so that your legs are over your midsection and relaxed. Slowly contract your abdominal muscles, lifting your hips 2 to 4 inches off the floor. Hold, then slowly lower. Repeat for 60 seconds. Rest 15 seconds before moving on to the next exercise.

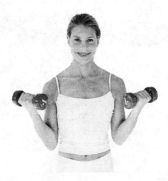

2. Biceps curl: Stand with your feet shoulder-width apart, holding dumbbells at your sides. Bending your elbows and turning your wrists upward, lift the dumbbells toward your shoulders. Don't move your upper arms. Stop when the dumbbells are at chest height, palms facing your body. Pause, then lower. Repeat for 60 seconds. Rest 15 seconds before moving on to the next exercise.

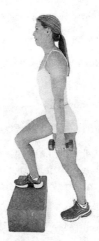

3. Step up: Stand facing an aerobic step or regular stairs, holding dumbbells at your sides. Place your right foot on the step, and lift yourself up. Just tap your left foot on the top of the step, slowly lower your left foot to the floor, then step off with your right foot. Repeat, alternating feet, for a total of 60 seconds. Rest 15 seconds before moving on to the next stretch.

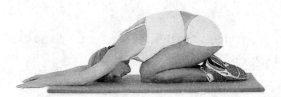

4. Praise pose stretch: Kneel with your toes pointed behind you. Sit back onto your heels, and lower your chest to your thighs. Stretch your arms overhead, and rest your palms and forehead on the floor (or as close as is comfortable). Hold for 15 seconds.

Circuit 3

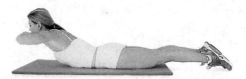

1. Chest lift: Lie facedown on the floor, your hands under your chin. Lift your head, chest, and arms about 5 to 6 inches off the floor. Hold, then lower. Repeat for 60 seconds. Rest 15 seconds before moving on to the next exercise.

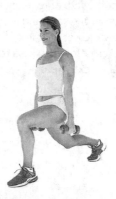

2. Lunge: Stand with your feet together, holding dumbbells down at your sides, your palms facing in. Take one big step forward with your left leg. Plant your left foot, then slowly lower your right knee toward the floor. Your left knee should be at a 90-degree angle, your back straight. Press into your left foot, and push yourself back to the starting position. Repeat, alternating legs, for a total of 60 seconds. Rest 15 seconds before moving on to the next exercise.

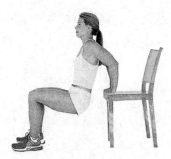

3. Dip: Sit on the edge of a sturdy chair, hands grasping the seat on either side of your rear. Walk your feet out slightly, and inch your butt off the chair. Keeping your shoulders down and your back straight, bend your elbows back, and lower your butt toward the floor as far as is comfortably possible. Slowly push back up. Repeat for 60 seconds. Rest 15 seconds before moving on to the next stretch.

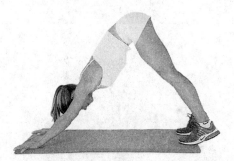

4. Downward dog stretch: Position yourself on the floor on your hands and knees, your feet flexed. Press your hands and feet into the floor, raising your hips toward the ceiling. Your body should look like an upside-down V. Keep lifting your tailbone toward the ceiling as you lower your heels to the floor as far as is comfortably possible. Hold for 15 seconds.

Circuit 4

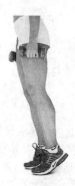

1. Calf raise: Stand with your feet about hip-width apart, holding dumbbells at your sides. Slowly rise onto your toes while keeping your torso and legs straight. Hold, then lower. Repeat for 60 seconds. Rest 15 seconds before moving on to the next exercise.

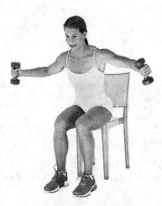

2. Back fly: Sit in a chair, your feet flat on the floor and about hip-width apart. Hold a dumbbell in each hand so the weights are about chest level and about 12 inches from your body. Your palms should be facing each other and your elbows slightly bent as if you were holding a beach ball. Bend forward from the hips about 3 to 5 inches. Keeping your back straight, squeeze your shoulder blades together, and pull your elbows back as far as is comfortably possible. Pause, then return to start. Repeat for 60 seconds. Rest 15 seconds before moving on to the next exercise.

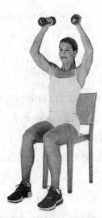

3. Overhead press: Sit in a chair, your feet flat on the floor. Hold dumbbells up at shoulder height, your palms facing your ears. Press the dumbbells straight overhead without locking your elbows. Hold, then lower. Repeat for 60 seconds. Rest 15 seconds before moving on to the next stretch.

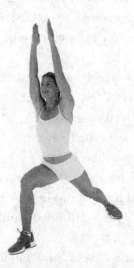

4. Warrior stretch: Stand tall, your feet about hip-width apart. Take a giant step forward with your right foot, bending that knee. (Be sure your knee does not jut out over your toes.) Turn your left foot to the side so your left arch faces the heel of your right foot. Raise your arms over your head, your palms facing each other, your chin slightly lifted. Hold for 15 seconds, then switch sides.

In addition, circuit training gives you a cardio workout. Because you move quickly from one exercise to the next, your heart rate stays up, and you burn more calories while you're lifting weights. (Traditional strength training has more rest time.)

To add flexibility benefits—an essential fitness component, especially as you get older—we've mixed in a few yoga poses. These easy moves stretch your muscles while also helping to further increase your strength. (Research shows that stretching while you lift weights can boost strength gains by 20 percent.)

"With circuit training, you can get a good cardiovascular workout and great muscle definition in a short time," says Vern Gambetta, a conditioning coach in Sarasota, Florida, who often trains Olympic and pro athletes using circuit training.

The Menopause Exercise Program Basics

The exercises in our circuits are bunched into groups of three, followed by a stretch. Perform each exercise for 60 seconds, doing as many repetitions as possible. (It helps to have a clock with a second hand or a timer nearby.)

You can use a lighter weight and perform more repetitions—or a heavier weight and perform fewer, slower repetitions—so long as you maintain good form and challenge yourself. The effort should feel tough during the final 10 to 15 seconds. To avoid injury, allow at least 3 seconds to lift and 3 seconds to lower the weight for each repetition.

Rest no more than 15 seconds between exercises. Before you start, always warm up with 5 minutes of moderate exercise, such as walking or stationary cycling. When you've finished, cool down with 5 minutes of easy activity.

Use this workout 3 days a week, and you'll see results in as little as 4 weeks. You'll get even greater results if you make it part of a cross-training, variety-packed program. For instance, you might try circuit training Monday, Wednesday, and Friday, cycling on Tuesdays, walking on Thursdays, and nature hiking on the weekends. For more cross-training ideas, see the opposite page.

CIRCUIT TRICKS

To make your circuit workouts feel more like play than work, try these circuit tricks during your next session.

Perform to a soundtrack. Because it's rhythmic and consistent, circuit training works well to music. Pick a CD with a steady groove that will keep you humming along. Anything R&B works well.

Form a circuit circle. First there were sewing circles, then book groups. Invite a friend or two to work out with you. Each person starts at a different point in the circuit; every 60 seconds, shout "Switch!" and move to the next exercise.

Do the shuffle. Keep the workout fresh and interesting by changing the order whenever it feels too familiar. Since the exercises are bundled in groups of three followed by a stretch, just rearrange the groups, one week starting with group two, the next week group three, and so on.

Create a Cross-Training Program— and Have Fun

In order to speed up the results of the Menopause Exercise Program, try to work in other fitness activities on the days that you don't circuit train. It really doesn't matter what you do, as long as you choose an activity that you enjoy. You might try singles tennis, cross-country skiing, swimming, a brisk walk with a friend, or inline or ice-skating. We've pulled together a menu of options to get you started.

Regardless of the activity you choose, make sure you start out at a comfortable speed and gradually increase your intensity within 5 minutes. You should break a light sweat and be slightly breathless but still able to hold a conversation.

Walking. Everyone knows that walking is as simple as putting one foot in front of the other. But if you want to lose weight, you'll have to walk like a woman on a mission—and pump your arms. In other words, power walk.

If you power walk regularly, your body will burn more calories and fat throughout the day because of the boost to your metabolism. You'll firm

EAT FOR SUCCESS

What you eat can speed up—or slow down—your success. For the best results from the Menopause Exercise Program for total-body toning, try this advice from Liz Applegate, Ph.D., of the University of California in Davis and author of *Eat Smart, Play Hard*.

Start with a snack. Too many women exercise on empty, hoping they'll burn more calories and lose more weight. The reality: You don't perform as well and can't lift as much when you're not well-fueled, so the workout is less effective.

If it's been more than 2 to 3 hours since your last meal, eat a small snack, such as a banana, about 30 minutes before lifting. Just make sure that you compensate for these additional calories (110 for a medium banana) by cutting back a little at a later meal.

Pump up your protein. Protein helps to repair your working muscles after a bout of lifting weights so that they get stronger. To make sure you're getting enough, plan on eating about ½ gram of protein per pound of body weight. So a 140-pound woman would aim for 70 grams of protein a day.

Make sure with a multi. People who exercise regularly have a higher demand for many vitamins and minerals than do sedentary folks. The best way to get them is to eat more fruits and vegetables. *Prevention* magazine recommends nine a day. It's also a good idea to take a standard multivitamin for insurance.

up the muscles in your buttocks, thighs, calves, back, upper arms, shoulders, and abdomen. You'll condition your cardiovascular system; reduce stress, heart disease, and stroke risk; help prevent osteoporosis; and elevate your mood. On average, walking burns 100 calories per mile, so you can burn 350 to 450 calories an hour, depending on how fast you walk and whether you hike on flat or hilly terrain.

Step aerobics. Choreographed to the beat of heart-pumping music, step aerobics are high-intensity, low-impact exercises that combine dance moves on and around an adjustable platform. The "step" exploded onto the fitness scene in the late 1980s and hasn't lost its popularity yet.

Aerobics can help tone and shape the muscles in your buttocks, hips, thighs, calves, and abs. Plus, the arm movements will sculpt your biceps, triceps, and shoulders. Depending on the intensity of your workout, you can burn 600 calories in an hour using a 6-inch-high step.

Jogging. Like walking, jogging is one of the most accessible—and enjoyable—aerobic activities. But that's where the similarities end. While

WHATEVER HAPPENED TO CALISTHENICS?

It's pretty easy to have mixed feelings about calisthenics. On the one hand, the word comes from two Greek roots meaning "beauty" and "strength"—qualities that are certainly worth saving from extinction! On the other, it will forever be associated with that sadistic physical education teacher you had in high school. No wonder it's an endangered exercise species.

Calisthenics usually refers to an exercise routine that you do without weights or any other equipment. Well-known calisthenics movements include pushups, situps, jumping jacks, running in place, and leg raises.

You can see from that partial list that calisthenics haven't entirely disappeared. The "legwork" that is tacked on to many aerobics classes is a lot like calisthenics. In any weight-training routine, workouts for your midsection will consist mostly of crunches and similar exercises. And pushups are still considered a pretty good upper-body strengthener.

Certain traditional calisthenics movements, however, have turned out to do more harm than good: Deep knee bends are a prime example. That's one reason for calisthenics' fade. Another is those negative associations. Yet another is that—let's face it—calisthenics are boring. And if you really want to be cynical, you can blame their demise on the fact that it's pretty hard to sell merchandise around such an equipment-free, no-frills mode of exercise.

But the main reason that you don't hear too much about calisthenics these days is that we've found better ways to get fit. In the last few decades, new knowledge about aerobic exercise has pushed jumping jacks into dinosaur land. More important (since strength and toning is the main goal of calisthenics), resistance training has been shown to get results more quickly, more thoroughly, and more easily than any calisthenics routine. Weights let you adjust the resistance so you can make steady progress. Weights also let you concentrate on individual muscles in a way that calisthenics can't.

And yes, weight training is a lot more fun.

jogging burns about the same number of calories per mile, you're moving a lot faster than with walking, so you burn calories faster, too (about 500 to 600 calories per hour). And afterward, your metabolic rate stays supercharged for hours.

In addition to strengthening and toning your abs and the muscles in your buttocks, hips, thighs, and calves, jogging is one of the quickest ways to achieve cardiovascular fitness.

Bowling. Who would have thought that bowling is actually a good workout? Well, repeatedly lifting and hurling a 6- to 14-pound ball, not to mention all that legwork, can do quite a bit for your figure. You'll tone your throwing arm, hand, and shoulder as you release the ball. And you'll strengthen your thighs, butt, and lower back during your approach, knee bend, and finish position.

Bowling burns 204 calories an hour. Intensity depends on the number of games you play and the number of people you bowl with. More people means longer time lapses between turns, while bowling alone or with just one or two others keeps you moving more. Aim to bowl about twice a week to see results.

Spinning. You'll be glad to know that twirling around in circles like a top is not the workout we're talking about here. Spinning is an aerobic, high-intensity indoor cycling class that conditions your cardiovascular system and tones the muscles in your thighs, calves, buttocks, and hips. With upbeat music jamming in the background, an instructor takes you through a routine that challenges you with intervals of fast and slow riding at various speeds and resistances. Throughout the workout, she helps you envision yourself riding through hill climbs, fast descents, and all kinds of thrilling cycling scenarios. And you'll burn 260 to 660 calories an hour, depending on your weight and how intensely you pedal.

Classes are held at various health clubs. You can buy your own stationary bike designed for spinning and work out in the comfort of your own home. But without the direction of a fitness trainer, you may not burn as many calories—or have as much fun. It's the environment you're in that makes spinning such great exercise. The instructor pushes you, the music pushes you, and the people in the class push you.

Kickboxing. The word may conjure up images of spindly martial arts champions waiting to knock out their opponents, or visions of David Carradine demonstrating kung fu in the Old West. But at your local health club or YMCA, kickboxing is a noncontact cardiovascular workout that combines aerobic exercise with shadowboxing to whip you into ring-side shape. A total-body cardiovascular workout, kickboxing sculpts and tones your arms, back, hips, thighs, calves, and abs and can improve your sense of coordination and balance.

Essentially, it involves a series of kicking, punching, and blocking movements against an imaginary opponent that are choreographed to high-energy music. Classes often go by the names Kwando, Cardio Kick-boxing, Cardio Kicks, Boxercise, Tae-Bo, or just kickboxing. Depending on the club, you may wear boxing gloves or hand mitts, use actual punching bags, or combine the movements with step aerobics. You can also buy or rent kickboxing videotapes and do the routines at home. Either way, you can burn 680 or more calories in a 1-hour session.

Table tennis. If you have a Ping-Pong table packed away in your basement or garage somewhere, take it out, dust it off, and call a friend. Hitting a small lightweight ball back and forth across a table actually counts as a real workout because it strengthens your quadriceps, hamstrings, inner and outer thighs, and hips.

Plus, you can burn 270 calories per hour of steady playing. The type of workout you get is directly related to the level of skill with which you and your partner play. If you really want to start incinerating some calories and improving your game, find a friend who would like to practice a minimum of three times a week for about an hour each time. Some tables fold up on one side so that you can play by yourself against the up-ended tabletop—a handy option if you can't find someone else to play as regularly as you'd like.

Feeling motivated? Great! Head for the gym, go for a walk, or climb on the exercise bike right now. Once you're back, cooled down, and ready to relax, turn to chapter 5 to find out all about the best supplements to help you stay healthy through menopause and beyond.

Chapter

5

SUPER MENOPAUSE SUPPLEMENTS

Experts assure us that menopause is a time of life, not a disease that can be "cured." If only it were that easy. Yes, we certainly agree: Menopause is not a disease. But the hormonal ebb and flow that characterizes the years before and during menopause creates a flood of symptoms that range from merely irritating to totally debilitating. And after menopause, women are at higher risk for three major diseases: heart disease, cancer (especially endometrial and breast cancers), and osteoporosis.

If you're like us, you'll want to do everything possible to strengthen your body against this onslaught—and that's where supplements can help. By making sure you're getting the right combination and amounts of vitamins, minerals, and other supplements, you can give your body a powerful weapon to ward off menopause's worst effects. And luckily doctors, herbalists, and other experts now know quite a lot about what to take specifically for menopause, as you'll see in this chapter.

What you choose to take depends on your situation, so we present the information in this chapter to help you customize a supplement program that meets your individual needs. We recommend that all women take the basic vitamins and minerals in the section called "Restoring Your Balance" on the opposite page. Menopause brings with it a lot of long-term mental, physical, and emotional stress. A well-nourished, well-rested, carefully supplemented body can help you minimize stress in all three areas.

If you find yourself experiencing uncomfortable or embarrassing menopausal symptoms, turn to "Menopausal Changes" on page 107, look up your symptom, and choose one or more of the supplements we suggest to combat it. And if you have a family history of or have personally experienced heart disease, cancer, or osteoporosis, you should read all your options in "Healing the Heart" on page 123, "Combating Cancer" on page 132, and "Outwitting Osteoporosis" on page 140.

To make it easier for you to remember what you'd like to take, we've included Super Supplement Checklists throughout the chapter. You can photocopy the ones that interest you (say, the ones on general supplements, menopausal symptoms, and osteoporosis), then check off the supplements you feel would be most helpful to you as you read about them in the chapter. We recommend that when you're finished making your list, but before you begin your shopping excursion, you discuss with your doctor the supplements you'd like to take. Then take your checklists to the health food store, pharmacy, or supermarket, and see at a glance what you need to buy. For more on supplements, see chapter 12.

Restoring Your Balance

Menopause is kind of like puberty in reverse. In puberty, your body started producing larger quantities of the hormones estrogen and progesterone, among others, and you started to menstruate. In menopause, your body produces less of these hormones, so you stop menstruating.

By now, your body has gotten used to higher hormone levels. Thus, for some women, menopause is like putting your body through withdrawal. Here are some supplements that can provide you with a good foundation for stemming the tides of time and helping you look and feel younger.

Multivitamin/mineral supplement. This is an easy way to make sure that you're getting enough of all the nutrients your body needs: folic acid, vitamins B_6 and B_{12}, chromium, selenium, and magnesium. As we age, we absorb less of the nutrients than we once did. We also tend to eat less, so a multivitamin is a great way to supplement your diet with the essentials. Look for a "mega" supplement that has 600 to 1,000 percent of the Daily Value (DV) for all your B vitamins, 100 to 200 milligrams of vitamin C, and a nice showing of trace minerals, says Connie Catellani, M.D., medical director of the Miro Center for the Integrative Medicine in Evanston, Illinois.

Note that only women who are still having periods or who are anemic should take iron supplements. (Acids and proteins increase iron absorption, so take your iron with some orange juice or milk.) If you aren't anemic and are past childbearing, look for an iron-free multivitamin/mineral formulation. (Most supplements targeted to men are iron-free, and more general iron-free supplements are becoming available.)

Vitamin C with bioflavonoids. As an antioxidant, vitamin C plays an important role in preventing disease. Antioxidants are protective substances that help destroy unstable molecules that can damage cells and make them more susceptible to cancer. Vitamin C also helps to lower blood pressure, which could also protect your arteries and heart. Bioflavonoids are compounds found in citrus fruits that have be shown to protect capillaries and other small blood vessels.

Vitamin E. Vitamin E is important for heart health. If your multivitamin supplement contains 200 IU or so, take an additional 200 to 400 IU

SUPER SUPPLEMENT CHECKLIST #1

Here's a checklist for general supplementation. Choose these supplements to help yourself stay in peak nutritional health throughout the menopausal years, from perimenopause straight through to postmenopause.

- ☐ "Mega" multivitamin/mineral supplement
- ☐ Vitamin C with bioflavonoids
- ☐ Vitamin E
- ☐ Calcium
- ☐ Vitamin D

as a separate supplement. Like vitamin C, vitamin E is an antioxidant and thus is important in the fight against aging and cancer.

Calcium and vitamin D. The calcium in your bones is like savings in a bank. You deposit calcium through the foods you eat, and when your body needs calcium—which it uses for many important functions, such as regulating muscle contraction, heartbeat and blood clotting—it's "withdrawn" from the bones. If withdrawals exceed deposits, bones eventually weaken and become fragile. Most of us begin to lose bone around age 35, but additional calcium may help slow that loss. The best way to meet your calcium needs is through various foods and beverages. However, older people, as well as people who consume few dairy products, may need to supplement.

Just as important to bone health is vitamin D, which your body needs in order to use calcium. Unfortunately, many women age 50 or older don't get enough to keep their bones strong. You should be getting 1,200 milligrams a day of calcium, including supplements if necessary, and 400 to 800 international units (IU) a day of vitamin D if you are age 50 or over.

Menopausal Changes

The changes that arise around the time of menopause may be predictable, but that certainly doesn't make them comfortable. Hot flashes and night sweats are just the beginning. Women may also experience vaginal dryness, loss of sex drive, mood swings, depression, and a host of related problems. There are a number of herbs and supplements that may help. Some address the whole range of discomforts, while others take aim at specific problems, such as vaginal dryness or low sex drive. Here is an overview of what these supplements can do for you.

Hot Flashes and Night Sweats

While we don't really know what causes hot flashes (sometimes called hot flushes), we do know that as many as 65 to 80 percent of women will experience them at some point during their transition to menopause. Whatever the cause, hot flashes are uncomfortable and unpredictable, sometimes disturbing a restful night's sleep. You wake drenched in sweat,

VITAMIN D:
THE "OTHER" BONE-FRIENDLY HORMONE

Way back in 1922, at the University of Wisconsin in Madison, professor Elmer McCollum discovered vitamin D in cod liver oil, earning himself the title "Father of Vitamin D." Over 70 years later, vitamin D is still a hot research topic on the Madison campus, where three generations of scientists have studied the nutrient.

Leading the latest wave of researchers is Hector DeLuca, Ph.D., chair of the biochemistry department, who has studied vitamin D since 1951. Five decades later, he remains intrigued by this vitamin and its benefits in the body.

Technically, vitamin D is a hormone, not a vitamin, says Dr. DeLuca. And while estrogen gets all the attention for protecting your bones, your body relies on vitamin D to fully absorb calcium, keep bones strong, and prevent osteoporosis. Vitamin D targets the intestines, kidneys, and bones, all of which respond by making calcium available for bone growth.

"In a sense, vitamin D acts like a chauffeur, driving calcium to where it is needed in the body," says Dr. DeLuca. "I believe all life originated in the sea, where calcium was abundant. Today we live on land, where calcium is not so abundant. I think vitamin D has evolved to help us with this calcium shortage."

Even if you drink milk, eat yogurt or other calcium-fortified foods, and take calcium supplements, you need to make sure you're getting enough vitamin D—

sometimes several times a night—hence the name "night sweats." Because night sweats disturb sleep, you're often tired during the day. Here are some suggestions to help you chill out.

Vitamin E. About 400 international units (IU) of vitamin E a day helps decrease hot flashes by balancing the levels of estrogen in your body. Not only that, but research shows that postmenopausal women who get at least this much vitamin E have a lower risk of death from heart disease. Getting enough vitamin E from a low-fat diet is a bit difficult. So take a vitamin E supplement with a little bit of fat to ensure absorption. It may not work right away, however. You may have to take vitamin E for at least 6 weeks before noticing any effects.

Vitamin C and bioflavonoids. Research has found that by strength-

400 International Units a day—especially in winter, says Dr. DeLuca. Your body uses sunlight to produce vitamin D. So spending as little as 10 minutes a day in the summer sun is enough to soak up a whole day's worth of D. Using sunscreen will interfere with the production of vitamin D, however, and sunblock will completely prevent it. Yet you don't want to forgo protection during peak hours. The best solution: Drink in those rays after 3:00 P.M., when the sun isn't so damaging, and wear sunblock the rest of the time.

If you live in northern areas of the country, squeezing out even 200 IU of vitamin D from the sun can be difficult, however. "If it's cold and snowy for weeks, and you don't get out, your vitamin D may be totally depleted by April," says Dr. DeLuca. Sunlight pouring through a window won't do because glass filters out the rays you need most for vitamin D. If you're not sure you're getting enough vitamin D, Dr. DeLuca recommends taking a supplement once a day that provides 400 IU of vitamin D, along with the recommended intake of 1,000 to 1,200 milligrams of calcium.

Avoid taking more than the recommended amount of vitamin D. Taking large amounts—2,000 IU or more of vitamin D a day over several months—can cause high blood levels of calcium, kidney damage, and calcium deposits in the heart and lungs, which can be fatal. And if you take combination calcium/vitamin D supplements, make sure you keep your daily calcium intake under 2,500 milligrams.

ening and stabilizing capillaries and other small blood vessels, these supplements in combination can prevent hot flashes from occurring. You can find supplements that combine vitamin C and bioflavonoids at most health food stores. Look for a supplement that contains 500 to 1,000 milligrams of vitamin C, and 200 to 500 milligrams of bioflavonoids, per capsule.

Pantothenic acid. This B vitamin boosts the functions of your adrenal glands, which take over most of the estrogen production when your reproductive system stops. If night sweats are causing insomnia, try taking 500 milligrams a day. Continue to take it until you get relief.

Black cohosh. This herb (*Actaea racemosa*) has estrogen–like effects, which enable it to quell hot flashes, says Beverly Whipple, Ph.D., professor at Rutgers University College of Nursing in Newark, New Jersey. Several

SUPER SUPPLEMENT CHECKLIST #2

If you're experiencing unpleasant menopause symptoms, here's an array of supplements to help you, organized by symptom. (Remember, we're not advising you to take them all at once! Read the descriptions of each and their effects, then pick the ones you think would work best for your situation.)

Hot Flashes and Night Sweats
- [ ] Vitamin E
- [ ] Vitamin C with bioflavonoids
- [ ] Pantothenic acid
- [ ] Black cohosh
- [ ] Flaxseed
- [ ] Sage
- [ ] Dang gui, damiana, and chasteberry
- [ ] Motherwort and chasteberry

Irregular Periods and Flooding
- [ ] Iron
- [ ] Yellow dock root
- [ ] Vitamin C with bioflavonoids
- [ ] Chasteberry
- [ ] Black cohosh
- [ ] Cinnamon
- [ ] Dang gui
- [ ] Lady's mantle

Vaginal Dryness
- [ ] Licorice
- [ ] Panax ginseng
- [ ] Black cohosh and dang gui

Mood Swings
- [ ] Calcium
- [ ] Magnesium and vitamin B_6
- [ ] Pantothenic acid
- [ ] Black cohosh
- [ ] Chamomile
- [ ] Skullcap
- [ ] Chasteberry

clinical trials found that black cohosh reduced hot flashes by up to 80 percent. To put your fire out, take 4 milligrams of black cohosh, either in one dose or in two 2-milligram tablets twice a day, but don't use it for more than 6 months, says Dr. Whipple.

Flaxseed. Flaxseed's essential fatty acids act like weak estrogens in your body, helping to relieve menopausal symptoms and lubricate vaginal tissues, writes Lana Lew, M.D., an Australian women's health specialist, in her book *The Natural Estrogen Diet.* Flaxseed also contains omega-3 fatty acids, which help protect your heart. You need 1 to 2 tablespoons of flaxseed a day to get the greatest benefit. Because your body can't absorb the healing properties of the whole seeds, buy ground flaxseeds at health food stores, or grind them in a coffee grinder. To get what you need each day, add a tablespoon to your cereal in the morning and another to yogurt, baked goods, or salads.

Sage. Garden sage is famed for the way it reduces or even eliminates night sweats. It acts fast—within a few hours—and a single cup of infusion can stave off the sweats for up to 2 days, says Susun S. Weed, an herbalist and herbal educator from Woodstock, New York, and author of the *Wise Woman* series of herbal health books. What's more, you probably have a bottle of sage sitting on your spice rack. Just make sure it's still nice and aromatic before you use it medicinally.

To make a sage infusion, put 4 heaping tablespoons of dried sage in a cup of hot water. Cover tightly and steep for 4 hours or more. Strain and drink hot or cold. Or, for a no-fuss infusion, look for sage tea bags at your health food store.

Herbal combinations. "My own standard recommendation for hot flashes and other symptoms of menopause is a trio of traditional herbs," says Andrew Weil, M.D., director of the program in integrative medicine at the University of Arizona College of Medicine in Tucson and author of *Spontaneous Healing*.

Dr. Weil recommends taking 1 dropperful each of tinctures of dang gui, chasteberry (also called vitex), and damiana once a day at midday. Continue taking the herbs until your hot flashes cease, then taper off gradually.

Dang gui is an herb that has been used for centuries in China. In fact,

DON'T USE HT AND BLACK COHOSH TOGETHER

Using prescription hormone therapy (HT, formerly known as hormone replacement therapy, HRT) and black cohosh together is not recommended. "Both of them work on your endocrine system, so it's best to err on the side of caution. Choose one or the other, but not both," recommends *Prevention* magazine advisor Douglas Schar, DipPhyt, MCPP, MNIMH, a European-trained clinical herbalist. "Think of it as double-dipping, using Tums and Rolaids together for indigestion or Motrin and Tylenol together for a headache."

it is Chinese medicine's leading remedy for gynecological ailments. Don't use dang gui while menstruating, spotting, or bleeding heavily because it can increase blood loss.

Damiana is a nervous system tonic said to ease depression and anxiety. Chasteberry may counteract the effectiveness of birth control pills, so if you're on them, skip this herb.

Motherwort and chasteberry. For some women, menopause follows surgical removal of the ovaries, or chemotherapy or radiation treatments that can destroy the ovaries, says Susun. If you're one of these women, your hot flashes may be especially frequent and intense. "Volcanic hot flashes are to a normal hot flash as a tidal wave is to a normal wave," Susun says. Twenty-five to 30 drops of motherwort tincture can stem the tide, she suggests. And for the long term, Susun recommends 30 to 90 drops of chasteberry tincture three times a day for at least 13 months.

Irregular Periods and Flooding

You might call the decade before menopause "period pause." Your period used to arrive like clockwork, every 28 days. Now it's early one month and late the next. Sometimes it doesn't show up for months. And when it does, it may last 2 weeks or more. Your periods may be very heavy or very light. What's going on here?

If you're in your forties but not yet menopausal, your hormones may be on the blink. Levels of estrogen and progesterone, which used to fluctuate on cue, may surge one month or be released at odd times the next. "It's a complex change in the symphony of hormones that are being played inside a woman's body. But it's a normal passage that every woman goes through," says Susun. Even so, that doesn't mean you have to put up with problem periods. Let these supplements and herbs help you navigate the transition from super tampons to none.

Iron. If you are experiencing heavy blood loss, iron may be the most important mineral you can take to help control it. Heavy menstrual flow can deplete your body's iron stores, and some researchers also believe that chronic iron deficiency may cause heavy bleeding. Do not take more than the Daily Value (DV) of iron (18 milligrams) on your own,

PERIMENOPAUSAL RELIEF TINCTURE TONIC

This combination of herb tinctures can help stabilize symptoms that occur during perimenopause, the 5 to 10 years before menstruation actually stops. Take this mixture to regulate off-kilter menstrual cycles or just to cool the occasional hot flash, says Virginia Frazer, N.D., a naturopathic physician and licensed midwife in Kennewick, Washington.

Use a dosing syringe (available at drugstores) to accurately measure your doses. Take 5 milliliters of the blend two or three times a day, depending on the severity of your symptoms, says Dr. Frazer. Tinctures tend to have a strong taste, so to make your herbal combo easier to swallow, add the measured amount to a half glass of water, tea, or juice.

  4 ounces black cohosh
  2 ounces partridgeberry
  2 ounces motherwort
  1 ounce chasteberry
  1 ounce wild yam

Pour the black cohosh, partridgeberry, motherwort, chasteberry, and wild yam into a glass mixing bowl, and set the empty bottles aside. Stir gently to blend, then use a small funnel to carefully rebottle your custom combination.

though. You must be tested for iron deficiency before supplementing with higher doses.

You might also consider including some iron-rich herbs in your diet. Try dandelion leaves, milk thistle seed, echinacea, and peppermint. Eating them on the days you are bleeding heavily is best. You'll feel the effects within 2 weeks, and your next period won't bring heavy floods, says Susun.

Yellow dock root. One problem with iron supplements is their tendency to cause constipation. That's why some popular herbal tonics include yellow dock root. While the herb is a source of iron, it also produces a gentle laxative effect. Thus, while it's contributing to your body's stores of iron, it can also help counter supplemental iron's constipating tendencies.

Yellow dock root also contains thiamin and vitamin C, which help the absorption of iron. It has 1 milligram of iron per 20-drop dose of alcohol tincture or 3-teaspoon dose of vinegar tincture, says Susun. Either an alcohol or a vinegar tincture is fine, taken daily in tea or water. Iron is absorbed a little at a time, so she suggests taking yellow dock root throughout the day.

Vitamin C and bioflavonoids. Vitamin C can significantly increase iron absorption, so you should take it with your iron supplement. But the combination of vitamin C and bioflavonoids is better yet, according to Liz Collins, N.D., a naturopathic doctor and co-owner of the Natural Childbirth and Family Clinic in Portland, Oregon.

If you're prone to excessive menstrual bleeding, it might be the result of fragile blood vessels. Vitamin C and bioflavonoids may strengthen those blood vessels, making them less susceptible to damage. In one study, for example, 14 out of 16 women who took supplements of 200 milligrams of vitamin C three times a day along with bioflavonoids found relief from heavy bleeding. Dr. Collins recommends taking 500 to 1,000 milligrams of vitamin C three times a day, and 500 to 1,000 milligrams of bioflavonoids once a day.

Chasteberry. "The single best herb for regulating the menstrual cycle is chasteberry," says Robert Rountree, M.D., a holistic physician at the Helios Health Center in Boulder, Colorado. When taken regularly, chasteberry regulates the timing of the menstrual cycle by acting on the pituitary gland, which in turn releases the hormones that regulate ovarian function. Recommended for a number of menstrual disorders by Germany's Commission E, which evaluates herbs for safety and effectiveness, chasteberry is now approved as a common treatment for menstrual irregularity. Take one or two 225-milligram capsules standardized for 0.5 percent agnuside (an active component) every day. (This information should be on the bottle, or ask at the health food store.) If you want to use the herb in a less medicinal way, grind the dried fruits and sprinkle them on your food for a peppery flavor.

Black cohosh. Among Native Americans, black cohosh was a widely used folk remedy for menstrual irregularities. As we mentioned earlier, black cohosh works as a mild estrogen, like chasteberry. If your estrogen levels are too low, plant estrogens in the root, called isoflavones, pick up the slack and help regulate your cycle. Drink 2 to 4 dropperfuls of tincture in a little water or tea three times a day, or take two capsules of standardized extract daily, recommends Beverly Yates, N.D., a naturopathic physician with the Natural Health Care Group in Portland, Oregon, and Seattle.

Cinnamon. Cinnamon is more than just a kitchen spice—it's been used medicinally for thousands of years. Ancient Chinese herbalists mention it as early as 2700 B.C., and Chinese herbalists today still recommend it for keeping menstrual cycles regular and stemming heavy bleeding. If you are bleeding heavily, sip a cup of cinnamon infusion, chew a cinnamon stick, or take 5 to 10 drops of tincture once or twice a day, says Susun.

Dang gui. As we mentioned earlier, dang gui is widely used in China and is commonly prescribed for menstrual irregularities. The phytoestrogens in this member of the carrot family help regulate and balance the menstrual cycle, especially if your periods are scanty, says Dr. Yates. Take ½ teaspoon of alcohol-based tincture in a glass of water up to four times a day. Women who are prone to heavy menstrual bleeding should avoid using this herb. Be especially cautious if you have uterine fibroids or endometriosis, as anything that might promote uterine bleeding could aggravate these conditions.

Lady's mantle. It's believed that this herb can prevent excessive bleeding when taken 1 to 2 weeks before menstruation. In a clinical study, lady's mantle tincture controlled menstrual flooding in virtually all of the 300 women who participated. When taken after flooding began, lady's mantle took 3 to 5 days to become effective. Susun suggests using 5 to 10 drops of the fresh plant tincture three times a day for up to 2 weeks out of every month.

Vaginal Dryness

After menopause, your vaginal lining may begin to thin and dry out due to the lack of estrogen. This can make sex painful or even undesirable. Surveys indicate that this happens in 8 to 25 percent of postmenopausal women. While premenopausal women can generally lubricate in 6 to 20 seconds when aroused, it can take 1 to 3 minutes for a postmenopausal woman. Also, the thinning of the vaginal tissues makes the tissue more susceptible to irritation or trauma, which may provide a gateway for infection. Here are some ways to get relief.

Vitamin E. Take 400 international units of vitamin E each day. Recent research has paid little attention to the effects of vitamin E on vaginal dryness. But two studies done in the 1940s indicated that vitamin E supplements can improve symptoms of vaginal atrophy, says Michael T. Murray, N.D., a naturopathic doctor in Bellevue, Washington, and author of *Menopause: How You Can Benefit from Diet, Vitamins, Minerals, Herbs, Exercise, and Other Natural Methods.* These days, many doctors recommend vitamin E for vaginal dryness and other physical changes associated with menopause. If you decide to try vitamin E, give yourself at least 4 weeks to see results. You can also use vitamin E topically. Simply pop open the capsule, put the oil on your finger, and apply where it's needed. Do this twice a day or whenever you need relief.

Licorice. Chew two tablets (a total of 380 milligrams) of deglycyrrhizinated licorice root about 30 minutes before each meal. (Deglycyrrhizinated means that the compounds that elevate blood pressure have been removed; look for "DGL" on the package.) Licorice root targets vaginal dryness in two ways, according to Helen Healy, N.D., a naturopathic physician and director of the Wellspring Naturopathic Clinic in St. Paul, Minnesota. For starters, the herb stimulates mucous production in your body and even increases the number of goblet cells (cells that manufacture mucus). Plus, licorice root contains compounds that act as weak forms of estrogen.

You can buy chewable tablets of deglycyrrhizinated licorice root in health food stores. The tablets work so well, says Dr. Healy, that you may find yourself having to blow your nose as you chew them. Forget about munching on licorice candy, though—it doesn't even contain real licorice.

Panax ginseng. Take 100 milligrams of panax ginseng (sometimes called Asian ginseng), in the form of a standardized extract, once or twice a day. The active compounds in ginseng apparently have an estrogen-like effect on vaginal tissue, helping it stay moist and supple. "In traditional Chinese medicine, ginseng is often prescribed to women in their menopausal and postmenopausal years as a general tonic," explains James E. Williams, O.M.D., a doctor of oriental medicine affiliated with the Center for Women's Medicine in San Diego.

A standardized extract ensures that you are getting a consistent amount of the active compounds in ginseng—unlike most teas and herbal formulas, which contain very little of the compounds. Ask a medical professional who is knowledgeable about herbs to recommend a product to you, Dr. Williams suggests. You can buy the extracts in health food stores. Just look for the words *standardized extract* on the label.

Black cohosh and dang gui. You'd be right if you guessed at this point that the all-around best herb for menopausal symptoms seems to be black cohosh. Along with its many other attributes, it also helps relieve vaginal dryness. You can combine black cohosh with dang gui to get better results, if taking the herb individually doesn't relieve the dryness. Take 250 to 300 milligrams of black cohosh three times a day, says Dr. Collins. If you combine it with dang gui, take up to 4,000 milligrams of each per day for up to 6 months. Some women start with 4,000 milligrams per day and then, once their symptoms are under control, decrease the dose slowly to find the minimum dose that maintains control.

Mood Swings

In menopause, you can be merry one moment and maniacal the next—without any rhyme or reason, it seems. According to one theory, the hormonal downdrafts and upsurges of menopause trigger mood swings in an unpredictable and sometimes indirect way. Here's how to take the "menace" out of menopause.

Calcium. Boosting your calcium intake may be the ticket to relief from irritability. In a 5½-month study at the Grand Forks Human Nutrition Research Center of the U.S. Department of Agriculture in North Dakota, women who got 1,300 milligrams of calcium daily reported far fewer woes than those who got 600 milligrams daily. Nine of the 10 women had fewer mood changes, such as irritability and depression, says James G. Penland, Ph.D., a research psychologist at the center. Taking calcium supplements can also lead to less difficulty concentrating. In one of the largest studies of calcium for PMS, researchers found that women taking 1,200 milligrams of calcium daily for three menstrual cycles experienced a more positive mood. Researchers suspect that calcium relieves PMS by easing depression, but they have not yet discovered how.

HERBAL FORMULAS COVER ALL THE BASES

Many herbalists have their own special herbal tonics that that they've used over the years to treat a spectrum of menopausal symptoms. Hot flashes bedevil you. Your sleep isn't very deep or very restful. Your moods are a touch volcanic. And the periods you're still having could be less, well, bloodily intense. Nothing you can't live with, but life could be a whole lot more comfortable without this cluster of annoyances. Here's what highly respected herbalists have to offer.

Keep in mind, though, that when it comes to menopause, each woman is different. One of these formulas may work better for you than another, so you may have to experiment to find the best blend. Remember, too, that herbs work slowly, so you might not feel any results at all for 3 weeks or so. Susun S. Weed, an herbalist and herbal educator from Woodstock, New York, and author of the *Wise Woman* series of herbal health books, urges women to begin with one herb if they are novices. If you take a lot of herbs at once and one of them doesn't agree with you, you won't know which one it is.

Try the menopause formula. Created by herbalists Cascade Anderson Geller and Valerie Perrine for the National College of Naturopathic Medicine in Portland, Oregon, "this formula has helped women who are experiencing menopausal changes," says Cascade, who is a consulting herbal practitioner and herbal educator in Portland.

"If menopausal changes become increasingly intolerable, first consider improving your diet and lifestyle. Stick to a low-fat, high-fiber diet, drink lots of water, and exercise for at least 30 minutes every other day," she advises. "If these changes don't bring relief, try my herbal formula. It has helped countless women ease the effects of menopause." She adds, "Have your doctor monitor your progress. Tell her precisely what you're taking. Suggest that you may be able to take less estrogen as a result. Ask her to monitor you closely as you ease off your estrogen. Most M.Ds are more and more open-minded about herbs these days, and it's very important that you let your doctor know that you're taking herbs in hopes of taking less estrogen."

Menopause Formula

To make this formula, use the following herbal tinctures.

- 2 parts licorice
- 2 parts dandelion root
- 1 part motherwort
- 1 part true unicorn root or false unicorn root
- 1 part wild yam

Using a funnel, pour the tinctures into a bottle large enough to hold 7 ounces (nearly a cup). Add 1 to 3 dropperfuls of the tincture mixture to a little water, and drink two or three times a day 3 to 5 days a week.

Always take the lowest dose possible, and taper off as quickly as possible when symptoms diminish, Cascade advises.

Take one mixture for many ills. Chasteberry helps balance hormones, motherwort has antianxiety and antispasmodic effects, and false unicorn has hormonal and digestive benefits, says Silena Heron, N.D., vice president of the Botanical Medicine Academy in Sedona, Arizona. Dang gui, licorice, black cohosh, and alfalfa help enhance estrogen activity. Black haw reduces the spasticity that can promote hot flashes, and black cohosh relieves cramps. Sage decreases secretions, including sweat, which makes it useful for reducing both the frequency and severity of hot flashes. As a bonus, sage helps improve digestion, it's a source of zinc, and it kills germs, too. Dr. Heron includes St. John's wort in her menopause formula because of its ability to ease pelvic complaints and depression.

"A woman benefits most from herbal therapy when the formula is adjusted to her specific needs," says Dr. Heron. "But this basic formula has been so successful in relieving menopausal discomforts that many women return to my clinic just to have the prescription refilled."

Dr. Heron's Menopause Mixture

Dr. Heron's formula is made by mixing the following herbal tinctures.

- 2   parts chasteberry
- 1   part motherwort
- 1   part false unicorn root
- 1   part dang gui
- 1–2   parts sage
- 1   part St. John's wort
- 1–2   parts black cohosh
- ½–1   part licorice
- ½–1   part black haw
- ½–1   part alfalfa

Blend the herbal tinctures together in a jar. Take ½ to 1 teaspoon three times a day on an empty stomach, straight up or mixed with a little water, advises Dr. Heron.

(continued on page 120)

HERBAL FORMULAS COVER ALL THE BASES
—Continued

Opt for a hormone helper. Rosemary Gladstar's Menopause Tincture will strengthen and tone the endocrine system, which is responsible for manufacturing your body's hormones. During menopause, the adrenal glands take on the role of producing estrogen after the ovaries cease doing so, and they often need a boost during the transition, says herbalist Rosemary Gladstar, author of *The Family Herbal*. Each of the herbs in the formula helps revitalize the adrenal glands, she says. In addition, wild yam is known for its powerful effect on regulating hormone production, sarsaparilla is said to aid body functioning as a whole, and black cohosh has traditionally been recommended for menopausal pains and discomfort.

Rosemary recommends using high-quality dried herbs that you tincture yourself, in good brandy or vodka. You can also make this formula from store-bought tinctures. The formula will last you a very long time. Use the tonic consistently over an extended period of time to assure steady, long-lasting results, she adds.

Rosemary Gladstar's Menopause Tincture

- 2 parts wild yam
- 1 part sarsaparilla
- 1 part black cohosh
- 2 parts Siberian ginseng
- 1 part dang gui
- 3 parts sage
- 3 parts licorice
- 3 parts dandelion root

Magnesium and vitamin B$_6$. These nutrients help assure a healthy supply of serotonin and dopamine, two mood-regulating neurotransmitters. Women can supplement their diets with 350 milligrams of magnesium and 100 milligrams of vitamin B$_6$, says George J. Kallins, M.D., assistant clinical professor in the department of obstetrics and gynecology at the Keck School of Medicine of the University of Southern California in Los Angeles. However, you should get your dose of B$_6$ through a mul-

Mix the herbs together. Put 4 tablespoons of the mixture into a wide-mouth bottle and cover with 1 pint of good-quality brandy or vodka. Cover with a tight-fitting lid, place in a warm, shaded area, and let stand for 4 to 6 weeks. Shake daily to mix the herbs with the alcohol. After 4 to 6 weeks, strain into a clean bottle through a strainer lined with cheesecloth. The recommended dose is ¼ teaspoon three times a day for 3 months or longer. Rosemary suggests that you dilute the tincture in water, juice, or decaffeinated or herb tea before drinking.

To avoid irritability, you should avoid consuming caffeine and other stimulants while using ginseng.

Sip some menopause tea. If you prefer drinking tea, rather than taking an alcohol-based tincture, try this blend, created by herbalist Amanda McQuade Crawford, author of the *Herbal Menopause Book* and an herbalist at the Ojai Center of Phytotherapy in Ojai, California. Use high-quality dried herbs. All quantities are dry weight, not liquid.

Amanda's Menopause Tea

- 3 ounces chasteberry
- 2 ounces dang gui
- 1 organic orange or lemon rind (for flavor)
- 1 ounce Siberian ginseng or licorice
- 2 ounces St. John's wort
- 2 ounces horsetail
- 3 ounces motherwort

Mix the herbs together well. Infuse 1 ounce of herb blend in 2 pints of boiling water, cover and steep for 20 minutes, then strain. Amanda recommends that you drink one large glass three times a day.

tivitamin or B complex supplement, he says. The B vitamins work together, which means that supplemental B$_6$ won't be helpful unless you also have adequate amounts of the other B vitamins.

Pantothenic acid. Some studies indicate that some people in the United States aren't getting enough of this B vitamin. The Daily Value (DV) is 10 milligrams, and studies have shown that the average intake of most Americans is 5 to 10 milligrams a day. Deficiencies have been known to produce depression and fatigue. Taking 500 milligrams a day may bolster your mood, says Willow Moore, D.C., N.D., a chiropractor and naturopathic doctor in Owings Mills, Maryland. Pantothenic acid is sometimes labeled as vitamin B$_5$. (Other forms include calcium pantothenate and pantethine.)

Black cohosh. Once again, black cohosh is voted the herb most likely to succeed by natural practitioners. German physicians have been recommending it since the 1940s for hormone disturbances. Herbalists suggest taking ½ to 1 milliliter of tincture two to four times daily for relief of hormone-related mood swings.

Chamomile. "I've had high-powered executives say, 'My doctor wants to put me on Xanax,'" says Patricia Howell, a professional member of the American Herbalists Guild (AHG) and director of the Living with Herbs Institute in Atlanta. "Instead, I put them on chamomile tea, and they've told me that they felt their lives were theirs again."

But the chamomile tea that Howell recommends is much stronger than the average brew. To make this chamomile infusion, put 2 to 3 ounces of dried chamomile flowers in a jar and cover it with freshly boiled water. Let it steep overnight. Then strain out the herb and drink about ¼ cup of this fairly strong infusion, hot or cold, as needed for anxiety and accompanying digestive upset.

"It is a very strong preparation and can be taken as often as needed," she says. "It can be diluted with hot water to make a weaker tea." (For an easier method, use two or three chamomile tea bags rather than the loose herb.)

Skullcap. Skullcap tincture strengthens the nerves, eases oversensitivity, and helps promote deep, sound sleep, says Susun. She uses 4 to 8 drops of the tincture mornings and evenings when she's feeling "fried, stressed-out, wired, or just wound up." (Do not confuse it with Chinese skullcap, though, which has entirely different properties.)

Chasteberry. Take 5 to 15 drops of chasteberry tincture, mixed with a few ounces of water, three times a day. Chasteberry is commonly prescribed in European countries for PMS. The herb appears to work through the pituitary, your body's master gland, to help reestablish hormonal balance, says Daniel Mowrey, Ph.D., in his book *Herbal Tonic Therapies*. If you prefer to take vitex, which is the fruit of the chaste tree, try taking two 500-milligram tablets twice a day for a few months to see if it helps. If it does, you should keep taking it: In a German study, women who took vitex and then gave it up had a return of symptoms within 3 months.

Healing the Heart

By now, we all know that once a woman enters menopause, her estrogen production begins to slow down. A woman's risk of heart disease rises every year after menopause. Fortunately, there are many ways to minimize and even reverse any existing damage by living a heart-friendly lifestyle that includes managing high blood pressure and high cholesterol through a balanced diet. Women with a nutritious diet will get most of the nutrients that they need for long-term heart health, but herbs and supplements can provide some extra insurance.

Vitamin E. Studies have shown that women who take vitamin E supplements reduce their risk of heart attack by up to 41 percent. Vitamin E

SUPER SUPPLEMENT CHECKLIST #3

If you're concerned about heart disease, try these supplements. As you can see, the list is extensive, so make sure you read the descriptions, choose the ones you think are right for you, and check with your doctor before beginning a supplement program.

☐ Vitamin E   ☐ Amino acids
☐ Fat-soluble vitamin C   ☐ Garlic supplements
☐ Folic acid   ☐ Guggul
☐ Vitamin B_{12} ☐ Magnesium
☐ Vitamin B_6 ☐ Potassium
☐ Niacin   ☐ Calcium
☐ Fish oils   ☐ Ginger
☐ Coenzyme Q_{10} ☐ Fenugreek
☐ Aspirin   ☐ Turmeric
☐ Fiber   ☐ Dandelion root
☐ Black tea

VITAMIN E: NATURAL SUPPLEMENTS ARE TWICE AS GOOD

A generation ago, vitamin C topped the hit parade of vitamins, says Maret Traber, Ph.D., associate professor in the department of nutrition and food management at Oregon State University in Corvallis. These days vitamin E gets all the attention.

Dr. Traber ought to know: She's principal investigator for the Linus Pauling Institute, and she rates vitamin E an "E for excellent" when it comes to helping to prevent heart disease and cancer. It can also clear the lungs of air pollutants— *if* you get enough vitamin E, that is.

As premier member of a class of nutrients known as antioxidants, vitamin E protects your body against destructive oxygen molecules in your body by taking a spare electron from the harmful "free radicals" inside your cells. In your lungs, vitamin E protects you against nitrogen dioxide, ozone, and other pollutants that can oxidize cells in your lungs, allowing you to breathe more easily.

The Daily Value (DV) for vitamin E is 30 International Units (IU), but medical experts who have studied the benefits of E recommend 100 to 200 IU a day—more than you can realistically expect to get from even the richest dietary sources, so make sure you take a supplement. You'd have to eat 6 cups of peanuts or 39 cups of boiled spinach to get 100 IU. "Even in the healthiest

may help prevent heart disease in several ways. Its most important role may be helping to prevent ravages of free radicals—harmful oxygen molecules your body produces that damage tissues throughout the body. These molecules cause cholesterol to cling to artery walls and clog them up. Vitamin E can help prevent the cholesterol buildup by getting rid of free radicals before they do any damage. Slowing this oxidation process may limit cholesterol's propensity to clog up arteries. Vitamin E may also help prevent platelets from aggregating along the blood vessel walls, which promotes blood clotting.

Many doctors advise women to take 100 to 400 IU vitamin E daily. At the same time, it's helpful to take a multivitamin that also contains vitamin C, another antioxidant that "recharges" vitamin E in the body and increases its effectiveness.

of diets, we don't get enough vitamin E," says Dr. Traber. "So supplements are important."

Which vitamin E supplements are better, natural or synthetic? Several studies support the use of vitamin E in its natural form, d-alpha tocopherol, over its synthetic form, dl-alpha tocopherol. (Natural vitamin E supplements start with the letter "d," such as "d-alpha tocopherol." Synthetic vitamin E products start with the letters "dl.") For one thing, it's twice as active—you'd need 400 IU of synthetic vitamin E to equal 200 IU of natural vitamin E. But your body also retains natural vitamin E three times as long as the synthetic, which means it can build up to and maintain higher levels of protection.

Foods contain not one but eight types of vitamin E molecules—alpha, beta, gamma, and delta tocopherols, and alpha, beta, gamma, and delta tocotrienols. So experts say that even if you rely partially on supplements, you should aim to include good sources of vitamin E in your diet: soybean, corn, and canola oils and avocados, peanut butter, wheat germ, and sunflower seeds.

Large doses of vitamin E may increase the risk of bleeding problems and lead to strokes. So before taking vitamin E supplements, check with your doctor, especially if you have high blood pressure, if you smoke, if you have had a stroke, or if you take blood thinners (anticoagulants) or regular doses of aspirin for a heart condition.

Fat-soluble vitamin C. Vitamin C keeps our arterial walls from thinning as we age, says Maria Sulindro, M.D., president and founder of eAntiAging.com, an Internet organization that provides scientific information about antiaging approaches. When the walls thin, they have a tendency to crack and leak. This process causes inflammation, enabling the undesirable, LDL cholesterol to accumulate along the inner walls of the coronary arteries.

The most common form of vitamin C, ascorbic acid, is water-soluble and won't reach the vascular wall, says Dr. Sulindro. "Instead, take 1,000 to 2,000 milligrams of fat-soluble vitamin C, ascorbyl palmitate. This form stays in the body longer, having more chance to get to the arterial wall," she says. (If you are on a cholesterol-lowering drug, check with your doctor before taking supplemental vitamin C.)

Even in people with healthy intakes of vitamin C, additional vitamin C seems to help increase HDL levels. In one study at the Jean Mayer USDA Human Nutrition Research Center on Aging at Tufts University in Boston, men and women with low blood levels of vitamin C who took 1,000 milligrams of supplemental vitamin C a day for 8 months averaged a 7 percent increase in their HDL readings.

Folic acid. Unless you eat fortified breakfast cereals, you'd have to eat the equivalent of more than 5 cups of romaine lettuce daily to meet the daily requirement of folic acid. Take 800 micrograms to help lower your cholesterol, says Stephen T. Sinatra, M.D., a cardiologist at New England Heart Center in Manchester, Connecticut, and assistant clinical professor at the University of Connecticut School of Medicine in Farmington.

B vitamins. This family of vitamins is heart-friendly because they help your body chew up homocysteine, a substance that you can easily do without. Homocysteine is an amino acid by-product that can damage arteries. It creates rough spots on artery walls, and those roughened areas can pick up fatty deposits that harden into artery-clogging plaque. Taking the vitamins we recommend below can help keep your artery walls smooth.

Vitamin B_{12}. Your options for getting this vitamin through your diet are limited. It is found in red meat, but our hearts can do without the artery-clogging fats that come with the whole package. Take 20 micrograms of vitamin B_{12}, recommends Dr. Sinatra.

Vitamin B_6. Even if your homocysteine levels are low, a deficiency of vitamin B_6 will still put you at risk for heart disease. You need this nutrient to help your body use protein, fats, and carbohydrates properly. B_6 also helps convert the amino acid tryptophan into another essential B vitamin, niacin. Dr. Sinatra recommends taking 20 milligrams of B_6.

Niacin. In large doses, niacin raises HDL, the good cholesterol, and can lower LDL cholesterol, HDL's evil twin. It also lowers fibrinogen, a blood protein that causes clot formation. However, niacin is not universally effective, and it is also not a supplement you safely take with cholesterol-lowering drugs. You need to talk to your doctor before taking niacin, to make sure it's right for you.

Fish oils. If you are at risk for heart disease, your doctor has probably told you to cut back on saturated fats, including animal fat, butter, and the kind that's in many baked goods. Instead of those unhealthy fats, get more essential fatty acids, says Decker Weiss, N.M.D., a naturopathic doctor at Arizona Heart Institute in Phoenix. Omega-3 and omega-6 fatty acids change your body chemistry so that you produce less of the harmful prostaglandins, hormonelike substances that can narrow the arteries, cause excessive blood clotting, and jack up blood pressure. "I recommend 1,000 to 3,000 milligrams a day of a mixture of these two essential fatty acids," he says.

Coenzyme Q$_{10}$. This nutrient boosts the heart's pumping ability by improving energy supplies to the heart muscle cells, so it helps the heart to pump more efficiently with less effort. It may also help your liver withstand the toxicity of statin drugs, and it reduces their side effects, such as liver problems and muscle aches. However, a number of medications, including antidepressants and cholesterol-lowering drugs, can deplete coenzyme Q$_{10}$ from your body. As for how much to take, Dr. Weiss suggests a dosage ranging from 30 to 50 milligrams a day. (See "Super Supplement Checklist #3" on page 123.)

Aspirin. Those humble little aspirins you thought were good only to dull your headaches are such valuable weapons against heart attacks that even some doctors are popping them daily. And when you team up aspirin with another common item on your shelf—vitamin E—you've got an anti–heart attack combo that's about as safe, cheap, and simple as it is effective.

Aspirin helps prevent heart attacks by discouraging blood cells known as platelets from sticking together. This is great for women because heart attacks experienced by women are likelier to be caused by blood clots than by blocked arteries, which usually trigger heart attacks in men.

How much aspirin will your doctor recommend? It depends.

If you've been diagnosed with coronary heart disease but have not had a heart attack. You might reduce your chances of a heart attack by a third by taking aspirin regularly. "Women with coronary disease should be taking an aspirin every day," says Nanette Wenger, M.D., professor of medicine (cardiology) at Emory University School of Medicine and chief of cardiology at Grady Memorial Hospital in Atlanta.

If you've had a heart attack. Taking anywhere from 80 milligrams (a baby aspirin) to one adult aspirin (325 milligrams) daily may prevent another one.

If you're having a heart attack. Taking a 325-milligram adult aspirin right away may improve your survival chances by 25 percent. (If it's coated, chew it for more rapid results.) Yale researchers found that one reason top hospitals save more heart attack patients may be that they're more forthcoming with the aspirin.

If you don't have coronary heart disease but do have risk factors such as diabetes or high cholesterol. Follow your doctor's recommendation. A woman without heart disease or without multiple risk factors runs such a low risk of heart attack that it's not worth risking minor or unlikely complications of taking aspirin, like stomach irritation, bleeding, and, rarely, hemorrhagic stroke.

Fiber. Fiber is routinely prescribed for people concerned about heart disease because it binds with bile, which is secreted by your liver into the small intestine, and escorts it from your body. That means fats won't be reabsorbed into your system.

There is also some evidence that fiber can help reduce high blood pressure. In a study of more than 40,000 nurses whose lifestyles and diet patterns were followed for 4 years, researchers discovered that those who got the highest amounts of fiber were least likely to develop high blood pressure. In another study, with animals whose blood pressures had been elevated by high-fat diets, switching to a low-fat diet and taking fiber supplements reduced blood pressure by 10 to 15 points.

Of the two kinds of fiber—soluble and insoluble—it's the soluble type that is more important for reducing cholesterol and lowering blood pressure. This fiber is found in fruits, beans, and oats. If you want additional fiber, look for a supplement that contains mixed soluble fibers, such as psyllium, oat bran, gums, and pectin.

Black tea. If you're at risk for a heart attack, your doctor may prescribe daily aspirin and vitamin E supplements. If so, consider washing them down with tea.

When researchers considered the coffee- and tea-drinking habits of several hundred men and women, people who drank tea regularly had about

GINGER-GARLIC SUPER SOUP

Both ginger and garlic are great for boosting the immune system, says Mary Bove, N.D., a naturopathic physician at the Brattleboro Naturopathic Clinic in Vermont. Here's Dr. Bove's recipe for protecting and strengthening your immunity. (The mung bean sprouts are added for extra doses of folate, potassium, and magnesium for overall good health—not to mention a little added texture!)

    4   cups chicken broth
    ½   cup finely chopped fresh garlic
    ½   cup finely sliced fresh ginger
    ½   cup mung bean sprouts

Place the broth in a large saucepan and warm over medium-high heat. In a medium saucepan, sauté the garlic and ginger for 3 or 4 minutes, or until soft. Add to the broth. Stir in the sprouts and simmer for 2 or 3 minutes, or until heated through. Enjoy!

half the heart attack risk of those who didn't drink tea. (Coffee consumption had no effect on the risk of heart attacks.) The tea in question is black tea. It's rich in flavonoids, natural antioxidants that researchers suspect may account for tea's apparent heart benefits. Moderate tea drinking—one or two cups a day—will do you no harm, and may do your heart a world of good, says Howard Sesso, Sc.D., the Harvard Medical School epidemiologist who led the study.

Amino acids. The amino acids L-lysine and L-proline can help clear the LDL cholesterol that clogs blood circulation. "This clogging represents half of all deaths of heart disease patients," says Dr. Sulindro. Get your doctor's approval before taking these amino acids.

Garlic supplements. The benefits of garlic are well-known, so if you are a garlic fan, go ahead and eat your fill. (Try our Ginger-Garlic Super Soup if you want a delicious dose of "medicine" for high cholesterol and blood pressure.) For many people, however, consistently eating five or more garlic cloves a day to lower cholesterol is more than they can relish. If you're among the lukewarm fans of whole garlic, the pills are worth a try before you take cholesterol-lowering drugs.

Look for dried garlic powder preparation in enteric-coated tablets or capsules. These are designed to pass through the stomach and then degrade in the alkaline environment of the intestine, where the beneficial conversion of one compound, alliin, into the active ingredient, allicin, takes place. In studies it's been found that with supplements, people can lower total cholesterol by 10 to 12 percent, and LDL and triglycerides by about 15 percent. HDL levels usually increased by about 10 percent. For those results, you'll need a preparation that provides a daily dose of at least 10 milligrams of alliin, or a total allicin potential of 4,000 micrograms. You'll probably need to allow 1 to 3 months before you begin seeing a change in your cholesterol levels.

Guggul. Guggul is a gum resin loosely related to myrrh. The herb has come into the spotlight for its ability to lower cholesterol. Guggul helps the liver create more receptors for LDL, which enables the liver to "catch" more LDL from the blood and excrete it. Look for products that offer it in standardized form, advises Tieraona Low Dog, M.D., a family practice physician at the University of New Mexico Hospital and member of the University of New Mexico School of Medicine in Albuquerque. The recommended standardized dosage is 25 milligrams three times a day. A person should take guggul until lipid levels normalize, and then should reduce the dose to 25 milligrams once a day, she says.

Magnesium. If you have high blood pressure (consistently higher than 140/90), you may be low in magnesium. Those who find that salt raises their blood pressure may be low in this mineral, as well as in potassium, calcium, and others. Magnesium helps to relax the smooth muscles in the blood vessels, which allows them to dilate.

If you are taking a diuretic for blood pressure control, it may be depleting your magnesium supply. The diuretic may actually stop working after 6 months if your magnesium stores are low. "Supplemental magnesium sometimes make the diuretic more effective again," says Dr. Weiss. It's safe for most people to use up to 350 milligrams a day, he says. The preferred forms are magnesium orotate and magnesium glycinate.

Potassium. Potassium affects blood volume because it helps you excrete sodium, says David B. Young, Ph.D., professor of physiology and biophysics at the University of Mississippi Medical Center in Jackson.

When you excrete sodium, you also excrete water, which reduces blood volume and in turn reduces blood pressure. The safest way to get potassium is from foods, he says. Baked potatoes, prune juice, avocados, and fat-free yogurt contain plentiful amounts of this mineral. In supplement form, a prescription is needed for dosages higher than 99 milligrams per tablet. If you are taking a diuretic for high blood pressure, that doesn't spare potassium though, you may need supplemental potassium, Dr. Young says. In this case, your doctor will monitor your blood levels.

Calcium. Like magnesium and potassium, calcium has a direct effect on blood volume or influences the ability of blood vessels to relax. The Daily Value (DV) for calcium is 1,000 milligrams, an amount that many of us fail to consume in our daily diets. Even if you're not getting the DV, though, if you already have high blood pressure, you should check with your doctor before taking supplemental calcium, Dr. Weiss says. "I don't normally recommend it for high blood pressure, unless I'm seeing an older woman who also has osteoporosis, because too much calcium can interfere with magnesium's muscle-relaxing ability."

Ginger. Ginger gives you a double bonus of protection because it temporarily lowers elevated blood pressure and reduces LDL while raising HDL levels, says Dr. Low Dog. "In addition, ginger can help ward off strokes and heart attacks because it keeps platelets from aggregating," she says.

Take one capsule of ginger, equivalent to 500 milligrams, three times a day. Then take less or more depending on what your lipid profile looks like after 8 weeks. Ginger remains medicinally potent when you cook with it, and crystallized ginger and pickled ginger (the kind you get in Japanese restaurants) are also effective *and* delicious, she says. (For a delicious way to pamper your heart, try the Ginger-Garlic Super Soup recipe on page 129.)

Fenugreek. Consume 1 to 2 tablespoons of ground fenugreek seeds three or four times a day, suggests Mary Bove, N.D., a naturopathic doctor and director of the Brattleboro Naturopathic Clinic in Vermont. In one study, at the National Institute of Nutrition in India, people who ingested roughly ¾ cup of the herb every day for 20 days cut their LDL levels by one-third. Even better, their HDL levels remained unchanged.

Fenugreek has a bittersweet licorice taste. Try sprinkling some of the ground seeds on food. Or make a tea by steeping a fenugreek tea bag (available at health food stores) or 1 teaspoon of ground seeds in 1 cup of freshly boiled water. If the taste of fenugreek doesn't appeal to you, take one or two 580-milligram capsules of the herb three or four times a day, advises Dr. Bove.

Turmeric. Researchers in India—where turmeric is a staple ingredient—have found that the herb enhances your body's ability to process cholesterol. As an alternative to using ground turmeric in your cooking, take 150 milligrams of the herb in capsule form three times a day, suggests Dr. Bove. Turmeric capsules are available at most health food stores.

Dandelion root. Natural healers often concentrate on the connection between blood cholesterol and your liver. "A neglected liver can really elevate cholesterol," says Pamela Sky Jeanne, R.N., N.D., a naturopathic family physician in Gresham, Oregon. "Your digestive system may not be eliminating the cholesterol, or your liver may be overproducing it." That's where dandelion can help. Although there's no direct evidence linking dandelion and reduced cholesterol levels, there's no doubt that it's a great herb for your liver, according to naturopathic doctors. It's easy to find, but make sure the tincture is made from the root, says Dr. Jeanne.

Use the bottle's dropper to fill a teaspoon, put the tincture in a small amount of water, and drink it down. It's best to take dandelion for about 2 months and then stop for about 2 weeks, says Dr. Jeanne. You can then take it for another 2 months and continue cycling until your cholesterol is lowered. Some doctors prescribe dandelion as a natural potassium-sparing diuretic for high blood pressure, but the dosage depends on your blood pressure. If you have high blood pressure, see your doctor first before trying dandelion.

Combating Cancer

For many of us, *cancer* is one of the scariest words in the English language. And it's one we never want to hear applied to us. Because menopause increases your risk of hormone-related cancers like endometrial and breast cancers (we'll tell you why in a minute), it's smart to do everything you can to prevent them. And supplements can help. Research has shown

SUPER SUPPLEMENT CHECKLIST #4

Add these supplements to your diet if you're concerned about cancer. They've been shown to have anticancer properties. Fortunately, many of them help with other menopause-related conditions as well!

- ☐ Vitamin E as oil (not dry)
- ☐ Water-soluble vitamin C
- ☐ Bioflavonoids
- ☐ Carotenoids
- ☐ Selenium
- ☐ Folic acid
- ☐ Calcium
- ☐ Green tea
- ☐ Garlic
- ☐ Fiber
- ☐ Flaxseed

that a host of supplements have anticancer properties. Read on to find out what they are and how to take them.

Endometrial Cancer

Endometrial cancer—cancer of the lining of the uterus—is the most common reproductive cancer in women. And menopause increases your risk. With low levels of estrogen and progesterone, the endometrium doesn't slough off as it did during menstruation. The endometrial cells are still there, and with maturity they become more vulnerable to cancer.

Estrogen therapy ups the risk because taking too much estrogen gets the endometrium growing again. The more growth and the more cells there are, the higher the likelihood that one cell will turn cancerous. That's why most hormone therapy (HT, formerly hormone replacement therapy, HRT) includes progestin (a synthetic form of progesterone) with the estrogen. Progesterone helps protect against endometrial cancer by "calming down" the estrogen-stimulated cells.

Breast Cancer

Few other places in the world have rates of breast cancer higher than those in the United States. Other than skin cancer, it is the most common form of malignancy diagnosed among women in this country, affecting 175,000 of us and claiming 43,000 lives each year. Only lung cancer is more lethal. Since 1973, the number of breast cancers diagnosed has increased about 2 percent annually, although much of that increase is the result of better methods of detection.

Doctors aren't certain what makes the breast so susceptible to cancer, but a number of factors are known to increase a woman's risk of developing the disease, including age and estrogen exposure.

Age. A woman's risk of breast cancer increases gradually as she gets older. It is rarely diagnosed in women under age 35, but all women ages 40 and over are at increased risk. Most cases occur in women over age 50, and the risk is particularly high among women over age 60.

Estrogen exposure. Women who experience menopause after age 55, or who have taken hormone therapy for a number of years, may be at a higher risk for breast cancer. And the longer you are exposed to estrogen, the likelier you are to develop it.

Risk factors are important, but paying too much attention to them may be misleading, as the odds that any one of them will trigger breast cancer are less than 1 percent, says Deborah Capko, M.D., a breast surgeon and associate medical director of the Institute for Breast Care at Hackensack University Medical Center in New Jersey. In fact, many women with known risk factors do not get breast cancer. And many women who have no factors develop the disease. Doctors are hard-pressed to explain this paradox. That is why diligence is critical.

There are no known surefire ways to prevent breast cancer, but some supplements and herbs may help reduce your risk.

Antioxidants. Researchers speculate that up to 30 percent of cancers are affected simply by what we eat. Vegetables and fruits supply your body with an armory of antioxidants. Getting the requisite five or more servings a day of fruits and vegetables is the first step in defending yourself against cancer. But while prevention may start at your plate, you can go even further with specific antioxidant supplements known for their anti-cancer actions, says Keith Berndtson, M.D., medical director of the American Wholehealth Centers of Integrative Medicine in Chicago. In addition to a healthy diet, he says, "I'd stick to a high-potency multiple vitamin with additional antioxidants for cancer prevention."

Vitamins E and C. Two of the most important antioxidants are also the most well-known—vitamin E and vitamin C. These two are favorites when it comes to improving overall health, and for cancer prevention, they seem to be all-stars.

Oily vitamin E is hard to get in abundance from dietary sources alone. Supplemental amounts from 400 to 800 international units (IU) a day are recommended by W. John Diamond, M.D., medical director of the Triad Medical Center in Reno, Nevada, and coauthor of *An Alternative Medicine Definitive Guide to Cancer.*

Water-soluble vitamin C is relatively easy to find in foods. Although the Daily Value (DV) for C is only 60 milligrams, Dr. Diamond suggests much more for the prevention and treatment of cancer. He recommends between 1,000 and 8,000 milligrams in divided doses throughout the day.

Bioflavonoids. Hidden inside vegetables, fruits, flowers, herbs, and grains are compounds commonly known as bioflavonoids. Researchers regard them as powerful antioxidants because they provide protection against free radicals. These compounds may have anticancer properties. Bioflavonoids are widely available in supplements as quercetin, rutin, or hesperidin. You'll also see supplements called proanthocyanidins, or PCOs, which are derived primarily from red wines and grapeseed extracts. These multitalented substances may have remarkable effects, one of which could be their ability to convert malignant cells into normal cells.

While the many benefits of bioflavonoids are being explored, experts are still trying to decide whether most of us can benefit from supplementation. Some say that we get all the bioflavonoids we need from our diets and that supplementing provides no additional benefits. Others argue that supplements provide extra protection and help fill the gaps when our diets are lacking. If you decide you would like to supplement your diet with bioflavonoids, talk to your doctor first before you do.

Carotenoids. Nutrition researchers have distinguished another group of antioxidants, called carotenoids. These substances are also associated with a reduced risk of cancer. In most studies, however, researchers studied the effects of carotenoid-rich foods rather than supplements. The most studied has been beta-carotene. In early studies, researchers found that the group of people who got the largest amount of this nutrient from foods also had substantially fewer cancers. Beta-carotene was hailed as the newest antioxidant

VITAMIN C: YOUR ALL-DAY POLLUTION SHIELD

Back in grade school, we all learned that scientists discovered our need for vitamin C by accident, when British sailors deprived of fresh fruits and vegetables developed scurvy. Today we need more vitamin C than ever. Vitamin C naturally battles toxins, fortifying us against cigarette smoke, exhaust fumes, smog, and other pollutants that—except for the occasional volcanic eruption—didn't exist back in the past.

"Smokers need more vitamin C than nonsmokers because what they are inhaling is essentially highly polluted air," says Robert A. Jacob, Ph.D., a research chemist for the USDA Western Human Nutrition Research Center in Davis, California.

Even if you don't live in a smog capital like Los Angeles or spend hours in bumper-to-bumper traffic, you need vitamin C. This water-soluble antioxidant helps to detoxify your system by activating glutathione, a sulfurlike antioxidant, inside the body. Antioxidants eliminate cell-damaging molecules known as free radicals.

"Vitamin C not only neutralizes free radicals by itself but works with glutathione to eliminate other potential toxins you might take in through food or drugs," says Dr. Jacob. Vitamin C also helps your immune system protect you against infectious and chronic illnesses.

Pound for pound, women need less vitamin C than men. That's because vitamin C is used by muscle, not fat, and since women typically have less muscle mass, we need less vitamin C to derive the same benefits. However, Dr. Jacob recommends that women and men both get at least 60 milligrams of vitamin C a day, and smokers 100 milligrams a day. Your body can absorb only so much vitamin C at a time. So if you take supplements, try to spread out your vitamin C supplements throughout the day.

vitamin, able to protect not only the outsides of cells against free radicals, but also the insides, providing a stronger defense against damage.

When researchers started studying supplements of beta-carotene, however, they observed that the benefits didn't apply to everyone who upped their consumption. For smokers, beta-carotene might have a negative effect. This has led experts to be wary of recommending supplemental beta-carotene to everyone. True, a nutrient that poses a risk to smokers might be beneficial rather than harmful to nonsmokers. Smokers are already at high risk for cancer, and perhaps because of that, they react differently to beta-carotene than do nonsmokers. Researchers are wondering, though, whether it might be harmful to take beta-carotene in isolation from the rest of carotenoids, and with that question still hanging, a beta-carotene supplement can't be recommended as an across-the-board preventive. The moderate doses of carotenoids that come from foods, however, continue to show substantial anticancer promise.

If you want to add carotenoids to your diet, you might try a supplement called mixed carotenoids, says Dr. Berndtson. Look for one that supplies beta-carotene as well as the carotenoids gamma-carotene, lycopene, lutein, and zeaxanthin, he advises.

Selenium. Supplementing your diet with a small amount of the trace mineral selenium may make a huge dent in your cancer risk. A 10-year study found that men and women who took selenium supplements had a 37 percent lower incidence of cancer than those who took a placebo. The supplements appeared to have a significant impact on colon cancer, cutting incidence of the disease by 58 percent, and lung cancer, cutting incidence by 46 percent. It's possible that selenium may encourage abnormal cells and small, undetected tumors to self-destruct before they can cause trouble. The people who participated in the study took 200 micrograms daily. Check with your doctor, however, before you start taking this much.

Folic acid. Cancer can be the result of an accumulation of damage to DNA over time. Smoking, exposure to harmful chemicals, frequent exposure to x-rays, and certain viruses can damage a cell's genetic material. Add the injury of folic acid shortage to any one of these insults, and "you are turning up the speed of damage severalfold," explains Patrick Stover, Ph.D., assistant professor of nutritional biochemistry and cell biology at Cornell University in Ithaca, New York.

In several studies, folic acid deficiency has been strongly linked to DNA damage. In one, researchers at the University of California at Berkeley found that even a mild deficiency caused a large increase in the amount of damaged DNA. Other studies have shown a link between folic acid deficiency and dysplasia (abnormal, precancerous cells) in the cervix, colon, and lungs.

Most people get about 200 micrograms of folate a day, about half the daily value (DV). With folic acid–fortified foods, such as breads and breakfast cereals now on the market, daily intake could increase on average to about 300 micrograms a day, leaving a 100-microgram deficit. Most over-the-counter multivitamins contain 400 micrograms, and a few super-potency vitamins provide 800 micrograms. You should never take more than 1,000 micrograms without checking with your doctor first.

Calcium. This mineral is found in broccoli, grapefruit, brussels sprouts, apples, and of course milk. But you don't have to drink three glasses of milk a day if you don't want to. In its supplement form, calcium is a real power-house against cancer. "It has been found to fight cancers of the skin, breasts, ovaries, lungs, and bones," says Dr. Sulindro. It's also being studied as a way to prevent breast cancer in high-risk women.

Calcium works in the liver to chemically change cancer-causing substances so they pass quickly through the body without doing any harm. Dosage recommendations are anywhere from 200 to 2,000 milligrams daily, says Dr. Sulindro, so check with your doctor. For better absorption, spread your doses out over the day, and take no more than 500 milligrams at once. If you use calcium citrate, lactate, or gluconate, you can take it between meals without absorption problems, and it won't interfere with iron and other trace minerals. All other forms of supplemental calcium are best absorbed with taken with food.

Green tea. The traditional pale green brew that accompanies Japanese food appears to have potent anticancer properties, according to Jerzy Jankun, M.D., a cancer researcher and associate professor in the department of urology at the Medical College of Ohio in Toledo.

Green tea contains a substance called epigallocathechin-3 gallate (EGCG). Dr. Jankun's research shows that EGCG inhibits urokinase, an enzyme that allows tumors to grow and spread. "By inhibiting urokinase, those processes *could* be stopped," says Dr. Jankun. "EGCG has been known to possess other anticancer activity, but inhibition of urokinase seems to be the most important factor."

How much green tea should you sip? You can follow the lead from the East: Asian tea lovers commonly drink up to 10 cups a day. While this may seem like a lot, research suggests that consuming such a large quantity may be necessary to reap green tea's anticancer benefits. If you prefer your protection in capsules rather than cups, green tea extract is available in supplement form, says Dr. Jankun. Sometimes an equivalent in cups will be noted on the label, or the label will give the concentration of green tea in milligrams. Since potencies are different, follow the directions on the label. Most brands advise taking one or two capsules two or three times a day.

Garlic. Research suggests that garlic and other members of the onion family can cut your odds of developing cancer. In once study, women who ate garlic at least once a week cut their colon cancer risks by one-third, compared with women who never ate the stuff. If you avoid fresh garlic because you don't like it or it doesn't agree with you, look for dried garlic powder preparation in enteric-coated tablets or capsules. Follow the directions on the label.

Fiber. Women whose diets include lots of fibrous foods—like fruits, veggies, and whole wheat cereals and breads—may have fewer breast, colon, and rectal cancers than those who don't eat those foods. Fiber reduces the amount of estrogen in the blood. Estrogen possibly alters cell structure and promotes breast cancer. In addition, fiber helps speed stool through your body, reducing exposure of your digestive tract to carcinogens.

Fiber may also help prevent other cancers. In a study of 399 women with endometrial cancer and 296 disease-free women, researchers found that women who ate more than two servings of high-fiber breads and cereals a day had 40 percent less risk of developing endometrial cancer.

If you aren't getting the 20 to 30 grams of fiber a day recommended by the National Cancer Institute, then consider taking a fiber supplement, like Metamucil.

Flaxseed. Flaxseed is an incredibly rich source of a group of compounds called lignans. While many plant foods also contain lignans, flaxseed has the absolute most—at least 75 times more than any other plant food. This is important because lignans may have powerful antioxidant properties that can help block the damaging effects of free radicals. Lignans show particular promise for battling breast cancer. They do this by blocking the effects of estrogen; exposure to estrogen over time seems to increase breast cancer risk in some women. Even when estrogen-sensitive tumors get a chance to grow, lignans exert a restraining influence that can slow or even halt their growth.

In a laboratory study, breast tumors in animals given flaxseed shrank by 50 percent in 7 weeks. In addition, it is rich in polyunsaturated fats, including omega-3 fatty acids. These appear to limit the body's production of prostaglandins, which, in large amounts, are thought to speed up tumor growths. And flaxseed is high in fiber, which quickly ushers harmful compounds out of the body.

Flaxseed oil comes in liquid and gelatin capsules, but you may want to skip the oil and just add flaxseed to your diet. The oil contains only trace amounts of the cancer-protective lignans because they are removed during processing. However, if you do decide to go with the supplement, stick with oil from the refrigerated section of your health food store. Flaxseed oil degrades quickly when exposed to heat and light. Buy only oil that comes in an opaque bottle, and store it in the refrigerator as soon as you get home. Or, if you don't plan to use it right away, keep it in the freezer. Look for oils certified by a third party as organic. Also, high-quality oils have a "pressing date" listed on the bottles. If the oil was pressed more than 6 months ago, don't buy it.

Outwitting Osteoporosis

If you've ever pitied "big-boned" women, save your sympathy. Their strength may protect them from osteoporosis, one of the most devastating age- and hormone-related processes women experience. It's a condition where the hormone-controlled process of bone breakdown speeds up as the bone-rebuilding process slows down. After age 50, half of all American women have bones weak enough to fracture. By age 90, one-third of all women will have suffered a hip fracture.

The more bone we build by the time we're in our twenties, the better prepared we are for bone loss that occurs with aging and menopause. While our bones do begin to weaken as we age, osteoporosis is not inevitable. Doctors are sending the message to women that this is not really an illness of aging, but rather an indication that the body isn't receiving enough calcium. Experts agree that that is never too late to strengthen

---

SUPER SUPPLEMENT CHECKLIST #5

By now, you know to take your calcium and vitamin D for strong, healthy bones. (And don't forget those weight-bearing exercises!) But there are plenty of other supplements that can help in the fight against osteoporosis and brittle bones. Here they are.

☐ Calcium   ☐ Nettle
☐ Vitamin D   ☐ Oatstraw
☐ Magnesium   ☐ Dandelion leaf
☐ Vitamin K   ☐ Asian ginseng and ginger
☐ Horsetail   ☐ Alfalfa

---

your skeleton. Here are some supplements to help you avoid osteoporosis or, if you already have it, to slow its progress.

Calcium. Most women get about 500 milligrams of calcium a day from food. Much of that comes from dairy sources. If you happen to be lactose intolerant and therefore avoid most dairy products, you're probably getting even less than the average. In any case, you should probably have two or three times as much calcium as you're getting from food.

Almost every bit of calcium in your body is stored in your bones. There is also some in your blood, where it's used to regulate your heartbeat and keep muscle and nerve function and blood clotting at optimal levels. Your body's top priority is to maintain adequate levels of blood calcium. When these levels decline, your body will begin mining calcium from the next available source—your bones.

Knowing this, researchers have been probing to discover the optimal amount of calcium supplementation that most women need. At University Hospital in Ghent, Belgium, doctors found that a calcium intake of 1,500 milligrams a day helped protect postmenopausal women from bone loss. Another study, at Winthrop-University Hospital in Mineola, New York, showed that giving 1,700 milligrams a day of calcium to women who were past menopause significantly slowed their rates of bone loss. Other studies show calcium's protective role against osteoporosis, but there are varying estimates of how much you need to take.

Lorilee Schoenbeck, M.D., a naturopathic doctor with the Champlain Centers for Natural Medicine in Shelburne and Middlebury, Vermont, recommends 1,000 milligrams a day for women who are in menopause or have passed through it. Whatever amount you're taking, you want a supplement that provides the most easily absorbed form. Your body is better able to absorb and use calcium if it's in the form of citrate or aspartate. While some doctors say that you can get what you need from antacid tablets, Dr. Schoenbeck notes that the calcium in antacids is less absorbable than calcium citrate. Another form you'll see on drugstore shelves is calcium carbonate, but that's the least absorbable, she says. (Taking this form with meals can increase absorption, however.)

Vitamin D. Vitamin D helps your body absorb supplemental calcium. A deficiency of D can lead to soft bones, which in turn can lead to fractures. Studies suggest that vitamin D is related to bone mineral density. Researchers at the Jean Mayer USDA Human Nutritional Research Center on Aging at Tufts University in Boston concluded that anywhere from 400 to 800 IU of vitamin D a day (taken with 1,000 to 1,500 milligrams of calcium) is necessary to minimize bone loss. For more information, see "Vitamin D: The 'Other' Bone-Friendly Hormone" on page 108.

Magnesium. With regard to bone health, this mineral serves a different function from vitamin D. Magnesium is important because it transports calcium to the bones. It also helps convert vitamin D in the body to its active form.

A study in Israel found that 22 of 31 postmenopausal women who were given from 250 to 750 milligrams of magnesium for 6 months, then 250 milligrams a day for 18 months, increased their bone density by 1 to 8 percent. Comparatively, a group of women who received no magnesium supplementation over the same period had rapid loss of bone density.

To figure out how much magnesium you need, just take your calcium dosage and divide it in half. If you're taking 1,000 milligrams of calcium, for instance, you should take about 500 milligrams of magnesium. The least absorbable form of magnesium is magnesium oxide. You'll do better with magnesium aspartate.

Vitamin K. Vitamin K doesn't get much mention in the media, but it's very important for maintaining bone health. It helps reduce the amount of calcium you lose through urine. Vitamin K is also crucial to the formation of osteocalcin, a protein that is the matrix upon which calcium is put into the bone. "Vitamin K is kind of like the foundation that calcium builds on," says Dr. Schoenbeck.

This vitamin is abundant in green leafy vegetables and whole grains. If your diet isn't rich in these foods, take a supplement that supplies the Daily Value (DV) of 80 micrograms.

Horsetail. Horsetail is a reasonable source of silicon, one of the minerals that help give bones flexibility as well as strength, says C. Leigh Broadhurst, Ph.D., a nutrition consultant and herbal researcher based in Clovery, Maryland. To ensure that you get a pure, strong dose, she recommends using the liquid extract. Take 2 dropperfuls of extract in 1 cup of water twice a day. Take it on an empty stomach, if possible, in the morning and in the evening.

Horsetail is also available in capsules, says Allan Warshowsky, M.D., a gynecologist on staff at the Long Island Jewish Medical Center in New Hyde Park, New York. He recommends using capsules of standardized extract. Take 700 to 800 milligrams in capsule form twice a day.

Nettle. Nettle is an excellent source of magnesium and calcium, says Dr. Warshowsky. Drink 1 dropperful of extract in 1 cup of water once or twice a day. Another way to take nettle is to buy standardized extract in capsule form. Take a 500-milligram capsule twice a day. People who have already developed signs of osteoporosis can double either dosage, he adds. Nettle tea is also available in health food stores.

Oatstraw. Oatstraw infusion is an excellent source of calcium and magnesium, according to herbalist Susun Weed. One particularly effective way to extract those minerals from the herb is to make a strong infusion, rather than a tea. Here are Susun's instructions. Put 1 ounce (by weight) of dried oatstraw in a quart mason jar. (If you don't have a scale, fill the jar approximately one-third full of herb.) Pour boiling water into the jar right to the top (approximately 4 cups), put a tight lid on it, and let stand for at least 4 hours. Strain out the plant material and drink from 1 cup to 1 quart a day as you like it, either hot or cold, she says. The taste is mild and mellow, but you can mix it with anything, even tea or coffee, if you wish. Drink 1 to 4 cups of infusion a day. Refrigerate right away what you don't drink, but use it within 48 hours.

Dandelion leaf. Dandelion leaf has an abundance of minerals, including calcium, according to Dr. Warshowsky. Take the extract according to the package directions twice a day. He recommends looking for a standardized extract.

Panax (Asian) ginseng and ginger. Like other root plants, ginseng and ginger can absorb plenty of minerals, especially boron, from the soil, says Dr. Broadhurst, the nutrition consultant and herbal researcher. Ginseng has the added benefit of being an energy booster. Having energy can boost your enthusiasm for exercise, another important element of bone health. Take one 500-milligram capsule of each herb three times a day.

Alfalfa. The freshest way to ingest leafy green plants—your prime sources of bone-helping vitamin K—is to frequent the salad bar, but an alfalfa supplement can help salad-phobic people get the green nutrients they need. Take four 500-milligram capsules of extract daily. Take two capsules in the morning and two at night, Dr. Broadhurst suggests.

Another easy way to get more leafy greens in your diet, she adds, is to use the "green drink" mixtures sold in health food stores, which combine everything from barley grass to various types of seaweed.

Congratulations! You've made it to the end of that long list of supplements. But we hope you noticed how many supplements fight several menopausal problems. And that means you don't have to take as many as it might seem at first. We suggest that you go back through this chapter, checklists in hand, and reread the sections that are most important to you. Note carefully how much, how often, and what form of each supplement to take for maximum effectiveness. Choose which supplements you want to try. (Of course, we hope *all* of you will take the basic vitamin/mineral supplement recommended on page 105, which gives you a great basis to begin adding specific supplements according to your needs.) Once you've made your list and checked it twice, it's time to move on to something that's a lot more fun, and every bit as important: looking great.

Chapter
6

LOOKING FABULOUS

The menopausal years pose some unique beauty challenges. Hormonal fluctuations can make our skin and hair drier. Our bodies tend to become more voluptuous. But in general, our generation of women take these exterior changes in stride because we know something that our mothers didn't: Growing older doesn't mean growing *old*.

In fact, it may mean exactly the opposite.

Studies of older women find that for many of them, midlife and beyond means more choices, more opportunities, more freedom—perks in short supply in our younger days. With this optimistic outlook and full-speed-ahead mentality, it's natural that we would want our outward appearance to mirror our inner vitality and passion for life. But we don't need to look like Goldie Hawn to celebrate our own unique beauty.

Of course, we can't promise you that we can give you back your 25-year-old face and body. But you'll find tips and advice in this chapter for a head-to-toe, vibrant glow—like how to achieve softer, smoother skin; adding shine and luster to your hair; revitalizing workworn hands and nails. You'll also find simple ways to give your makeup and clothing a youthful "makeover" by updating your personal style.

Here are the new easy-to-follow rules for putting your best face and figure forward.

KNOW THY BEAUTY ENEMY: THE SUN

We know how glorious the sun feels on bare skin and how sexy a golden tan can make you feel. But make no mistake: Baking in the sun will—repeat, *will*—accelerate your skin's aging process. Worse, it might lead to skin cancer. Here's how to help prevent both.

Avoid peak sunburn hours. The sun's rays are strongest between 10:00 A.M. and 3:00 P.M.. So if you can, avoid outdoor activities during these hours—or make sure to pile on the sunscreen. Use a broad-spectrum sunscreen, which blocks both ultraviolet A (UVA) rays and ultraviolet B (UVB) rays daily, year-round.

Give your sunscreen "soak-in time." Apply sunscreen 30 to 45 minutes before sun exposure. Your skin needs this time to absorb it.

Be aware of skin changes. If you see changes such as a new spot, a little notch, darker pigmentation, or a change in a lesion, wart, or mole, consult a dermatologist.

Consider a yearly screening. Even if you don't see changes, get a skin screening from a dermatologist once a year, especially if you're fair-skinned. "A yearly screening is likely to pick up early skin cancer at its most treatable, entirely curable stages," says Evelyn Placek, M.D., a dermatologist in Scarsdale, New York.

Get-Glowing Rule #1:
Follow the Skin-Care Commandments

During the years leading up to and during menopause, our skin can be drier than a stale rice cake, more fragile than a newly painted fingernail, and duller than an accountant explaining the tax code. There are several reasons for these troublesome skin changes.

• Our estrogen levels decline, which causes a reduction in the skin's content of collagen. This structural protein gives skin its youthful plumpness and resiliency. Basically, the collagen in our skin is less able to maintain an adequate water supply, which tends to leave it drier.

• Our skin's protective outside layer, the epidermis, becomes thinner and more fragile.

- The oil glands in our skin produce less oil, which can leave skin drier and more sensitive.

- Our skin doesn't replace old, dead cells with fresh new ones as quickly as it once did.

- The number of blood vessels in our skin decreases, as does the rosy glow of youth.

Genetics, too, plays a role in how skin ages. The skin of fair women shows signs of aging faster than that of their darker-skinned sisters. That's because lighter skin contains less melanin, the substance that gives skin its pigment and helps protect it from the sun.

But to a large extent, your skin's "age" depends on how well you take care of it. A lifetime of basking in the sun and smoking can accelerate the breakdown of both collagen and another structural protein called elastin, which can result in premature wrinkling, sagging, blotches, and age spots. Chronic stress, poor nutrition, and excessive dieting, all of which plague many women of menopausal age, also can add years to a woman's appearance.

Happily, though, it's fairly simple to baby your menopausal skin. If you make just a few tweaks in your skin care routine and lifestyle, you're likely to be rewarded with smoother, softer, younger-looking skin. Try our 11 skin-care commandments and see for yourself!

1. **Scrub away the years.** Dry, thin skin needs a bit of help in re-newing itself. Exfoliation can speed this process. To reduce the dead outer layers of skin, gently rub with a washcloth or Buf-Puf once or twice a week. Then hydrate with a rich cream.

2. **Splurge on sunscreen.** Even if you spent years basting your skin with baby oil and iodine, starting to use sunscreen now can help prevent future sun damage and possibly the formation of wrinkles. For everyday protection, use a sunscreen with a sun protection factor (SPF) of at least 15, and apply it at least 30 minutes before you leave the house.

   Don't apply sunscreen just to your face. Slather it on your neck, ears, and whatever other parts of you are being exposed to the sun. If you'll be on the beach, boat, tennis court, golf course, or ski slope, use a sunscreen with an SPF of 30.

3. **Buy a built-in sunscreen.** If you prefer, you can use a moisturizer with added SPF 15. Apply the equivalent of 1 teaspoon to assure the SPF promised. You can also use a foundation with SPF 15, but unless you use a teaspoon of the stuff, you probably won't get the protection you need.

4. **Make your eyes a crow's-feet-free zone.** To protect the delicate skin around your eyes, don wraparound sunglasses designed to block 95 to 100 percent of both types of the sun's ultraviolet rays, called UVA and UVB.

5. **Ban the booths.** Never use a tanning booth. Ever. Ignore tanning salons that claim to use "safe" tanning rays; there's no such thing.

6. **Moisturize your interior.** To stay hydrated from the inside out, drink eight 8-ounce glasses of water a day.

7. **Say no to yo-yo dieting.** Gaining and losing weight over and over again can cause wear and tear on collagen. Steer clear of starvation diets, too. Very low calorie diets deprive your skin of the nutrients it needs—and may thin your hair, too.

8. **Lock in moisture.** If your skin is severely dry, use ointments made with camphor and menthol, such as Lac-Hydrin and Aquaphor. Slather them on damp skin so moisture is "locked in."

9. **If you smoke, quit.** Smokers are two or three times likelier than nonsmokers to develop premature wrinkles, research has shown. That's because smoking causes the fibers of the skin to lose their elasticity sooner, which makes skin more susceptible to wrinkling. What's more, the nicotine in cigarettes narrows blood vessels, preventing oxygen-rich blood from reaching the tiny capillaries in the skin's top layers. This oxygen deprivation makes for dull, gray, leathery skin.

10. **Sleep on your back.** (If you can't, learn.) Smushing your face into your pillow every night for 40 years will eventually press wrinkles into your skin.

11. **Winterize your skin.** In the colder winter months, use a humidifier and lower your thermostat to below 70°F. Both will

help retain moisture in the air. Also, when temperatures are colder and the air is dry, opt for quick showers rather than lingering baths. Use warm water instead of hot, which can strip away the thin moisturizing layer on your skin.

Get-Glowing Rule #2: Wrinkle-Proof Your Skin

As you get older, it's tempting to believe that those moisturizers, creams, and other skin care items really will erase years from your face. And it's true that some over-the-counter potions do contain specific ingredients that can help skin look better—temporarily. But before you spend another dime on an ultra-expensive cream, check this primer on wrinkle cream ingredients. They're listed in order of potential effectiveness.

Just one thing first: If you use any of these products, please pair them with sunscreen. Some of these ingredients (such as retinoids, AHAs, and BHAs) make skin more sensitive to sunlight.

Tretinoin. The active ingredient in Renova and Retin-A, prescription-only creams, tretinoin is proven to rejuvenate the skin structure—if you use it continuously. Tretinoin helps your skin produce new collagen, form new blood vessels, and shed layers of dead skin. It can be irritating, though, causing peeling, flaking, sun sensitivity, and redness.

Retinol. Retinol is a retinoid (a vitamin A derivative) used as an ingredient in some over-the-counter wrinkle creams. "We don't know yet if the effects are comparable, but it's worth a try for a woman whose skin can't tolerate tretinoin," says Grace Pak, M.D., a cosmetic dermatologist in New York City.

Alpha hydroxy acids (AHAs). Basically exfoliating agents, alpha hydroxy acids "help to 'unglue' the layer of dead skin cells that tends to accumulate and give skin a lackluster appearance," Dr. Pak explains. With continued use, they, like Renova, also stimulate the development of new collagen, which is what makes your skin look and feel "plumper." Glycolic acid is the most common AHA.

If you've found AHAs to be too harsh for your skin, or if you've always had sensitive or delicate skin, look for products that contain amphoteric

REACH FOR THE "FAKE BAKE"

Want a healthy-looking tan without damaging your skin? Consider an artificial tanning gel. Used correctly, self-tanners look remarkably convincing, says Leslie S. Baumann, M.D., director of cosmetic dermatology at the University of Miami. They're especially convenient for women who want to go without stockings in summer but hate the pasty white way their legs look without a tan.

All self-tanners use the same active ingredient—dihydroxyacetone (DHA)—although the amount varies from product to product. Lotions are easier to apply than sprays. Here's how to get the best results:

- Use an alpha hydroxy body lotion for 1 week prior to applying the self-tanning product. The lotion will eliminate dead skin, so the self-tanner will go on more smoothly.
- For the most natural-looking tan, don't be tempted to buy the darkest tanner you find. If your skin is very pale, use a lighter formula. If you have a dark or olive complexion, select a medium or dark shade. Or start with a light shade and work up gradually.
- Remove your rings or other jewelry. Next, take a shower or bath, using an exfoliating scrub and giving special attention to your arms, legs, elbows, and knees. Then shave your legs. Your goal is to get rid of all the dead skin and hair that can cause an uneven application, says Dr. Baumann.
- Apply the self-tanner to any area that you would normally tan—your arms, legs, tops of feet and hands, neck, and face. Don't apply it to your underarms, though, because it will look unnatural. And go easy on your elbows and knees, to keep them from getting too dark.
- Blend lightly on your face. Feather the tanner into your hairline and eyebrows.
- To eliminate tan palms, wash your hands thoroughly with an exfoliating scrub after applying to arms and legs.
- If you want tan hands, go back and apply the tanner to the tops of your hands with a cotton ball or a finger. Blend the edges of your hands and fingers.
- Apply a moisturizer after the tanner has dried—usually within a few minutes but up to a half hour—to avoid uneven patches of color. Allow the lotion to dry thoroughly before you get dressed.
- Continue to use sunscreen with an SPF of 15 or higher. Artificial tanners won't protect your skin from sun damage.

hydroxy acids (AHCs). Researchers say they give you all the benefits of AHAs, minus the stinging, irritation, and redness.

Beta hydroxy acids (BHAs). BHAs (salicylic acid is the most well-known) have been used in acne treatment for years. They also help reduce wrinkling by sloughing off layers of dead skin, which in turn stimulates healthy cell turnover. However, they may not have the same tightening effect as AHAs, Dr. Pak says.

Vitamin C. Vitamin C is an antioxidant and theoretically protects your skin against sun damage from ultraviolet rays and the unstable molecules known as free radicals they introduce. The problem is, vitamin C breaks down when exposed to light—making it tough to package and effectively deliver topically to your skin. It's best used in conjunction with retinoids, AHAs or BHAs, and sunscreen, which have proven antiaging results, says Dr. Pak. To ensure the freshest, most effective product and to extend its shelf life, choose one packaged in a dark container you can't see through, with a pump dispenser that seals out oxygen.

Vitamin E. As an antioxidant, vitamin E should have the same effect on skin as vitamin C. However, there's no proof vitamin E does anything more for your wrinkles than moisturize them, says Dr. Pak. If your skin is dry and crinkly, any lotion—even Crisco—will temporarily reduce the appearance of your fine lines and wrinkles.

Coenzyme Q$_{10}$. This nutrient also acts as an antioxidant, neutralizing free radicals that lead to skin damage. While no published studies exist on the effectiveness of CoQ$_{10}$-supplemented wrinkle creams, "there's good reason to believe CoQ$_{10}$ might be helpful," according to Valerian Kagan, Ph.D., a biochemist at the University of Pittsburgh.

Furfuryladenine. Use of this plant growth hormone results in skin that looks and feels better, with some improvement in fine lines but without irritation, says Kathy Fields, M.D., clinical instructor of dermatology at the University of California in San Francisco. However, no independent research has yet verified how it compares with tretinoin.

Melibiose. This sugar molecule can temporarily help skin appear firmer, but no one knows if melibiose can make a long-term difference, Dr. Pak says.

Collagen and elastin. Derived from animal sources or produced synthetically, collagen and elastin molecules are too big to penetrate the skin. They work only if they're injected into the skin, which requires an office visit.

Get-Glowing Rule #3:
Try Surgery-Free Age Erasers

Hormone therapy (HT, formerly hormone replacement therapy, HRT), hormonal shifts, and the extended use of oral contraceptives all cause problems in the years surrounding menopause. But you needn't put up with them—nor do you need to go under the knife. Here's what to do if your skin starts to act up.

Sallow skin. To brighten up, ask a dermatologist about whether prescription-strength glycolic acid might be right for your skin. This AHA, derived from sugarcane, removes complexion-dulling dead cells from the

CHOOSE THE RIGHT HAIR REMOVAL METHOD

Unwanted facial hair is one unwelcome harbinger of the menopausal years. But that doesn't mean you have to live with it. Your options include:

Plucking is the fastest way to tame unruly brows. To tone down the sting, desensitize the brow area with an ice pack for 15 seconds before you begin.

Bleaching disguises the hair, drawing less attention to the area. This method is best for light facial hair, rather than heavy growth.

Waxing pulls hair out by the roots and is mildly to moderately painful, depending on your tolerance. Again, this method works best on light fuzz. Prewaxed plastic strips aren't as painful to use as warm wax, which hardens as it cools. A variation of waxing, called sugaring, coats hair with a paste of sugar and wax that is easier to pull off than wax alone and less traumatizing to the skin. You'll find both methods at drug and beauty supply stores. Don't choose waxing if you take Accutane or use Retin-A or Renova. These medications can make skin more sensitive.

Chemical depilatories are creams that dissolve hair. You usually leave the cream on for 10 minutes, then wipe it off. This isn't the best method for delicate or sensitive skin. Look for creams with hair growth inhibitors and fruit enzymes—ingredients that interfere with the protein that lets hair grow—so hair

skin's top layer, revealing the fresh new skin beneath. You can see results in as little as 2 weeks.

Dark circles. Use a yellow tone concealer one shade lighter than your skin tone.

Puffy eyes. To send the bags packing—temporarily—consider dabbing them with a little Preparation H. The product contains hydrocortisone, a topical steroid that reduces inflammation. Don't use Prep H every day, though. Long-term use can lead to acne, premature wrinkling, and broken blood vessels.

Less-than-firm skin. Try DMAE (dimethylaminoethanol). Research showed skin-firming effects after use for 8 weeks. Products containing this cream can be pricey, though—anywhere from $20 to $100.

Age spots. If you're bothered by these flat brown patches of darker pigmentation on your face, neck, hands, or upper chest, which are caused

grows back less quickly. Apply aloe if your skin is irritated afterward. And next time, choose a method that's easier on your skin.

Vaniqa (eflornithine) slows the metabolism of the hair follicle. It is applied twice a day. By slowing new growth, Vaniqa can decrease how often hair needs to be removed. (It is FDA-approved for treatment of facial hair.)

Lasers send a beam of concentrated light into the hair follicle, damaging it so hair falls out. Hair grows back in 3 to 9 months. This method works best on women with pale skin and dark, coarse hair. (Lasers zap pigment as well as hair. So if you're dark-complexioned, you could end up with light spots.) A dermatologist is apt to be better trained at laser hair removal than a spa attendant. Always perform a skin test first. Also, avoid sun exposure; it makes skin more vulnerable to laser burns.

Electrolysis is the only permanent hair removal option. You can't do it yourself: It's performed in a salon or a hair removal office and involves inserting a probe into each individual hair follicle and passing an electric current through it. Removal of all the hair on your upper lip may take several sessions. If done improperly, electrolysis can leave scars, so choose a highly experienced technician. The technician should be a member of a state or national electrolysis association and be a certified professional electrolysist (CPE).

For other options, see page 293.

by sun damage, ask your doctor about azelaic acid. This medication, available by prescription, has been found to inhibit melanin production, fade age spots and freckles, and prevent new pigment from forming. You might also try AHAs, vitamin C, and dermatologist-prescribed creams, such as Lustra, Allustra, Glyquin, or TriLuma.

Ruddy skin/breakouts/broken capillaries. If your face becomes reddened, especially if the ruddiness is accompanied by hot flashes, talk to a dermatologist. Hot flashes often trigger rosacea, a common inflammatory skin problem in menopausal women.

Out-and-out wrinkles. There are several options. Botox (recommended for the upper forehead only) can smooth deep furrows on the forehead. With nonablative laser therapy, laser light stimulates collagen production while avoiding the kind of damage that standard laser treatment can do to your skin's top layers. Cost: $400 to $1,500 for a full-face treatment. With chemical peels, a chemical solution is applied to the face to improve and smooth the skin's tone and texture. Costs run from $200 to $5,000, for the more abrasive peels.

Get-Glowing Rule #4:
Put Your Best Face Forward

Not every menopausal woman feels the need to wear cosmetics. But most would agree that it's the simplest way to minimize or conceal age-related imperfections. Foundation softens the appearance of fine lines and brightens skin, while blush returns the bloom of youth to a tired-looking complexion, and lipstick delivers a welcome jolt of color to pale skin. What's more, there's a wide selection of cosmetics formulated specifically for dry and aging skin.

If you wear little or no makeup, you might be afraid to start now. But rest assured, you'll look great. Makeup is virtually goof-proof once you learn the Three Rules of Cosmetic Wizardry:

• Less makeup is more.

• Blend your makeup carefully.

• Color is your friend. Just use it artfully.

STOP MAKEUP ABUSE NOW!

Makeup can help us erase the years—unless we apply it incorrectly. Then it can *add* years. Check the list below to see if you're committing "cosmetic abuse."

Wearing too much makeup. Some of us try to hide the years beneath layers of foundation and eye shadow. But the truth is, using too much makeup makes us look older. (Just ask any 14-year-old girl.) Look at your reflection critically. Could you lose some of that foundation, blush, or eye makeup?

Not blending in. Too many of us end our foundation at the jawline or don't blend the blush into the foundation. Blend both until you can't see where they begin and end.

Using too much eyeliner. It makes eyes look smaller.

Being stuck in the past. Would you be caught dead in a pair of gaucho pants or leg warmers today? We thought not. So don't apply makeup the same way you did when the Beatles broke up. Makeup styles change, and to look more youthful, we have to keep up.

Flattering Foundation and Concealer

Let's start with the basics here: what you wear *under* your "showy" makeup. With these tips, everyone will think they're seeing your own flawless skin.

Pick your perfect weight. Foundations come in three weights, or amounts of coverage: sheer, medium, and full. Generally speaking, mature skin is most flattered by a sheer- or medium-weight foundation.

Foundations also come in two basic formulas: oil and water. Oil-based foundations are best for dry or mature skin. Avoid matte finish foundations, which can accentuate lines and wrinkles. Some of the new light-reflective foundations (without the sparkles) can diminish signs of aging.

Perform this foolproof color test. To many women, finding a foundation to match their skin color can be nearly impossible. To pick the right color, you must first find out whether your skin contains more red (ruddy) or more yellow (sallow).

To do this, hold a piece of very white paper against your skin, which will help you see those red or yellow tones. Yellow-based shades such as gold beige or honey beige are most flattering to ruddy skin, while rosier shades such as rose beige and ivory beige can perk up a sallow complexion.

Use the right tool. Apply an oil-based foundation with a wet cosmetic sponge. It goes on more thinly and evenly that way.

Just say no to stick concealer. When choosing a concealer, opt for one that comes in a pot or wand, rather than in a stick. They're sheerer and lighter than stick formulations, so they won't look thick or chalky. If the skin under your eyes is very dry, pat on a light eye cream before you apply concealer. It will make even a sheer concealer sheerer.

Blooming Blush and Powder

Restore the blush of youth to your cheeks and get rid of hot flash–induced shine with these tricks.

Go creamy. Cream or cream-powder blushers are most flattering to dry or mature skin. Powder formulations tend to accentuate lines and wrinkles.

Pick the perfect shade. Warm shades that contain more yellow than red are more forgiving of mature skin. Virtually any woman will look great in warm shades of peach and pink.

Opt for moisturizing powder. Whether you choose pressed powder or loose powder, choose a product formulated specifically for mature skin. They contain added moisturizers.

Lighten up. Select a powder three shades lighter than your foundation.

Apply powder the right way. Dust on loose powder with a big, fluffy makeup brush. To apply pressed powder, "tap" it into your foundation, using the puff that comes with the compact.

Luscious Lip Color

As we age, our lips tend to become paler. And worse, they also become thinner. To keep them from disappearing completely, we're often tempted to smear on the darkest lipsticks we can find. Don't go there! Rather than looking like an Elvira impersonator, you'll restore your lips' color and fullness with these proven tips.

Opt for cream. To keep your lips moist and supple, use cream lipsticks, which contain added moisturizers. As a bonus, cream formulations soften the appearance of mature skin and draw attention away from lines and wrinkles.

Try a tried-and-true hue. Regardless of your hair or skin color, all women can wear what is called a true red, which contains equal amounts of yellow and blue.

Nix dark sticks. Don't wear very dark lipsticks. Lips get thinner with age, and darker hues can make them look even thinner.

Keep your lips in place. If you have vertical lines on your upper lip, use an anti-feathering cream to help keep lipstick in place. Outlining the lips with a lipstick pencil as well will further help keep lipstick from feathering.

Enviable Eyes

Make your eyes look large and impressive with these simple techniques.

Opt for the essentials. You don't have to use eye makeup like Tammy Faye Bakker. A soft smudge of liner around your upper lids and a coat or two of mascara is all you need to make your eyes look bigger and brighter.

Choose powder power. Opt for a powder eyeliner pencil. They make the eyes look smoky and soft, and they're easy to apply. Extra-hard wax-based eye pencils tend to drag across delicate skin.

Give your brows the brush. To give yourself an instant eyelift, brush brows down, using a toothbrush or lash comb. Fill in with a soft pencil. Spray a toothbrush with hair spray and brush brows back up and into place.

Choose a fiber-free mascara. Most brands are fiber-free, but the ones that aren't will be labeled "with fibers." Mascaras that contain fibers tend to clump, cake, and look goopy, which draws attention to aging eyes.

Fatten up your lashes. To make your lashes extra-thick, hold a metal eyelash curler under your blow-dryer for 5 to 10 seconds. The heat will help your lashes hold their curl. (Test the metal against your hand before touching it to your eye area.)

Get-Glowing Rule #5:
Reclaim Your Youthful Mane

Fluctuating hormones can affect hair as well as skin. So if your hair seems drier than it used to, and the grays are coming in thick and fast, don't despair. A new style and, possibly, color can make your locks look more youthful.

While we don't recommend selecting a new coiffure from an MTV video, most newer hairstyles can be adjusted to suit your own style and personality. As you seat yourself in the stylist's chair, keep these guidelines in mind.

HAIR LOSS: HOPE—AND HELP

Not all women experience hair loss, or alopecia, at menopause. But it can be devastating for those who do. Again, the culprit is estrogen or, more specifically, the lack thereof.

Estrogen lengthens the life cycle of each hair so that it stays on the head longer, which results in thicker hair. (This is why you may have marveled at your lush locks during pregnancy, then mourned their passing several weeks after your children were born.) What is called estrogen deficiency alopecia generally starts some months before or just after menopause. Because estrogen levels start to fall before periods stop, this form of hair loss can be the first sign of approaching menopause.

"Women definitely disguise hair loss better than men," says Marty Sawaya, M.D., Ph.D., a dermatologist in Ocala, Florida, who specializes in hair loss. Yet the quest can be a tough one, given the number of factors besides falling estrogen levels that can cause temporary and long-term hair loss, including hereditary hormonal imbalances, stress, oral contraceptives, and other medications.

So what can you do, besides shopping for a wig? It depends.

If you've just gone through a divorce, a move, or some other major stress, relax. All of these factors can cause your roots to close down and rest for 3 months. But after that, your hair should return to normal without help.

If your hair is coming out in patches but you haven't experienced any of those life stresses, think about other changes. Have you started taking a new medication or changed your eating habits? Antithyroid drugs, anticonvulsants, diuretics, and even ibuprofen can trigger hair loss in some people, and chemotherapy causes temporary hair loss in many women. (It will grow back within 1 to 3 months after your last treatment.)

If you have no idea why you're losing your hair, promptly consult a dermatologist who deals with hair problems. "It's better to arrest the process as soon

A Cut Above

Just because you've worn the same haircut for the past 20 years doesn't mean you're condemned to wear it forever. Or, if you find that you've succumbed to a more "mature" style because you thought it was the right thing to do but now feel dowdy, be bold and make a change. Choose a new style that looks right to you, and go for it! Your hair will always grow out.

as possible, instead of waiting for years, because it becomes more difficult to treat over time," says Dr. Sawaya.

Meanwhile, take these steps to conserve what you've got.

- If you use birth control pills, ask your doctor to prescribe only those that contain desogestrel or norgestimate, and avoid those that contain norgestrel or norethindrone, which promote hair loss, says Dr. Sawaya.
- Abstain from perming, straightening, or coloring your hair until it is back to normal. Chemical treatments can inflame and irritate your scalp.
- Give your hair a rest from tight braids and rollers, which can break the hair.
- Apply minoxidil, an over-the-counter hair-restoring treatment, to your scalp twice a day. It has been proven effective especially for the 25 to 30 percent of women who lose their hair due to hereditary factors.
- Have patience. "Nothing restores hair loss in 6 weeks. It usually takes 6 months for the process to turn around," says Dr. Sawaya.
- If you have no intention (or possibility) of becoming pregnant, ask your doctor if you would benefit from Propecia, a prescription drug that restores hair in men but is marketed only to men because it can cause birth defects. Some doctors prescribe it to women who are not trying to become pregnant. Some doctors also prescribe the diuretic spironolactone, which has anti-androgenetic properties.
- Beware of miracle hair restorers. People often spend a lot of money on over-the-counter products advertised to help with hair loss. Says Dr. Sawaya, "Spend your money only on approved products that have been tested and that we know will work."

For more options on handling hair loss, see page 265.

Go on a "style safari." Collect several photos of models with hair-styles that you like. Don't worry that the styles won't look good on you. Pictures can give stylists a better idea of what you're looking for. Without specific examples, they may not understand what you mean by an updated or youthful new hairstyle.

Talk about it first. If you already have a stylist that you like, call a couple of days before your next appointment and tell him or her that you want to try something new. And don't get shampooed immediately upon walking into the salon. Talk over what you want while your hair is dry so that your stylist can see your hair in its natural state.

Keep an open mind. Get a good idea of what you want, but keep in mind your stylist's advice on what might work well for you. Discussing your lifestyle with her can help. For example, how much time are you willing to devote to styling in the morning? Are you all thumbs with styling tools, or a pro?

Don't make a snap judgment. Once you have your new style, give it some time before you make your final decision: It takes a while to get used to something new. But if after a few days you're still not sure, go right back to your stylist to get help on how to make the style work better for you.

Soften flaws with the right style. If your jawline is softened by a double chin, consider a bob that's slightly raised in the back. Or to give the illusion of a narrower jaw, put more weight near your temples.

Choosing a Color

Color can take years from your face—or, if you go too dark, *add* years, even if your hair was raven black as a young woman. Keep these tips in mind when choosing a color.

Sneak up on gray. When those first gray strands appear, try using a process that covers gray—like a semi- or demi-permanent color—rather than one that removes pigment from the hair. While it won't pro-vide total coverage, it will camouflage the gray so it blends into your natural color.

Go warmer and lighter. If you are coloring all your hair, be aware of which colors and shades work best with your coloring. As you age, your skin lightens, so you might not be able to carry off the strong blue-black of your youth. Also keep in mind that warm hair colors are usually more flattering. The tones reflect on the face to give it a glow, rather than wash out the complexion as cool colors tend to do. If you have white or gray hair, consider highlighting with lighter shades of blond, platinum, or steel to give you a more vibrant look.

Adding Texture

Combat thinning hair—another consequence of menopause's estrogen drain—with these effective techniques.

Oil up. To infuse dry hair with much-needed moisture, apply a *moderate* amount of olive oil to towel-dried or slightly damp hair. Work it through your hair, paying special attention to the ends. Style as usual. If you find that your hair has become too greasy, wash the oil out with your regular shampoo. Your hair will still feel significantly softer.

Try a secret from the East. *Wear* your yogurt, as the Indian and Pakistani owners of unbelievably long, thick tresses do. Work plain yogurt into your hair, cover it with a towel, and let it work for ½ hour. Then shampoo as usual. Yogurt is a rich natural conditioner for hair.

Feast on fish . . . "Eat fish at least twice a week," suggests Earl Mindell, R.Ph., Ph.D., author of many books, including *Dr. Earl Mindell's Natural Remedies for 101 Ailments* and *Earl Mindell's New Herb Bible*. The oil in salmon, herring, and other cold-water fish is rich in omega-3 fatty acids, which help replenish lost moisture in dry skin and hair, according to Dr. Mindell.

. . . And on flax. Eating up to 2 tablespoons of flaxseed oil a day can also help replenish hair and skin oils, says Julian Whitaker, M.D., founder and director of the Whitaker Wellness Institute in Newport Beach, California, and author more than 20 books, including *Dr. Whitaker's Guide to Natural Healing*. It has a nutty-buttery taste, so you can use it as a topping on popcorn, potatoes, or other foods you might otherwise flavor with butter, he says. Flaxseed oil is available in most health food stores.

Get-Glowing Rule #6:
Nurture Your Hands and Nails

At any age, having soft, smooth hands and well-groomed nails can add to your allure. But as we grow older, achieving them may take a bit more work.

During this time, our fingernails (and toenails!) grow more slowly. They may also become dull and brittle, take on a yellowish cast, or split and break more easily. Also, the soft, thin skin on the backs of the hands is prone to roughness and wrinkles.

Prolonged, repeated contact with water is one of the leading con-

10 STEPS TO MORE BEAUTIFUL NAILS

You don't need to spend a bundle at a nail salon. Keep your hands looking great with this guide to at-home manicures.

1. If you polish your nails, remove the old polish with a nonacetone remover, which is less drying to nails.
2. File nails to desired shape. What looks modern now is a shortish nail, straight across the top, with rounded edges. File your nails in one direction, starting at the edges and moving toward the top.
3. Soak your nails in soapy water for a few minutes to soften cuticles.
4. Dot a cuticle cream on the cuticles and rub it in.
5. Use an orangewood stick (available in drugstores) to push back cuticles. Be sure not to cut your cuticles, which can cause infection and damage the nail.
6. Massage hands with a hand lotion for extra moisture.
7. Wipe nails with a damp cloth to remove excess oils.
8. Apply a base coat. Let dry for 1 minute.
9. Apply two coats of your favorite color. Always apply polish by starting on the side of the nail. You should be able to cover the nail in three stokes, one on each side and one in the middle.
10. Apply a top coat. Don't use a fast-dry top coat; your polish will not last as long.

tributors to split, brittle or peeling nails, says Amy Newberger, M.D., an associate in clinical dermatology at Columbia University College of Physicians and Surgeons in New York City and author of *Looking Good at Any Age*. What's more, the problem gets worse with age as nail thickness diminishes and nail growth slows.

Here's what happens. Nails expand when they absorb water and contract when it evaporates. As water moves in and out of the nail, the weak areas, especially at the nail tips, become weaker and tend to separate, peel, and crack. The effect is similar to what happens when you get split ends in your hair.

Fortunately, your hands and nails will respond to TLC. Here are some ways to make them softer, smoother, and more youthful.

Wear gloves indoors and out. Use latex or rubber gloves for doing dishes, cleaning, or other wet work, especially if you're working with harsh solvents or detergents. If your hands *must* be in and out of water frequently, apply a silicone or a similarly based protectant film that sheds water over the hands and nails, such as Prevex, Atrixo, or Barriere Cream.

Wear sunscreen "gloves," too. Slather your hands with SPF 15 before you leave the house each day. It can help prevent age spots and a leathery texture.

Replenish lost oils. Keep a bottle of moisturizer by each sink in the house. Smooth some on after your hands hit the water. Take the time to massage the lotion into your nails and cuticles as well.

Give your hands an oil treatment. For an extra-special treat, fill a teacup with warm olive oil, dip your fingers in, and let them soak for a minute or two. Remove your fingers, then rub the oil into the skin of your hands. Allow as much of it as possible to be absorbed before rinsing away the excess.

Wear polish. There's virtually nothing more indulgent than treating yourself to a manicure. What's more, nail polish acts as a barrier against water diffusion. Choose polishes with lacquers that contain polyester resins, which won't dry out nails. And use acetone-free remover—it's not as harsh or drying as acetone.

Hydrate thirsty nails. To give nails added moisture, soak them for 10 minutes twice daily in warm water, pat dry, and immediately apply one of the chemically enhanced moisturizers that contain urea, lactic acid, or glycerin oil.

Whiten with citrus. If your nails take on a yellowish cast, massage them with a drop (just a drop!) of lemon oil twice a week. Don't overdo it—you may dry the nail and surrounding skin.

File correctly. When you drag an emery board back and forth along your nails, it frays and weakens them, causing splitting. After filing, use a buffer to gently smooth the edge of the nail, in one direction only.

Try biotin. Two milligrams a day have been shown to improve nail thickness by as much as 25 percent.

Get-Glowing Rule #7: Revamp Your Style

If you think the secret to looking good in the menopausal years is to dress your age, think again. The key is dressing for your *shape*.

Even if you're wearing the same size you did 10 years ago, you may notice that your clothes have become too tight in some places and too loose in others. From the mid-forties on, women's tummy measurements can begin to exceed the circumference of their hips.

The best way to determine what works for you is to experiment. In our teens, many of us spent hours trying on clothes. Now it's time to rediscover that fun. Don't get preconceived ideas of what looks good on you and what doesn't. Try on different styles constantly, just like you did when you were younger.

These tips can help make sure you're dressed to show off your assets, and camouflage your figure flaws. You'll feel more confident and more attractive, and the compliments will start pouring in!

Before You Buy

Have a little fun—and get caught up on the latest trends—*before* you put your money down. Here's how.

5 WAYS TO UPDATE YOUR LOOK— AND KEEP IT THAT WAY

What you wear says a lot about who—and how old—you are. Here are five ways to keep yourself in style while staying comfortable with yourself.

1. At least twice a year, leaf through women's fashion magazines, such as *Elle*, *Vogue*, and *Harper's Bazaar*.
2. Go to different stores and try on new labels, even if the style is similar to something you already own. You might be surprised at what you're missing if you rely only on certain merchants and brands.
3. Color up your wardrobe. With every fashion season comes a trendy color palette. Use it to add inexpensive punch to your wardrobe—a bright scarf, a camisole under a suit. Staying in style colorwise will also make you look younger.
4. From a new bag to a pair of sexy sandals, accessories are the easiest ways to update a look. If you're not sure what's modern, ask a sales associate for her suggestions. She'll know what others are asking for.
5. Don't try to radically change your look. Make subtle changes over a period of time.

Leaf through fashion magazines. What are the models wearing? Notice the details, like color and cut. What do you like—and dislike—about the current trends? Chances are, the youthful trends you see in the magazines will be reinterpreted for the more mature woman.

Go on a fashion safari—solo. Give yourself a Saturday or Sunday to browse through clothing stores. Don't plan to spend—just try things on. Go alone so that you won't be influenced by your friend's or sister's opinion.

Look for mature styles that interpret junior trends. For example, a few years ago, the younger crowd was wearing fitted, waist-length leather jackets. Designer Dana Buchman offered her customers leather jackets that looked fitted but weren't quite so tight. They also had lower hemlines.

Four Fashion Basics

You'll look and feel better (and younger!) if you make these four fashion changes.

Buy the best clothing you can afford. Generally, clothing that's more expensive is designed to fit the body better.

Update your jeans. We're not saying you should wear hip huggers, but do give a nod to current trends—it shows you're up-to-date. As you look for jeans that fit comfortably, try to look for some fun extras, like cargo pockets. Or try low-rise or boot-cut jeans.

Toss the Church Lady purse. Don't kill a youthful-looking outfit with a matronly handbag. Look for a bag that's a departure for you—a livelier color, perhaps, or a different shape. Just be sure to choose a bag that's a good proportion for your size. Shoulder bags that fit under the armpit (not too tiny or huge) are generally the most flattering.

Express your sensual side. We might not be able to dress like J.Lo or Britney Spears, but we can indulge in luxurious fabrics like silk, leather, cashmere, and fur.

Fabulous Fit

If clothes fit well, they'll look good. And if they don't—even if they're perfect for you—they won't. Read on to avoid these common fit mistakes.

Don't buy a size too small. Squeezing into a size that's too small for you will not make *you* look smaller. Looser clothes will do a better job at hiding those extra pounds. You should be able to insert two fingers into a waistband. And if you can't pinch out 2 inches of fabric from a pair of pants or a skirt, it's too small.

Avoid "tucking in." It emphasizes a thick waist or tummy bulge. Instead, consider an overshirt with narrow pants or a T-shirt dress in a fabric that has drape without cling. For added camouflage, slip on a jacket with set-in sleeves (the top of the seam that joins the sleeve to the jacket is positioned at the upper arm/shoulder hinge).

Splurge on bras that really *fit*. A sagging bustline can add years to your figure, so opt for bras built-in support, such as underwires, nonstretch straps, and pushup pads. You should be able to slip a finger inside the elastic band. If you have a bulge at each side of the bra band between the underarm and top of the shoulder, you need a larger cup.

Camouflaging Figure Flaws

To hide a few extra pounds, try these easy tricks.

Slim down in the dark. Choose darker colors as the basis of your wardrobe—navy, black, charcoal gray.

Slip on a bodyshaper. Undergarment foundations, from all-in-one shapers to control-top panty hose, really can make a difference.

Pair your pants with heels. They'll give your legs added length and sleekness. Heels of 2½ to 3 inches will work beautifully.

Dress in one color. Choose longer jackets to hide larger bottoms; add a sexier cami or blouse to soften the look and draw attention to the face.

Play up your best features. For example, show off shapely legs with a knee-length skirt, or a long, graceful neck with scoop-neck shirts.

We hope you've had fun reading all the makeover options in this chapter. Choose the ones that appeal to you, and start brushing up your look—and brushing off the years. In the next two chapters, we'll look at the mental side of menopause—how to cope with stress and manage your moods. Please join us!

Chapter

7

GETTING RID
OF STRESS

STRESSED-OUT. FOR MANY OF US, THOSE TWO WORDS DESCRIBE
our state of being. The pace of our society—running, running, running,
from morning till night; always doing something (or 20 things); never
feeling really caught up with anything—is stress inducing. Add menopause, with its discomforts, anxieties, and mood swings, and you have
stress upon stress. Now you not only have a ton to handle at work, the
house to clean, the kids to take care of, shopping to do, and outings to organize, but you're wondering if you're looking old, you're so cranky that
your spouse claims he doesn't know you, you can't sleep, you're gaining
weight . . . good grief!

These problems are bad enough. But stress makes them worse because
stress is bad for your body. When you're stressed-out, it takes longer to
spring back from an illness, injury, or personal problem. And stress triggers hormonal reactions (as if you weren't already having enough problems with those!) that can cause serious health problems. We'll discuss in
detail how stress affects your health in "How Stress Can Hurt Your
Health" on page 178.

But first, since just reading this is probably raising your stress levels,
we'll give you some proven ways to bring it under control. Armed with

them, you can begin right away to bring yourself—body, mind, and soul—back into balance. You'll start to feel your stress and tension drain away, you'll be energized and engaged, your self-esteem will soar, and—surprise!—you'll discover that you feel really good about yourself, perhaps for the first time in years. So set your stress aside, read on, and do something good for yourself today.

DOWNSIZE YOUR STRESS, UPSIZE YOUR LIFE

Don't let stress get the better of you! Our lives are set up in ways that make stress hard to avoid, even without menopause's adding to the strain. No matter what, the mortgage will come due each month, the kids will have to get into college (and that college will have to be paid for somehow), the job requirements will change with each new boss and each corporate merger. You may be facing a divorce, the serious illness or death of a spouse, or older parents requiring special care. Your grown kids may be moving back into the house—and bringing their own kids with them. Life isn't easy, and the lack of supportive communities makes it still harder. But there are ways you can form your own communities, reconnect to others, and do other important things that have been proven to reduce stress. Here are some of the best.

Look Out for Number One

You may be world's most generous caregiver, but finding ways to indulge yourself is not only well-deserved but also imperative for your well-being. Mood swings, crying spells, and irritability shouldn't all be chalked up to hormones. Have you stopped to consider your lifestyle? Women of menopausal age have sometimes been called the sandwich generation, caught between the demands of raising their own children and the responsibility of caring for aging or ill parents. Being tugged in so many directions (children, husband, parents, housework, job) often leaves little or no time for the self.

Taking care of yourself will help you replenish your energy and your soul. Without that refueling, you can become depleted emotionally and won't be able to take care of anyone, including yourself.

Schedule time for nurturing opportunities like these.

- If you are always everyone else's sympathetic ear, it's time to be your own, too. Buy a cassette recorder and some audiotapes. Talk into it about the anxiety or confusion you may feel. It helps to get worry, anxiety, or frustration out of your head and your body.

- Start a weekly bath ritual. Light some candles or incense and play your favorite relaxing music. Savor a glass of wine or mug of herbal tea while you bask. Afterward, send love and appreciation to each part of your body as you rub it with lotion. This is a little thing, but it can make a marvelous difference in your life.

- Whether it's an attic guest room, the bedroom of a child who has moved out of the house, or a tree house, claim your own sacred space in the world. Make it beautiful. Hang pictures and paint the walls with colors that inspire you. Bring in plants or flowers. Buy art supplies to play with and a radio or CD player. Into this space, let out the meditation maven, poet, sculptress, storyteller, or spoon player who has always lived latently within you. If you don't have space in your house to devote an entire room to yourself, carve out a corner somewhere, but make sure it's entirely your own.

- Take yourself on a date to a museum, a movie, a garden, the library. Do all the things for yourself that really make you feel loved and content, like buying yourself flowers, picking up roasted chestnuts from a street vendor along the way, or pausing to watch geese pass overhead.

- Play hooky from work once every few months if you have a really stressful job.

- Treat yourself to a country bed-and-breakfast or retreat center for the weekend.

- Learn to say no if you really don't feel like doing something for someone else that day.

Write Off the Stress of Self-Criticism

Stress isn't just a product of what's happening around you. Many times, you're swirling in negativity because of your deepest thoughts and opinions about your life, the choices you've made, and what your future holds both personally and professionally. The best way to challenge self-defeating thoughts is to try writing down the logic—or lack of it—behind them.

In order to erase negative attitudes, you must uncover their messages, which may sound and seem true—until you really put them to the test of reason.

Here is a sampling of the negative thoughts that menopausal women frequently express.

- "I'll never feel attractive again."
- "My husband (or partner) does not want me anymore."
- "In terms of my career, it's downhill from here."
- "It's too late for me to realize my creative self."
- "My sex drive has declined, and it will only decline further."
- "My children don't need me anymore."
- "I've gained weight, and I can't get it off."
- "I'm useless to my family and society."

Once you've determined what thoughts are bothering you, subject each of your negative thoughts to our four-part logic test, below. You will be surprised at how responding to these four questions can help you quickly overcome negative thoughts.

1. Where did I learn this thought?
2. Is this thought logical?
3. Is this thought true and fair?
4. How does this thought contribute to my stress?

Start by writing down the four responses to all the negative thoughts that you feel relate to you. If you feel it benefits you, make this an ongoing process by keeping a "diary of distortions," in which you write down your automatic negative thoughts every day, always putting them to the logic test.

Just writing down negative thoughts has therapeutic value. It's a relief when you can say to yourself, "There it is, the cause of so much suffering." Better yet, once you are liberated from your distortions, your mind is free to restructure unjustified self-criticism into well-deserved self-respect.

Stand Up for Yourself During Menopause

Feeling better during menopause may be as simple as standing up. Believe it or not, self-confidence is a by-product of good posture. That's because by standing correctly, you increase your body's supply of oxygen and improve your blood circulation, which can bring a heightened sense of well-being. You may also become more mentally focused and emotionally grounded when you stand tall and sure.

On the other hand, poor posture may compress your internal organs, impeding circulation and digestion. If you're feeling lethargic or insecure, slumping in your chair or on your feet will only enhance the effect.

Using yoga to improve posture may bring multiple mind–body benefits to menopausal women. Try this simple yoga exercise, the mountain pose (also known as Tadasana), and you can feel for yourself what a difference it makes to stand upright.

Here's how to practice the mountain pose.

- Stand with your feet turned slightly inward, the joints of your big toes about 1 inch apart and your heels slightly farther apart (about 2 inches). Allow your arms to hang naturally at your sides.

- Bring your chin back a bit, lift the crown of your head, and lengthen the back of your neck so that, from the side, your ears are in alignment with your shoulders. Your forehead will be parallel with the wall in front of you.

- Allow your face to soften and relax.

- Broaden your chest from the center, almost as if it were "blooming" like a flower. Don't stick your ribs out. The bottom ribs move down slightly toward your hipbones.

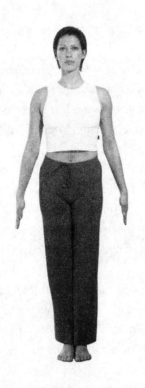

The mountain pose is a great exercise to do while waiting in line or when you need a few minutes to de-stress. It may seem like a lot to remember at first, but keep practicing and it will become second nature.

- Place your pelvis in a neutral position. To find this position, imagine that you have a long tail, and place the tail on the floor between your heels. This will align the pelvis nicely.

- Spread your toes and stand firmly on your feet. Keep your legs straight without gripping your thighs, and move your thighbones back slightly.

- Breathe normally. Close your eyes for a few moments and pause. Become still. Then open your eyes slowly.

(See the Alexander Technique on page 353 and yoga on page 363.)

Give of Yourself and Get Rid of Stress

You may find that entering a new phase in your life brings with it a readiness to share time, talent, and wisdom. It may surprise you to learn that while volunteering is noble and worthwhile, it can also be one of life's most richly indulgent activities, especially for a menopausal woman whose life is changing rapidly.

Sure, your motivation may be respect for humanity, but the bonus is that in the end, volunteering truly heightens your own sense of self-worth. Get involved in making a difference in someone's life. In the process, you will discover your talents and abilities, and develop interests and skills you might never have had a chance to explore. It is also a great way to meet new people that share similar interests.

In a study called the Women's Roles and Well-Being Project, researchers observed the lifestyles of 427 wives and mothers from upstate New York for 30 years. An exciting outcome: Women who belonged to volunteer organizations had significantly lower rates of illness, better mental health, and greater longevity.

What could be a better way to use retirement leisure time or make one of your free weeknights meaningful? There are many volunteer opportunities everywhere you go. Animal shelters, women's clinics, museums, children's sporting events, and environmental groups are just a few places to consider. Or you can volunteer to help senior citizens or to read to children.

You can also go on a "volunteer vacation," where volunteers participate in community projects for local people. Projects through the Global Citizens Network can be anything from painting, decorating, or construction to helping out at village clinics and schools in places such as Nepal, Guatemala, or Native American reservations.

If you're not ready for a global adventure, you can start spreading happiness right at home. Look in your local paper for a weekly listing of needs in the community. Or contact the Volunteers of America (VOA) for information on local, national, and international opportunities. Call VOA toll-free at (800) 899-0089, or log on to www.voa.org, www.consciouschoice.com, or www.volunteermatch.org. For volunteer vacations, contact www.globalcitizens.org, or call the Global Citizens Network toll-free at (800) 644-9292.

Pray for Peace (or Health, or Happiness)

Menopause might be prime time to come into or discover a mature spirituality. More than 250 studies published in the medical literature show statistical relationships between spiritual practices and health benefits—mental health included. For many menopausal women, prayer offers a dimension of inner peace that cannot be achieved in any other way.

Prayer, of course, comes in many forms. Practice prayer in any way that is comfortable and meaningful for you, given your religious history and proclivities. The bottom line is to do some seeking. Make a commitment to finding your own spiritual perspective and a form of prayer that acknowledges and honors your most personal beliefs.

Science has discovered that we don't need a formal or complex prayer to reap health benefits. Studies have shown that simply repeating a sacred or meaningful word or phrase produces a relaxation response. Here are some common focus words or phrases you can use to begin your practice.

Christian

Come, Lord
Lord, have mercy
Our Father, who art in Heaven
Hail Mary, full of grace
The Lord is my shepherd

Jewish

Sh'ma ("Hear, O Israel")
Echod ("One")
Shalom ("Peace")
Hashem ("The Name")
Shekhinah ("The Feminine Face of God")

Eastern

Om (the universal sound)
Shanti ("Peace")

Aramaic

Maranatha ("Come, Lord")
Abba ("Father")

Islamic

Allah

Empowering Yourself and Others

The many changes that take place during menopause may make you feel as if no one else understands what you're going through emotionally or physically. But others out there are experiencing exactly what you're experiencing, and now may be the time to reach out for support and friendship.

Can't find a local support group? Take the initiative to start your own. You will benefit in countless ways. Leading a group can be a real inspiration as it will remind you of your connection with all women. You may uncover leadership abilities that will help you and your group to discover who you really are: beautiful, wise, wonderful, powerful women.

Try these suggestions if you're interested in starting a support group.

- Create an environment that's safe for deep sharing. Ways to do this include asking everyone to make a commitment to confidentiality and making it clear that the group is a place to let down the masks we often wear. No one is expected to have a perfect life.

- Establish guidelines at the first meeting, such as make a commitment to attend all sessions; be respectful of the time and the need to give others a chance to share; do not cross-talk while someone is speaking; focus sharing on the issue, not the whole "story"; try to use responsible language such as using "I" statements like "I feel . . . " rather than "They made me. . . . "

- If the group is large, you can have people form smaller groups of five or six.

- Cultivate a nonjudgmental, accepting attitude. Do not tell anyone what she "should" do. Offer suggestions for ways that she could change her thoughts and perspectives. If people sense judgment, they will immediately go into resistance mode.

- Each group is different, and each session will be different. Learn to flow with the energy of the current group and session.

- If someone is trying to dominate the group, tell her in private that you appreciate all that she shares with the group, but your concern is that others who are not as assertive might feel inhibited. Finding some task that this woman could assist you with may also be helpful.

- Don't argue with someone who seems to want to stay stuck. Try not to allow yourself to get depressed by someone else's drama. As a group leader, you must learn to hold on to that sense of knowing that healing is available to all, whether or not they claim it.

- Develop a sense of humor. Laughter is a marvelous way of gaining a different perspective.

- After each group session, go to the mirror and tell yourself how well you're doing, especially if you are new to leading groups.

- Begin and end each session with a meditation or centering process. It can be as simple as having everyone close her eyes or hold hands and breathe for a moment or two.

Find Yourself in Women's Literature

Take yourself to the place where can you *Walk the Long Quiet Highway* in the light of your full creativity, learn to demand *A Room of Your Own* from the world, and release your spirit to *Run with the Wolves*. Sound esoteric? It's not. It's women's lit.

Share in the vicissitudes and grand transformations of sisters all over the planet through multiethnic short-story anthologies. Invoke your inherent creative force through Alice Notley's poetry, experience a midlife erotic awakening along with novelist Edith Wharton, or reinvent a more empowering use of language for yourself through Mary Daly's feminist writings. Or just have fun and get some attitude with *The Sweet Potato Queens' Book of Love* or *Maxine: Yelling It Like It Is*.

Women's literature brings you into an infinite family of heroines and may give you the first opportunity in your life to deeply discuss certain dimensions of womanhood. The students of Heather Thomas, Ph.D., professor of writing at Kutztown University in Kutztown, Pennsylvania, have commented that reading women's literature has given them a powerful boost to their self-esteem as well as a newfound sense of groundedness.

Consider signing up for a course in women's literature. If getting homework and being graded are too much pressure, ask to audit the class. (Auditing is participating without being graded.) Or, for a less formal sharing of women's words, consider starting a women's reading circle. Invite your female friends, relatives, and colleagues, or post an invitation at local libraries, grocery stores, coffee shops, and bookstores.

HOW STRESS CAN HURT YOUR HEALTH

We all know that stress is bad for our nerves, our mental clarity, our attitude, and our relationships. But did you know that it is literally bad for your health? You might picture a stressed-out guy at the end of his rope, heading for a heart attack or a stroke. But stress affects women's health on a lot of levels, starting with our hormones and our reproductive systems. Stress can also make us gain weight (and not just because we're eating comfort foods to cope!), predisposing us to diseases like diabetes and heart disease; depress our immune systems, making us prey to everything from allergic outbreaks to colds and flu and lengthening our recovery time from illness and surgery; and worsen cancer, if we've developed the disease.

Let's take these stress-related health problems one by one and see how stress plays a role and what we can do about it.

Stress, Hormones, and a Whole Lot More

Menopause is already wreaking havoc—or about to wreak havoc—on our hormones. What does stress have to do with hormones, and why does it matter? Well, it matters because hormones aren't just about sex. (Not that sex isn't important!) The reality is that nearly every system in our bodies is controlled by hormones. From estrogen to insulin, serotonin to cortisol, these critical chemical messengers determine the state of our physical and emotional health. When things are calm, they work like the proverbial well-oiled machine. But throw chronic stress into the mix, and it's like tossing a pile of rocks into that machine.

Hormones may also partly account for the fact that stress seems to be a greater problem for women than for men. Not only do we report higher

HORMONES AND HOMEOSTASIS

Hormones are highly specific agents released when a gland receives a signal from another part of the body that a hormone is required. For example, stress hormones are released when the nervous system detects a potential threat—anything from a charging tiger to a nasty coworker.

These hormones can then trigger—or interfere with—the release of other hormones from other parts of the body. For example, the stress hormones, which include adrenaline and cortisol, can affect the amount of sex hormones, such as estrogen and progesterone, we produce, creating problems in the reproductive system.

When your body is functioning normally, it's in a state of homeostasis, or balance, and all systems work to maintain this balance. Chronic stress destroys homeostasis by keeping levels of stress hormones high—which in turn creates imbalances in other hormone levels. For instance, stress affects insulin and thus blood sugar. Additionally, stress—or more precisely stress hormones—can create problems in your bones, muscles, and connective tissue. In fact, chronic stress, which results in chronically elevated levels of stress hormones, has been linked to osteoporosis and serious loss of muscle, according to Pamela M. Peeke, M.D., assistant clinical professor of medicine at the University of Maryland School of Medicine in Baltimore, *Prevention* magazine advisor, and author of *Fight Fat after Forty*.

levels of stress and more depression and anxiety than men, but our nervous systems also tend to react more to stress than men's, possibly setting us up for greater health consequences. Experts are still researching all the reasons behind these gender differences.

Two areas that are particularly important to women—reproduction and metabolism—are regulated by hormones that are especially sensitive to stress.

Stress, Reproduction, and Menopause

While the effects of stress on estrogen and the other sex hormones aren't yet fully understood, researchers know that stress can have a debilitating effect on reproductive health. Stress can make it harder for women to conceive, by causing erratic menstruation or even stopping menstruation altogether. For example, the menstrual cycles of women who eat poor diets and are socially isolated—two forms of stress—are less regular.

One theory suggests that chronic stress reduces the amount of estrogen in your body. In addition to affecting the menstrual cycle, lower levels of estrogen may rob you of many of the hormone's protective effects on your bones, your heart, and even your emotional health.

While it's not known whether stress can accelerate the onset of menopause, researchers find that women who are experiencing stress report more frequent and more severe menopause symptoms, perhaps because of unusually low estrogen levels. In fact, long before the onset of "the change," stress in perimenopausal women has been shown to trigger the same dramatic estrogen drop associated with the elevated risk of heart disease that women face after menopause.

Stress and Immunity

The effects of stress on the immune system have probably been around as long as we have. The experts suspect that the immune system's natural tendency to take a hiatus during stressful periods may be left over from the days when stress was acute and external, such as when a hungry lion decided that you were dinner.

"It was adaptive to temporarily divert energy away from the immune system to the brain and muscles in order to respond to the stressful situation—when running from a lion, it's more essential to have energy than to fight off bacteria," says Christopher Coe, Ph.D., professor of psychology at the University of Wisconsin in Madison.

But today this system tends to backfire. Stressors don't go away as quickly as a sprinting lion, resulting in long-term suppression of the immune system, says Dr. Coe.

Stress sets off a chain reaction in the body. For instance, say you narrowly escape a car accident. When you see the car coming at you, the fight-or-flight response kicks in and your adrenal glands (located on top of your kidneys) release the stress hormone cortisol. Cortisol prepares your body to deal with the stress—immune cells prepare to fight, blood sugar

A CRASH COURSE ON THE IMMUNE SYSTEM

Immunity is a lifelong concern, and the stresses involved in the menopausal process can affect how well your immune system functions. Basically, the immune system works like this: The immune cells move from the lymph nodes, bone marrow, spleen, and thymus (a gland in the lower neck) through the body's lymphatic ducts and blood vessels to patrol nearly all the body's organs in search of enemy bacteria, viruses, parasites, or cancer cells. The immune cells can differentiate between your normal body's cells ("self") and enemy cells ("nonself"). Under normal circumstances, if they find an enemy (like bacteria), they attack it, and if they bump into one of your own cells (like a muscle cell), they move on.

There are several types of immune cells, all of which are white blood cells: phagocytes, B cells, T cells, and NK (natural killer) cells. The B cells make antibodies to fight infection, the T cells help to distinguish self from nonself cells, and the NK cells fight cancer cells. Phagocytes help destroy invader cells and assist in controlling inflammation.

But the immune system isn't flawless, and sometimes it misses invaders, which is why we get sick. Sometimes it mistakes the body's own cells for invaders and attacks them, which is why we get autoimmune diseases. Stress often acts as a catalyst in both these scenarios, lowering the number of B, T, or NK cells.

rushes to the muscles to give them energy, breathing and heart rates quicken, and blood pressure rises. Cortisol also then helps undo the stress-preparing actions after the car misses you by inches.

We have some cortisol in our bodies at all times, even when we're not stressed (levels are high in the morning, and they steadily decrease throughout the day). But when stressors don't decline after a few minutes, as is the case with chronic marital tension, the cortisol curve changes. The morning peak is absent or much lower, and overall levels are higher. Exposure to too much cortisol for too long suppresses the immune system. In HIV patients, for instance, it has been found that an increase in cortisol in the blood nearly doubles the risk that a patient will progress to full-blown AIDS.

How Stress Affects Immunity

Multiple factors determine our own stress–immunity reactions, including genetics and life changes like menopause, the number of stress triggers in our lives, and the ways we deal with illness. Here are other important stress–immunity factors.

The type of stress you have. Your boss comes in and fires you, then says, "April fool!" You laugh shakily, but the hairs on your arms are standing upright and your legs are wobbly. In a few minutes, however, you're fine. This is acute stress. But if you hate your job, and for the past year you've been coming home with a tension headache, that's chronic or prolonged stress, from which you might not recover so quickly. Prolonged stress decreases nearly all aspects of immune function.

The way you perceive stress. Losing a job may be a major stressor for one woman, while another views it as a relief and a chance to make a fresh start. The brain is in the driver's seat—it determines how much of a change there is in hormonal stress response, which in turn has a bearing on any changes in the immune system.

Your support system. If you have friends and family galore supporting you, the effects of your stress will be lowered; but if you have no one to call, stress's effects will be magnified. One study showed that compared with patients who had social support, lonely patients had higher cortisol levels and decreased numbers of certain white blood cells called natural killer cells.

How much control you have over the stress. Studies show that a single session of inescapable electric shock in rats made their tumors grow faster than rats exposed to a shock they could get away from. Although experimental evidence is rather scarce, it's commonly thought that a stressor you can't control, such as a relative with a terminal illness, has a much worse effect on your immune system than one you can control, such as a malfunctioning refrigerator.

Stress and Cancer

You don't *really* know stress until you've been told you have cancer, says Dorothy Leone-Glasser, R.N. And she should know. She's survived three different cancers—melanoma, vaginal, and cervical cancers.

DOES STRESS CAUSE CANCER?

Scientists know that stress triggers certain reactions in the nervous and endocrine systems that in turn affect immunity by altering the release of antibodies and natural killer cells. But there's no proof that stress weakens the immune system enough to let cancer grab a toehold.

In fact, some research disputes *any* link between personal stress and the development of cancer. For example:

- A study of 332 women at the Leeds General Infirmary in England found that women with breast cancer were no likelier to have experienced a major stressful life event than women diagnosed with a benign lump.
- A study of 8,000 healthy women followed for more than 15 years by the University of Peace at the United Nations found that stress factors alone had little effect on whether or not women developed cancer.

The bottom line: If you're blaming your workaholic schedule or bad marriage for your cancer, stop. The only definitive way stress can contribute to the onset of cancer is through lifestyle choices. Some people who experience a lot of stress start smoking or drinking, which leaves them more open to developing cancer. However, once you *have* cancer, stress can make things worse.

"Sure, life is stressful to begin with. But cancer goes beyond stress. It's something that permeates every aspect of your life," says Dorothy, a holistic health counselor in Atlanta and founder of the Coping Program, which integrates traditional and holistic concepts of wellness to help people deal with cancer or other serious illness.

Stress is as much a part of cancer as chemotherapy and radiation. There's even some suspicion that stress may have something to do with the formation of cancer, and numerous studies suggest that it affects the disease's progression.

Once You Have Cancer

When a doctor says you have cancer, all the uncertainty about stress and cancer dissolves like cotton candy in the rain. As much as the cancer itself, anxiety becomes a constant companion. One day you're fine; the next you're dealing with a life-threatening illness. It happens that suddenly for many people.

The stress and uncertainty of cancer are enough to stop even the most "together" people in their tracks. Stress can really limit your ability to listen, understand, and make decisions on a vast amount of new information that can affect her life.

Once you move beyond the initial shock, the reality of living with cancer hits—and the stress can be even more overpowering than that of the initial diagnosis. The questions come from all sides: What kind of treatment will I choose? Will it make me sick? Will I lose my hair? Who will take care of me? How do I tell people at work?

There's more to cancer-related stress than sleepless nights and constant worrying. While stress might not weaken your immune system to the point of causing cancer, once you're sick, the effects of stress on your immune system could make things worse. The hormone cortisol—which your body produces in response to stress—may stimulate tumor growth. In one study of patients operated on for breast and stomach cancers, those whose cortisol levels did not decrease within 2 weeks of surgery had shorter survival times than those whose levels did decline. Stress also elevates the hormone prolactin, known to help tumors grow.

It's thought that stress affects natural killer (NK) cells, which seek out and destroy cancer cells. In one study from Ohio State University, researchers found that women with breast cancer who reported high stress levels actually had fewer NK cells and didn't respond as well to gamma interferon—a compound the body produces to enhance killer cell activity.

And, of course, when you're stressed, you don't sleep well, you don't eat right, and you often don't do the very things you need to do to get better. The better care you take of yourself, both physically and emotionally, the stronger you will feel as you face the many challenges brought about by cancer and its treatment.

Coping with Cancer Stress

If there's any positive news, it's this: Studies show that controlling cancer-related stress not only is doable but also can improve your well-being and hasten your recovery. An Ohio State University study of 115 women with Stage II and Stage III breast cancers found that women who participated in a stress reduction program had significantly lower levels of the stress hormone cortisol and 25 percent higher levels of an antibody known to fight breast tumors.

Any stress-reducing exercise—such as deep breathing, reiki, and guided imagery—can help you deal with the cancer anxiety. But as science and the women who have fought these battles themselves can attest, there are some stress reduction techniques unique to cancer.

Get the Facts

As soon as patients connect to information, experts, and one another, develop a plan of action, and know what to expect, their stress is substantially reduced. One useful information tool is a Web site www.breastcancer.org, specifically created to help patients learn everything they can about the disease.

The Web is filled with information about cancer, but so are libraries, hospital reading rooms, and your own doctor's waiting room. The more you know, the more control over your disease and your life you'll feel you have.

Join a Support Group

For people with cancer, social support takes on a new level of importance. Three randomized trials have shown that people with breast cancer, melanoma, and lymphoma lived longer when they had high levels of social support.

Often that support comes from strangers as women with cancer join support groups of other women with cancer. These groups provide a safe place to talk about worries and fears, typically with a level of honesty that would be impossible to exhibit with well-meaning friends and family.

In a support group, just about everyone knows exactly what you're going through, says Dorothy Leone-Glasser. "These people understand how you feel from the moment you open your eyes in the morning till you close them at night." You can talk openly about throwing up after chemo, finding hunks of hair in your brush, and feeling so tired that the simple act of making your bed is enough to unhinge you.

Science bears out the benefits of support groups. In one study, conducted at Stanford University School of Medicine, women with metastatic breast cancer who were assigned to a support group where they were encouraged to express their feelings survived 18 months longer than those who weren't in any group.

There's another stress-relieving benefit to support groups: hope. "You'll meet other women who have not only survived but thrived," says Linda Burrowes, cofounder of Your Bosom Buddies, a support group in Miami. "You meet people who are longtime survivors. You need to know that there is life after cancer and that it can be a very fulfilling life."

Express Yourself

Are you ticked off that you got cancer? Good. Then let it be known. Scream, cry, yell, curse, vent. Expressing your true feelings is key to coping. In women with breast cancer there's evidence, for example, that those who express more "negative" emotions—even anger and uncooperativeness—actually live longer.

A study at the University of Kansas found that women with breast cancer who talked about their fears and emotions had more energy, less distress, and fewer cancer-related medical visits. It's thought that letting it all out discharges stress, anger, and other negative emotions and could positively influence both your hormones and your immune system.

The feelings have to come out. You need to work through them, and then the goal is to get to a place where you feel like you can move on. The last thing you want to do is shut down and cloak yourself in denial— what experts call "avoidance." A study at the University of Manitoba in Winnipeg found that women with breast cancer who faced their fears were significantly better adjusted than other women and took a more active role in their treatment decisions.

In addition to participating in a support group, you can write in a journal or just talk—to friends and family or to anyone who will listen.

Need someone to talk to but don't know where to turn? Call the Adelphi Breast Cancer Hotline at (800) 877-8077. Volunteers can put you in touch with resources in your area of the country.

And when you talk, talk honestly. Be blunt about what you want and need. Women think they can still do it all—even when they have cancer. They've also been taught to be polite, even if they're not getting what they need.

That all goes out the window when you have cancer. Be frank with yourself and others about your capabilities. If someone asks you to do a favor and you don't want to, say no. If you need someone to do an errand or paperwork while you recover, ask. And if an overbearing relative is hurting rather than helping, speak up—and then tell him exactly what would be helpful.

Use Your Illness to Grow

When Linda Burrowes was diagnosed with breast cancer in 1997, she didn't see it as a tragedy. In fact, she saw a need—and an opportunity.

Following reconstructive surgery after her mastectomy for breast cancer, she wanted to talk to other women who had undergone the procedure, and looked for a group that provided such support. She couldn't find any. So she started her own group, Your Bosom Buddies.

Even though she's been cancer-free since then, she still devotes most of her time to other women with breast cancer. "It is my way of coping. It's not that I am happy that I got breast cancer, but my life has been so enriched because of it. The people I have met will be my friends for the rest of my life," Linda says.

It's a theme you hear from many women with cancer: They wouldn't have chosen this road, but they have been enriched and changed by the experience.

Some experts believe that finding meaning in your cancer improves your psychological state, which enables you to handle the illness and its concurrent stress better. Often, a women who uses it as a catalyst for change finds she comes out of it a more enriched—and less stressed— person.

Many women find that their cancer awakens a need to help other people. They start to volunteer with various organizations or help other women with cancer. For others, it's a call to do what they've always wanted—travel, go back to school, begin to paint. Basically, they're nurturing themselves. And that has a positive impact on their emotional and physical well-being.

Stress and Your Weight

Stress affects how we metabolize fat, and research suggests that chronic stress causes us to develop dangerous levels of fat. And it's not just any fat that develops, but fat deep within the belly, which leads to central, or visceral, obesity. Unlike any other kind of fat, this fat is directly linked to heart disease, diabetes, and cancer. These particular fat cells are especially sensitive to stress hormones, meaning that the extra calories you consume when you're stressed go directly to these cells. And they can be lethal.

A woman doesn't have to be obese to have this kind of fat. Lots of times, a woman will be of average weight and just carry some extra pounds around the middle. And, as you read in chapter 3, this type of midsection weight gain is characteristic of menopause.

Stress, and the hormones it produces, also can inhibit our ability to process the foods we eat. Many of the stress-induced problems involving metabolism are created by the actions of stress hormones, both on their own and through their effects on the hormone insulin. Insulin helps move glucose, the body's primary source of fuel, and amino acids, required to build muscle and other tissues, into cells.

When we're stressed, the stress hormones cortisol and corticosterone increase glucose levels in the blood and liver. This occurs because the body is attempting to mobilize its resources, making available all the quick-burning fuel it can. But after a while, this exaggerated glucose synthesis can create real problems as the body continually produces more insulin to push the glucose into cells. Eventually, the cells may become resistant to insulin's shepherding actions, resulting in high levels of glucose in the blood and possibly leading to diabetes.

Additionally, physical stress, such as an infection, makes it more difficult for those who already have diabetes to manage their disease. This is true not only because of the effects stress hormones have on insulin but also because people who aren't stressed are generally better at maintaining the tight regimen of blood glucose monitoring and insulin injections required to control diabetes and prevent complications.

So when you're stressed and you find yourself reaching for the doughnuts, consider these points instead.

- When your stress hormones are high, you'll automatically crave carbohydrates and fat because those are the body's first choices to fuel its fight-or-flight response.

- Eating excessive carbohydrates and fat means you'll gain weight, with your stress hormones now ensuring that the extra calories go to the fat cells in your belly.

- Eating a lot of carbohydrates immediately elevates levels of insulin in your bloodstream—and insulin is among the most powerful appetite stimulants the body makes.

So when you're stressed, avoid cake and cookies, and opt for fresh fruit, whole grains, low-fat protein such as fish, chicken, or beans, and other healthy fare. It's the combination of high-quality protein and carbohydrate that cuts the cravings for sweets and fats.

Need more help fighting those stress-induced urges to pig out on fast food or reach for the Krispy Kremes? See "The 7 Commandments of Stress-Proof Eating" on page 190, and "Food and Your Mood" on page 210.

THE 7 COMMANDMENTS OF STRESS-PROOF EATING

Eating right when we're harried, under pressure, and generally stressed-out is particularly important because stress affects how we use what we eat. When you're stressed, your body absorbs fewer nutrients even as it excretes more, thus increasing your need for the vitamins and minerals found in nutrient-rich foods. It also ensures that we have the ammunition we need to fight their energy-draining effects. Not only can a well-balanced diet help during periods of stress, but how well we eat *before* a stressful occasion also plays a role in how we handle that event.

When you're frazzled, you might feel like you only have time to guzzle down a cup of coffee in the morning, while chocolate smothered in chocolate sounds like an appealing lunch. To avoid putting any more stress on you with complicated lists of nutritional guidelines, we've developed the following seven commandments.

Thou Shalt Forgo Coffee. Caffeine only aggravates stress. Just a cup or two of coffee, or any other caffeinated beverage, such as tea or cola, can escalate feelings of anxiety because caffeine directly affects the brain and central nervous system, producing changes in heart rate, respiration, and muscle coordination. That's why we get that jittery feeling when we drink too much caffeine. Coffee can also decrease absorption of certain minerals, like iron and stress-fighting magnesium.

Thou Shalt Not Skip Meals. When you miss meals, you deprive yourself of the essential building blocks you need to function at your best. Getting too little of just one nutrient amplifies the stress you feel by straining the processes in your body that depend on that nutrient. For example, if you deprive your body even slightly of iron, you may become irritable and tired because an iron deficiency decreases the amount of oxygen going to your tissues and brain.

Thou Shalt Eat Breakfast. It's arguably the most important meal. You've just awakened from a long period of fasting, starving your brain of the glucose it needs to function. Ergo, breakfast. It doesn't have to be complicated. A simple bowl of whole grain cereal topped with fresh fruit and skim milk is an energizing way to start the day.

Thou Shalt Strive for Balance. Research shows that when we eat meals with a high carbohydrate-to-protein ratio (lots of carbohydrates with a little protein), we increase the amount of tryptophan available to our brains. Tryptophan is an amino acid required to manufacture serotonin, a brain chemical that has a calming influence—a plus when we're under stress. Eating high-carbohydrate meals also helps keep levels of the stress hormone cortisol under control, while high-protein diets may increase cortisol levels, aggravating feelings of stress. Over the long term, elevated cortisol levels can reduce the brain's ability to use glucose, eventually affecting brain function. High cortisol levels can also lead to overeating because the hormone affects appetite control chemicals such as serotonin and dopamine.

Thou Shalt Choose the Right Carbohydrate. To get the right building blocks you need to function at peak levels, the focus should be on complex carbohydrates such as whole grains, fruits, and vegetables. Sugary simple carbohydrates, such as candy and sodas, provide little in the way of nutrients and are really just wasted calories. Also, as sugar intake rises, you enter dangerous territory because vitamin and mineral intake decreases, increasing your susceptibility to the negative effects of stress. Plus, diets high in sugar may increase the loss of calming minerals such as magnesium and chromium.

Thou Shalt Not Ignore Fats. All fat is not "bad" fat. In fact, our bodies actually require some fat in order to survive. But the type of fat you eat is important, especially when you're stressed. Saturated fats (found in red meat, full-fat dairy, and other animal products) and trans fatty acids (found in processed and fast foods, usually in the form of partially hydrogenated oils) can suppress your immune system and raise levels of stress hormones such as cortisol. So when you're stressed, focus on healthy fats, like the monounsaturated fats found in olive and canola oils and the omega-3 fatty acids found in cold-water fish such as salmon and mackerel. These fats won't aggravate the stress response, and the omega-3s may even boost your immunity, a plus during tense times. Still, that's not a license to overindulge. Fat should make up only 30 percent or less of your total calories.

Thou Shalt Get the Right Vitamins and Minerals. The top three stress fighters are vitamin C, the B-complex vitamins, and magnesium. Vitamin C, by boosting your immune system, helps you fight back when stress hits. The best sources of vitamin C are dark green vegetables (like spinach and broccoli), strawberries, and citrus fruits. The B-complex vitamins provide added energy to help fight battle fatigue. B-complex vitamins include thiamin, riboflavin, niacin, pantothenic acid, and vitamins B_6 and B_{12} and are found in a wide variety of foods, including poultry, whole grains, and some vegetables. We tend to lose magnesium when we're stressed, and foods high in magnesium, like nuts, beans, and whole grains, can help replace lost supplies.

Calming Cuisine: A Week of Relaxing Foods

Here's how the basic principles of antistress eating during menopause—a mini-meal plan that concentrates on high-carbohydrate, moderate-protein, and low-fat meals—translates into a week's worth of eating. This meal plan packs a powerful punch of just the right ratio of carbohydrates and protein, and emphasizes foods that are high in stress-fighting nutrients like vitamins B and C and magnesium. For an added nutrient boost, we've included many foods rich in omega-3 fatty acids.

Monday

Breakfast

1 cup low-fat or fat-free granola topped with ¾ cup mixed berries (blueberries, strawberries, and raspberries)

¾ cup low-fat or fat-free plain yogurt

1 ounce chopped walnuts

Snack

6 ounces vegetable or carrot juice

Lunch

1 serving Tranquil Tuna Slaw with Creamy Lemon-Dill Dressing (see the accompanying recipe on the opposite page)

1 piece whole wheat bread drizzled with 1 teaspoon olive oil

Snack

1 apple

1 ounce reduced-fat cheese

2 rye crispbread crackers

Dinner

2 cups whole wheat pasta with 2 tablespoons Placid Pesto (see the accompanying recipe on the opposite page)

2 cups mixed salad greens with 1 tablespoon fat-free dressing

Snack

2 fig bars

8 ounces fat-free milk (or 1% milk or calcium-fortified soymilk)

NUTRITION TOTALS: **1,767** CALORIES, **83** G PROTEIN, **284** G CARBOHYDRATES, **42** G FAT, **52** MG CHOLESTEROL, **35** G DIETARY FIBER, **2,098** MG SODIUM

Tranquil Tuna Slaw with Creamy Lemon-Dill Dressing

¼ cup reduced-fat mayonnaise
1 tablespoon lemon juice
1 teaspoon dried dillweed
1 teaspoon Dijon mustard
2 cups packaged coleslaw mix (see note)
2 cans (6½ ounces each) water-packed albacore tuna, drained and flaked

In a medium bowl, mix the mayonnaise, lemon juice, dillweed, and mustard. Add the coleslaw mix and toss to coat. Gently stir in the tuna.

MAKES 4 SERVINGS

Per serving: 135 calories, 19 g protein, 7 g carbohydrates, 3 g fat, 30 mg cholesterol, 1 g dietary fiber, 449 mg sodium

Note: Buy a coleslaw mix that contains carrots and other vegetables, or add a shredded carrot.

Placid Pesto

⅓ cup chopped walnuts
2 cups packed fresh basil leaves
½ cup grated Parmesan cheese
⅓ cup extra-virgin olive oil
1 or 2 garlic cloves, halved
⅛ teaspoon ground black pepper

In a small skillet, stir the walnuts over low heat for 2 minutes, or until golden and fragrant. Let cool, then transfer to a blender or small food processor. Add the basil, cheese, oil, garlic, and pepper. Process until smooth, scraping down the sides of the container as necessary.

MAKES 1 CUP (ENOUGH FOR 1 POUND OF PASTA)

Per tablespoon: 73 calories, 2 g protein, 1 g carbohydrates, 7 g fat, 2 mg cholesterol, 0 g dietary fiber, 59 mg sodium

Note: Store the pesto in a covered container for up to 5 days in the refrigerator or up to 1 month in the freezer.

TUESDAY

Breakfast

1 small low-fat bran muffin

1 egg or 2 egg whites, scrambled

8 ounces fat-free milk (or 1% milk or calcium-fortified soymilk)

Snack

10 baby carrots (buy these ready to eat, or peel and slice regular carrots) dipped in yogurt dressing (mix 1 tablespoon fat-free yogurt with 1 teaspoon fresh chopped parsley, 1 teaspoon lime juice, and a dash of cayenne pepper, if desired)

Lunch

Tomato and mozzarella sandwich (layer about 2 ounces low-fat mozzarella, ½ ripe tomato, and a few fresh basil leaves on a slice of seven-grain bread; drizzle lightly with 1 teaspoon olive oil and 1 teaspoon balsamic vinegar, and top with another slice of bread)

1 cup low-sodium vegetable or minestrone soup

Snack

1 cup sliced fruit (try a tropical fruit like papaya or pineapple)

Orange juice spritzer (mix ½ cup orange juice with ½ cup plain seltzer water and add ice)

Dinner

2 cups Soothing Soybean Stew (see the accompanying recipe on the opposite page) served over 1 cup whole wheat couscous

1 cup steamed greens tossed with 1 teaspoon olive oil and 1 teaspoon fresh lemon juice

Snack

1 poached pear with ½ cup fat-free vanilla frozen yogurt (For poached pears: In a small saucepan, bring to a boil ¾ cup water, 2 teaspoons maple syrup, and 1 teaspoon vanilla extract. Boil for 5 minutes, or until syrupy. Reduce the heat and add 1 small peeled pear. Cover and cook, turning the pear and basting occasionally, for about 20 minutes, or until tender but not overdone. Cool in the refrigerator.)

1 tablespoon raisins

Nutrition totals: **1,803** calories, **87** g protein, **256** g carbohydrate, **56** g fat, **250** mg cholesterol, **30** g dietary fiber, **3,156** mg sodium

Soothing Soybean Stew

1	tablespoon olive oil
1	large onion, finely chopped
½	cup finely chopped green bell pepper
1	tablespoon finely chopped garlic
1½	teaspoon ground cumin
1½	teaspoon ground coriander
¾	teaspoon ground ginger
1	small butternut squash, peeled, seeded, and cut into ½" cubes
2	cup water
2	cans (15 ounces each) soybeans, rinsed and drained
1	can (8 ounces) tomato sauce
1½	teaspoon salt

In a large saucepan, warm the oil over medium heat. Add the onion and cook, stirring constantly, for 3 minutes. Add the pepper, garlic, cumin, coriander, and ginger. Cook, stirring constantly, for 2 minutes. Stir in the squash and 1 cup of the water. Bring to a boil. Reduce heat to medium-low, cover, and simmer for 5 minutes.

Stir in the soybeans, tomato sauce, salt, and the remaining cup of water. Simmer for 20 minutes, or until thick.

Makes 6 cups

Per cup: 192 calories, 12 g protein, 21 g carbohydrates, 8.2 g fat, 0 mg cholesterol, 4 g dietary fiber, 543 mg sodium

WEDNESDAY

Breakfast

1½ cups oatmeal topped with 1 tablespoon raisins and 2 teaspoons flaxseeds

1 pink grapefruit

8 ounces fat-free milk (or 1% milk or calcium-fortified soymilk)

Snack

1½ cups Truly Tropical Smoothie (See the accompanying recipe on the opposite page.)

Lunch

Jazzy Turkey Sandwich (Layer 3 ounces turkey breast, 1 slice reduced-fat cheddar cheese, and ¼ to ½ sliced Granny Smith apple on a slice of whole wheat bread. Top with another slice of bread spread with a mixture of 1 tablespoon prepared horseradish sauce and 2 teaspoons low-fat mayonnaise.)

¾ to ½ Granny Smith apple (remaining from sandwich recipe)

6 ounces cranberry-apple juice

Snack

1 cup lightly steamed vegetables dipped in low-fat dressing (Try zucchini or yellow squash; steam them anytime it's convenient, store in resealable plastic bags, and use within 3 days.)

Dinner

4 ounces grilled or baked salmon fillet

1 cup cooked brown rice (or other whole grain, such as quinoa or bulgur)

1½ cups Swiss chard (or other dark green leafy vegetable) sautéed with 2 teaspoons olive oil

Snack

1 large peach (or a serving of another orange-colored fruit, such as ½ mango or 2 apricots)

NUTRITION TOTALS: 1,834 CALORIES, 101 G PROTEIN, 288 G CARBOHYDRATE, 40 G FAT, 139 MG CHOLESTEROL, 36 G DIETARY FIBER, 1,949 MG SODIUM

Truly Tropical Smoothie

1 **cup low-fat plain yogurt**
1 **cup mango cubes**
1 **small banana, sliced**
½ **cup pineapple chunks**
¼ **cup nonfat dry milk**
1 **tablespoon lime juice**

In a blender, combine the yogurt, mango, banana, pineapple, dry milk, and lime juice. Blend until smooth.

MAKES 3 CUPS

Per 1½ cups: 230 calories, 10 g protein, 45 g carbohydrates, 2.5 g fat, 9 mg cholesterol, 3 g dietary fiber, 129 mg sodium

Note: For a thicker, icy-cold drink, freeze the fruit first (keep a supply of fruit chunks in the freezer for instant smoothies).

THURSDAY

Breakfast

1 cup bran cereal topped with 1 sliced medium banana and 8 ounces fat-free milk (or 1% milk or calcium-fortified soymilk)

Snack

¾ cup low-fat cottage cheese with ½ cup pineapple chunks (canned in natural juice), sprinkled with 2 teaspoons flaxseeds

Lunch

1 serving Calming Quiche (See the accompanying recipe on the opposite page.)

1 small garden salad (2 cups lettuce, 3 or 4 tomato wedges, and 4 or 5 cucumber slices) with fat-free dressing

Snack

2 tablespoons nut butter (try cashew or almond butter as a peanut butter alternative) spread on 2 whole grain crackers

Dinner

2 cups Tranquil Vegetarian Chili (See the accompanying recipe on page 200.)

1 cup cooked brown rice

Snack

2 graham crackers

8 ounces fat-free milk (or 1% milk or calcium-fortified soymilk) Try warming the milk and serving it with a dash of cinnamon and 1 teaspoon honey.

NUTRITIONAL TOTALS: **1,757** CALORIES, **108** G PROTEIN, **287** G CARBOHYDRATE, **36** G FAT, **190** MG CHOLESTEROL, **44** G DIETARY FIBER, **4,198** MG SODIUM (THIS TOTAL IS HIGH DUE TO TRANQUIL VEGETARIAN CHILI, BUT SINCE IT'S HIGH FOR ONLY ONE DAY, IT AVERAGES OUT FINE OVER THE WEEK.)

Calming Quiche

Crust

 2½ cups brown rice

 ⅓ cup grated Parmesan cheese

 2 egg whites, lightly beaten, or ¼ cup liquid egg substitute

Filling

 12 ounces low-fat silken tofu

 4 eggs, lightly beaten, or 1 cup liquid egg substitute

 1 tablespoon cornstarch

 ½ teaspoon salt

 ⅛ teaspoon ground nutmeg

 1 pound asparagus, trimmed, cut into 1" pieces, and steamed

 3 ounces reduced-fat Swiss cheese, shredded

 2 ounces ham-flavored soy deli slices, finely chopped

 2 scallions, finely chopped

Cook the rice according to package directions. Refrigerate until cold. Preheat the oven to 350°F. Lightly coat a 10" deep-dish pie plate with cooking spray.

To make the crust: In a large bowl, mix the rice, cheese, and egg whites or egg substitute. Press evenly in the bottom and up the sides of the prepared pie plate. Bake for 15 minutes.

To make the filling: In a food processor, combine the tofu, eggs or egg substitute, cornstarch, salt, and nutmeg. Process until smooth, scraping down the sides of the container as necessary.

Sprinkle the asparagus, cheese, soy slices, and scallions over the baked crust. Pour in the tofu mixture, stirring gently to blend slightly.

Bake for 45 minutes, or until firm in the center. Let stand 5 minutes before slicing.

MAKES 6 SERVINGS

Per serving: 261 calories, 27 g protein, 25 g carbohydrates, 8.5 g fat, 151 mg cholesterol, 2 g dietary fiber, 524 mg sodium

Tranquil Vegetarian Chili

- 1 large onion, finely chopped
- 1 green bell pepper, finely chopped
- 1 small carrot, finely chopped
- 2 garlic cloves, finely chopped
- 1 tablespoon olive oil or canola oil
- 2 teaspoons chili powder
- 1 teaspoon ground cumin
- 1 can (15 ounces) red kidney beans, rinsed and drained
- 1 can (15 ounces) cannellini beans, rinsed and drained
- 1 can (14½ ounces) diced tomatoes
- 1 can (8 ounces) tomato sauce
- ¼ teaspoon salt
- ¾ cup low-fat plain yogurt or reduced-fat sour cream
- 2 tablespoons chopped fresh cilantro

In a large saucepan over medium heat, cook the onion, pepper, carrot, and garlic in the oil for 10 minutes, or until the vegetables are softened. Stir in the chili powder and cumin. Cook for 2 minutes, stirring often.

Add the beans, tomatoes (with juice), tomato sauce, and salt. Simmer for 45 minutes over medium-low heat, stirring often. If the mixture becomes too thick, add water as necessary.

Serve topped with a dollop of yogurt or sour cream and sprinkled with cilantro.

MAKES 6 CUPS

Per cup: 196 calories, 10 g protein, 33 g carbohydrates, 3.5 g fat, 2 mg cholesterol, 5 g dietary fiber, 1,167 mg sodium

FRIDAY

Breakfast

2 small whole grain toaster waffles with ½ cup Relaxing Raspberry-Melon Mélange (See the accompanying recipe on page 202.)

8 ounces fat-free milk (or 1% low-fat milk or calcium-fortified soymilk)

Snack

10 to 15 low-fat tortilla chips dipped in 1 tablespoon salsa

Lunch

Meditative Middle Eastern Pita Pocket (Stuff one whole wheat pita with 3 to 4 tablespoons hummus, ¼ cup chopped tomato, ¼ cup chopped cucumber, and ¼ cup chopped romaine lettuce. Add a dash or two of hot sauce if desired.)

1½ cups lentil soup with carrot

Snack

1 small orange cut into sections and dipped in low-fat chocolate syrup

Dinner

4 ounces baked trout (Marinate in 2 teaspoons olive oil and the juice of ½ lemon.)

1 cup kale (Steam, then sauté quickly in 1 teaspoon olive oil with ½ teaspoon chopped garlic.)

1 baked sweet potato

1 whole wheat dinner roll

Snack

1 bunch purple grapes (1 to 2 cups)

NUTRITION TOTALS: **1,735** CALORIES, **83** G PROTEIN, **296** G CARBOHYDRATE, **41** G FAT, **135** MG CHOLESTEROL, **51** G DIETARY FIBER, **2,060** MG SODIUM

Relaxing Raspberry-Melon Mélange

¼ cup honey or sugar
2 tablespoons orange juice
2 tablespoons finely chopped crystallized ginger
¼ teaspoon ground ginger
1 cantaloupe, cut into ½" cubes
1 cup raspberries
¼ cup toasted sliced almonds

In a large bowl, combine the honey or sugar, orange juice, crystallized ginger, and ground ginger. Add the cantaloupe and toss to coat. Refrigerate for at least 2 hours, stirring occasionally. Just before serving, gently stir in the raspberries and almonds.

MAKES 3 CUPS

Per ½ cup: 120 calories, 2 g protein, 23 g carbohydrates, 3.5 g fat, 0 mg cholesterol, 2 g dietary fiber, 10 mg sodium

SATURDAY

Breakfast

1 whole wheat bagel topped with 1 tablespoon reduced-fat cream cheese

2 slices fresh tomato

8 ounces fresh grapefruit juice

Snack

8 ounces fat-free milk (or 1% milk or calcium-fortified soymilk)

2 tablespoons walnuts and 2 tablespoons raisins mixed together

Lunch

Simple Chef's Salad (Tear 2 cups romaine lettuce into bite-size pieces and top with 1 cup cherry tomatoes, 2 ounces sliced skinless turkey breast, and 1 ounce grated reduced-fat Cheddar cheese.)

1 tablespoon low-fat or fat-free creamy dressing

1 piece whole grain toast

Snack

1 slice cantaloupe (about $\frac{1}{8}$ medium)

$\frac{1}{3}$ cup low-fat vanilla yogurt

Dinner

$1\frac{1}{2}$ servings Bucolic Beef and Broccoli Stir-Fry (See the accompanying recipe on page 204.)

Snack

1 cup fruit sorbet

NUTRITION TOTALS: **1,787** CALORIES, **105** G PROTEIN, **271** G CARBOHYDRATE, **40** G FAT, **140** MG CHOLESTEROL, **23** G DIETARY FIBER, **1,996** MG SODIUM

Bucolic Beef and Broccoli Stir-Fry

1   cup brown rice
1   tablespoon canola oil
¾   pound top round, thinly sliced
1   bunch scallions, cut into 1" pieces
2   cups broccoli florets
½   cup water
3   tablespoons reduced-sodium soy sauce
1½   teaspoons sesame oil

Cook the rice according to package directions. In a large nonstick skillet, warm the canola oil over medium-high heat. Add the beef and cook, stirring constantly, for 1 minute, or until browned on all sides. Remove from the pan and set aside.

Add the scallions to the pan. Cook, stirring, for 1 minute. Add the broccoli and cook, stirring, for 1 minute. Add the water, soy sauce, and sesame oil. Cook, stirring often, for 5 minutes, or until the vegetables are tender. Stir in the beef and heat through. Serve over the rice.

MAKES 4 SERVINGS

Per serving: 385 calories, 26 g protein, 47 g carbohydrates, 10.5 g fat, 40 mg cholesterol, 3 g dietary fiber, 464 mg sodium

SUNDAY

Breakfast

3 (4-inch) whole wheat banana pancakes (add ripe banana slices to whole wheat pancake mix) with ½ cup fat-free vanilla yogurt

6 to 8 ounces orange juice

Snack

2 cups air-popped popcorn

Lunch

1 to 1½ cups low-sodium black bean soup

1 serving Serenity Pizzas with Sun-Dried Tomatoes (See the accompanying recipe on page 206.)

Snack

8 ounces fat-free milk (or 1% milk or calcium-fortified soymilk)

2 tablespoons almond butter on whole grain bread

Dinner

4 grilled jumbo shrimp (or 6 large shrimp)

1 serving Relaxing Brown Rice with Spinach and Feta Cheese (See the accompanying recipe on page 206.)

Snack

1 serving Becalmed Berry Vanilla Pudding Parfaits (See the accompanying recipe on page 207.)

NUTRITION TOTALS: **1,809** CALORIES, **93** G PROTEIN, **263** G CARBOHYDRATE, **53** G FAT, **371** MG CHOLESTEROL (THIS TOTAL IS HIGH DUE TO RELAXING BROWN RICE WITH SPINACH AND FETA CHEESE, BUT IT AVERAGES OUT FINE OVER THE WEEK), **38** G DIETARY FIBER, **2,677** MG SODIUM

Serenity Pizzas with Sun-Dried Tomatoes

    4 whole wheat pitas
    1 cup water
    1 ounce dry-packed chopped sun-dried tomato halves
    ¼ cup tomato paste with Italian seasonings
    1 box (10 ounces) chopped frozen spinach, thawed and squeezed
       dry
    ½ cup reduced-fat ricotta cheese
    2 ounces shredded provolone cheese
    2 ounces shredded reduced-fat mozzarella cheese

Preheat the oven to 400°F. Arrange the pitas on a baking sheet.

In a small saucepan, stir together the water, tomatoes, and tomato paste. Bring to a boil over medium heat. Reduce the heat to low and simmer for 5 minutes. Spread evenly over the pitas.

In a small bowl, combine the spinach and ricotta. Spoon evenly over the pitas. Sprinkle with the provolone and mozzarella.

Bake for 10 to 12 minutes, or until the cheese is melted and the pitas are slightly crisp. Let stand 5 minutes before serving.

Makes 4

Per pizza: 279 calories, 18 g protein, 34 g carbohydrates, 8.5 g fat, 28 mg cholesterol, 3 g dietary fiber, 680 mg sodium

Relaxing Brown Rice with Spinach and Feta Cheese

    1   teaspoon olive oil
    1   large onion, finely chopped
    1   cup brown rice
    2½ cups water
    1   box (10 ounces) frozen chopped spinach, thawed and squeezed
        dry
    4   ounces reduced-fat feta cheese, finely crumbled
    8   kalamata olives, pitted and finely chopped
    4   eggs, lightly beaten, or 1 cup liquid egg substitute

In a large saucepan, warm the oil over medium heat. Add the onion and cook, stirring frequently, for 5 minutes. Stir in the rice and water. Bring to a boil, then cover, reduce the heat, and simmer for 45 minutes, or until the water has been absorbed. Remove from the heat.

Preheat the oven to 350°F. Coat an 8" × 8" glass baking dish with cooking spray.

Stir the spinach, feta, and olives into the rice. Stir in the eggs or egg substitute. Spoon into the prepared baking dish.

Bake for 25 to 30 minutes, or until a knife inserted in the center comes out clean. Let stand for 5 minutes before serving.

MAKES 4 SERVINGS

Per serving: 391 calories, 19 g protein, 49 g carbohydrates, 13.5 g fat, 213 mg cholesterol, 5 g dietary fiber, 677 mg sodium

Variation: To turn this into a hearty side dish, omit the eggs.

Becalmed Berry Vanilla Pudding Parfaits

   2 **large ripe bananas, sliced**
   1 **pint strawberries**
  16 **ounces fat-free plain yogurt**
      About 3 tablespoons superfine sugar

In a food processor, combine the bananas and strawberries and process until smooth. Add the yogurt and the sugar and process just until blended. (If your fruit is very sweet, cut back on the sugar. Taste the mixture before freezing to determine how much is needed.) Pour into an 8" × 8" metal baking pan. Freeze for 3 to 4 hours, or just until firm.

Break the frozen yogurt into chunks and return the mixture to the food processor. Process until smooth. Transfer to a freezer container and freeze until solid. Let stand at room temperature for 10 to 15 minutes to soften slightly before scooping.

MAKES 5 CUPS

Per ¹/₂ cup: 63 calories, 3 g protein, 13 g carbohydrates, 0.5 g fat, 1 mg cholesterol, 1 g dietary fiber, 35 mg sodium

THE LEPTIN CONNECTION

Although scientists are still investigating the connection between stress hormones and fat, some studies suggest that stress hormones may interfere with the body's ability to utilize leptin, a hormone that tells us when we're full. In laboratory experiments, rats with elevated levels of stress hormones overate and quickly became obese. When their stress hormone levels dropped, their appetites—and weight—returned to normal.

Now you have the story on stress, and from weight gain to cancer, it's an ugly picture. Fortunately, you also have the tools you need to combat it. So now it's time to move on to another menopausal bugbear: moodiness. Turn to chapter 8 to find out why menopause makes you moody and what you can do about it.

Chapter

8

MANAGING YOUR MOODS

To our mothers, menopause marked the beginning of the end, the doorstep to old age. To us, it often represents the beginning of a whole new chapter in our lives, the opportunity to once again remake ourselves.

But into what?

"When it comes to facing menopause, the generations of women before us left no road maps," says Stephanie DeGraff Bender, a licensed clinical psychologist, clinical director of Full Circle Women's Health in Boulder, Colorado, and author of *The Power of Perimenopause*. They handled "the Change" silently, privately, suffering through a bewildering range of symptoms, sometimes experiencing mood swings so unpredictable and severe that they feared for their sanity. At best, they might have taken some form of tranquilizer to get through unpredictable emotional swings.

Today we can do it differently. There are an assortment of modern-day, healthy ways to balance your moods and face the big "M" with confidence and composure.

Working the Swing Shift

Your body temperature isn't the only thing that can suddenly switch from one extreme to the other during menopause. Some women feel very short-tempered and somewhat depressed. Even women who have experienced mood swings from premenstrual syndrome all their lives note that these are a bit more intense. "They find it is much more noticeable than it used to be," says Lisa Domagalski, M.D., a gynecologist and assistant clinical professor at Brown University Medical School in Providence, Rhode Island.

Experts aren't sure what links mood changes to menopause. It could be an estrogen connection, or it may have something to do with mood-altering brain chemicals, such as serotonin. Part of the difficulty may lie in sleep deprivation due to hot flashes and night sweats.

If your mood changes last a long time or impair your ability to work or function, or if you feel that you are slipping into a deep depression, see a doctor immediately. He will help you explore options such as medication and therapy. But if your mood changes are causing you (and those around you) only minor grief, try the following strategies to get your emotions back on an even keel.

Food and Your Mood

It's hardly news that many of us, when we're feeling down or irritated, seek emotional comfort in foods, particularly such "comfort" foods as candy bars, snack cakes, or macaroni and cheese. But for some of us, comfort foods are anything but comforting. The very foods we eat to make ourselves feel better during mood swings may actually make us feel worse—listless, moody, and fatigued.

Researchers have learned that what you eat can lift your mood or, if you make the wrong choices, sink it. Moreover, what you *don't* eat can have as great an impact as what you do. Here are two types of food that have the ability to keep you balanced.

Carbohydrates. In a study conducted by researchers at Harvard University and the Massachusetts Institute of Technology, women suffering from premenstrual mood swings were asked to drink about 7½ ounces of a specially formulated high-carbohydrate drink once a month just before their periods. Within hours of having the drink, they experienced significant reductions in depression, anger, and confusion, the researchers found.

While the women in the study consumed a specially made drink, you can get a similar amount of high carbohydrates by eating a small portion of a carbohydrate-rich food such as a cup of low-fat yogurt, a baked potato, or ½ cup of raisins. (To learn more about incorporating carbohydrates in your diet and making your meal plans more resistant to turbulent emotional weather, see "The 7 Commandments of Stress-Proof Eating" on page 190 and "Calming Cuisine: A Week of Relaxing Foods" on page 192.)

Omega-3 fatty acids. These substances, which are found in fish and certain other foods, are known mostly for keeping hearts healthy, but they may also help mood disorders. "The brain is essentially made of fat," explains Joseph Hibbeln, M.D., a researcher at the National Institutes of Health in Bethesda, Maryland. "Some fats necessary for brain functioning—such as polyunsaturated fatty acids found in fish—cannot be manufactured by the

A "NAVEL" IDEA

The next time you feel yourself floating off into a bad mood, take a time-out. Consider what is going on around you. Are you or someone close to you going through some kind of crisis, large or small? You might or might not be able to do anything to resolve it on the spot, but at least you'll know why you feel the way you do. Then, to help even out your mood, try this easy relaxation technique.

This is a simple exercise from qigong, an Eastern belief system in which the navel is the center of existence. "Qigong can refresh the body in a short period of time," says Leah J. Dickstein, M.D., director of attitudinal and behavioral medicine at the University of Louisville School of Medicine in Kentucky.

Sit with your palms cupped, the heels of your hands together at your navel. Open them very slowly. "Think of pulling energy into your body," says Dr. Dickstein. "Feel softness moving into the center of your body, replacing bad feelings." Repeat entire process, beginning with the time-out, as often as you feel a need to.

body. You have to get them from diet." So try to include more seafood in your diet. Dr. Hibbeln also suggests using canola oil while cooking as another way to increase your intake of omega-3s.

Walk or Exercise Often

Okay, we've already told you to exercise in chapter 4, The Menopause Exercise Plan. But just in case you somehow, ahem, skipped that chapter, we're going to give you a second chance. Because exercise—even gentle, steady exercise like walking—really *can* work wonders on your mood. In a study conducted at Texas A&M University College of Medicine in College Station, women who walked for 20 minutes reported significant improvements in mood. "Walking and exercise naturally increase the body's endorphins, chemicals in the body that make you feel good. That's where the 'high' that people get from running comes from," says Dr. Domagalski.

But for exercise to work its magic, it has to be something you look forward to, not just another task on your already too long to-do list. Sharon Brown, Ph.D., assistant professor of physical education and exercise science at Transylvania University in Lexington, Kentucky, for example, says she isn't particularly flexible, so yoga would frustrate her and be stressful. A 4-mile run, however, is something she *does* do well, and it never fails to lift her spirits. "Even better," she says, "is running with friends. This encourages me to exercise; plus, my friends help me find healthy perspectives and solutions to situations at work and with relationships."

On the other side of the exercise equation is Peggy Elam, Ph.D., a New York City psychologist and yoga buff. She frequently recommends this ancient discipline to her clients as a way to deal with their own stress. The key is discovering what works best for you and finding the right balance.

Most important is doing something you like. If you're just starting out and aren't in very good shape, walking might be your best bet. If you're already fit and want to step up the pace a bit, you might consider a faster-paced aerobic workout such as kickboxing.

For safe, gentle ways to lift your spirits through exercise, a blend of meditation and relaxation techniques, like yoga and tai chi, may be the answer. Almost anyone, at any age or any fitness level, can do them. (If you have a chronic condition, such as heart disease or back pain, or if you are pregnant, consult your physician first. Once you get the go-ahead, let the instructor know your situation that so she can work with you.) For information on how to begin yoga or tai chi, see chapter 12.

Take Time to Relax

In the early 1970s, Herbert Benson, M.D., at the Harvard Medical School devised the "relaxation response." This tension-releasing technique can help you through mood swings or periods of anxiety. Here's how to do it: Sit or lie down in a comfortable position and breathe deeply. Relax all your muscles. Think of a phrase or word that evokes feelings of relaxation for you, perhaps a word like *serene* or *calm*. Repeat the word in your mind every time you exhale. Practice this for 20 minutes once a day or 10 minutes twice a day, as well as anytime you feel your mood beginning to change.

Master Mental Imagery

You can also use mental imagery to prevent shadows from darkening your days. Mental imagery is a quick and natural method to take control of the negative sensations that might arise during menopause. Gerald Epstein, M.D., director of the American Institute for Mental Imagery and author of *Healing Visualizations*, offers this classic technique to relieve anxiety and irritability.

Sit in a comfortable chair, preferably with a high back and armrests for support. Place your arms on the armrests and your feet flat on the floor. Close your eyes and breathe out and then in three times slowly. Imagine yourself on a beach.

As you are looking at the sky far over the ocean, it begins to cloud over. You are hearing claps of thunder and seeing streaks of lightning as the storm gets closer and closer, gradually intensifying. Then, instead of letting loose, the dark clouds roll behind you, the sounds stop, and the flashes cease. Looking out into the ocean, you see the sun come up in the sky and know that your symptoms have passed.

SOUND AWAY MENOPAUSAL MOODINESS

A mind–body technique called toning can help bring back harmony if you're experiencing menopausal mood swings and other symptoms.

"The use of the voice is a built-in tool that releases emotional tension from your body," says Don Campbell, a sound researcher and director of the Mozart Effect Resource Center in Boulder, Colorado. "A daily practice of toning, which is making a sound with an elongated vowel for an extended period, can improve your overall state of mind."

Toning is a great help for releasing and harmonizing your emotions during and following menopause because it moves your emotions through your body so that you don't feel pent-up, vulnerable, or ready to explode, he explains. When your body responds to the vibration you are creating, your hormone levels even out.

Don tells of a student who claims that she benefited so greatly from a toning practice that she could get off hormone replacement and say goodbye to her hot flashes.

Here is a brief outline of Don Campbell's 5-Day Toning Class. Do each exercise for about 5 minutes, holding the tone continually with natural breaths in between. If you enjoy the experience, repeat it whenever you need some relaxation or reviving.

Day 1—hum: Sit comfortably, close your eyes, and hum—not a melody, but

To stay in control of your emotions, do this imagery exercise three times a day at the same times each day. You can also practice it at the first sign of a symptom and continue until the difficulty is over.

If self-help techniques fail to control your mood swings—or if you experience mood swings on a daily basis—seek professional help. And don't be embarrassed to ask for medical or psychiatric advice; you might have an underlying condition whose treatment eliminates mood swings.

The Power of Positive Thinking

It's not a compliment to be called a Pollyanna. The little orphan girl who brimmed with boundless cheer has come to epitomize the cockeyed optimist who doesn't quite see reality for what it is. The fact is, positive

a pitch that feels comfortable. Relax your jaw and feel the energy of the hum warming up and energizing your entire body.

Day 2—ah sound: The *ah* sound immediately evokes a relaxation response. Whenever you feel a great deal of stress and tension, relax your jaw and make a quiet *ah*. In your office or other places where toning may disturb others, you can siimply close your eyes, breathe out, and think the *ah*.

Day 3—ee sound: The *ee* sound can awaken your mind and body, functioning as a kind of sonic caffeine. When you feel drowsy while driving or are sluggish in the afternoon, making a high *ee* sound will stimulate your brain and keep you alert. The *ee* tone is also good for releasing tension. Just don't practice it if you have a headache as the increased activity in your brain may make it worse.

Day 4—oh sound: The *oh* tone is a great tool for an instant tune-up. Your body responds to the *oh* by normalizing your skin temperature, breathing, and heart rate as well as releasing muscle tension and increasing brain waves.

Day 5—experimental singing: Start at the lowest part of your voice and let it glide upward, like a very slow elevator. Make vowel sounds that are relaxing and that arise effortlessly from your jaw or throat. Allow your voice to resonate throughout your body. Now explore the ways in which you can "massage" parts of your skull, throat, and chest with long vowel sounds.

thinking has gotten a bit of a bum rap. We tend to trivialize positive emotions like hope, joy, and contentment.

"People think they're goofing off or wasting their time when they're experiencing positive emotions," explains Barbara Fredrickson, Ph.D., associate professor of psychology at the University of Michigan in Ann Arbor. "The possible benefits of positive emotions seem undervalued in cultures like ours, which endorse the Protestant ethic and cast hard work and self-discipline as virtues, and leisure and pleasures as sinful."

But research shows that feeling good *is* good. And if we want to find our way to natural calm and balanced emotions, we need to nurture what is best in ourselves.

(continued on page 218)

ADOPT A "GLASS HALF-FULL" ATTITUDE

So how do we learn to become a "glass half-full" type of person instead of a "glass half-empty" person? First, understand what that means.

"Positive emotions are more than the absence of negative emotions," says Barbara Fredrickson, Ph.D., associate professor of psychology at the University of Michigan in Ann Arbor.

One of the misunderstandings about this way of thinking is that all you have to do is put on a happy face, says Dacher Keltner, Ph.D., associate professor of psychology at the University of California, Berkeley. But thinking positively involves taking an alternative approach, and that requires a great deal of hard work. It's difficult and taxing, he says, but ultimately rewarding.

These six simple steps will start your transformation.

Put on your rose-tinted glasses. Studies show that people in difficult situations who are able to reframe their circumstances in a more positive light cope with stress better. For instance, AIDS caregivers who focused on the value of their efforts and commented on how their caregiving activities demonstrated their love and preserved the dignity of their ill partners fared best, says Susan Folkman, Ph.D., professor of medicine and codirector of the Center for AIDS Prevention Studies at the University of California in San Francisco.

To get a rosier view of your own life, look at the lessons you've learned from a bad situation, suggests Dr. Folkman. Or simply give yourself a well-deserved pat on the back when you've just endured a very stressful situation. Say to yourself, "I didn't realize I could do that."

Act happy. We can *act* ourselves into a more positive frame of mind, says David G. Myers, Ph.D., author of *The Pursuit of Happiness*. Research has shown that simply manipulating your face into a smiling expression by holding a pen in your teeth can make you feel better. On the other hand, hold the pen in your lips, and you activate the frowning muscles. "Scowl and the whole world seems to scowl back," he says.

"Going through the motions can trigger the emotions," says Dr. Myers. "So . . . put on a happy face. Talk as if you feel positive, optimistic, and outgoing," even if you don't.

Take control of your time. Happy people feel in control of their lives. But stress makes you feel as if your life is out of control. "We often overestimate how much we will accomplish in any given day, which leaves us feeling frustrated," says Dr. Myers.

When you start feeling like this, it's best to focus on immediate goals, advises Dr. Folkman. Make a to-do list for the day. Sounds pretty basic, right? Here's the difference. Make sure the tasks are specific and small, such as "Mail letter to Aunt Hilda," not "Organize my closet." The more, the better. And then (and this is key) take *pleasure* in crossing each one off as you accomplish it. "It reduces anxiety and helps you regain a sense of control because you feel more effective. And that's no small thing," she says.

Laugh it up. "Laughter is a good thing in times of stress. That's why people often laugh at unlikely times—at a funeral, for example," explains Dr. Keltner. He interviewed mourners and noted how often they laughed and expressed positive emotions. Two years later, he interviewed them again and found that those who had displayed the most positive emotions were the least likely to have experienced depression and anxiety. In times of stress, laughter reduces the physiological reaction to stress and feelings of anxiety and helps people form stronger bonds with others.

Be social. We feel better when we're interacting with others, says Dr. Myers. So give priority to close relationships. If you're married, resolve to nurture your relationship, to not take your partner for granted. Treat your husband with the same kindness that you display to others. To rejuvenate your affections, act loving, play together, and share common interests, he says.

Savor positive moments. We might not realize it, but even when we're under stress, we also experience positive moments. In 1,794 interviews with AIDS caregivers, Dr. Folkman was surprised to find that 99.5 percent were able to recall a positive event—something that had made them feel good and helped them get through the day.

So tune in to those moments when they happen. "They give you a moment of relief—like relaxing a muscle that's been tense for a long time. That brief moment can be restorative," says Dr. Folkman. It could be receiving a compliment, observing a beautiful sunset, or hearing your teenager say, "Thanks, Mom." Or it could be something planned, such as a special meal or a get-together with friends.

Delight in those ordinary but positive moments in your day, and amplify them, says Dr. Folkman. For instance, pause when you see that sunset, and pay attention to this bright spot in your day. Or take time for a period of reflection at the end of the day and think about all the moments that day that made you feel good. This reinforces what's meaningful and valuable in your life, she says, motivating you and building self-confidence. In short, paying attention to positive emotions helps breed more positive emotion.

"Instead of focusing on what you might perceive as negative about menopause, you can say, 'Now is the time to take better care of myself, eat more healthfully, get enough sleep, and get rid of what is toxic in my life,'" she advises.

Positive psychology shifts the focus from what's *wrong* with us to what's *right* with us. The latest research in this fledgling field has shown that cultivating optimism, joy, contentment, interest, and other positive feelings and attitudes can help prevent and treat problems that can cause mood swings, such as anxiety, depression, and stress-related health problems. For tips on how to turn your thinking around, see "Adopt a 'Glass Half-Full' Attitude" on page 216.

Have the Last Laugh

Dwindling fertility hormones may be an unstoppable fact of life, but you can certainly boost your "feel good" hormones. Research shows that laughing produces beneficial physiological effects because it reduces the release of stress hormones from the adrenal gland while increasing the production of endorphins, the body's natural feel-good hormones.

"Humor can reduce anxiety, soften anger, lighten depression, and raise your tolerance for pain. In all seriousness, laughter is beneficial for your body, mind, and soul, particularly when you are going through difficult times," says David Simon, M.D., medical director of the Chopra Center for Well Being in La Jolla, California, and author of *Vital Energy*. (For tips on how to entertain your playful spirit, see "What's So Funny?" on the opposite page.)

Estrogen and Depression

"Estrogen makes women feel good," says Martha Louise Elks, M.D., professor of medicine at the Morehouse School of Medicine in Atlanta. It seems to raise levels of the feel-good hormone serotonin, making us mellower and more flexible in how we react to whatever life throws us. "We still notice life's injustices, but we're not so bothered by them," Dr. Elks says. "We say, 'Yeah, he's a jerk—men are jerks. So what?'"

Try that philosophy during a menopausal state, when your estrogen levels are low or erratic. Then your response is likely to be "Yeah, he's a jerk" as we slam the door/throw the plate/storm out of the room. Studies have shown that depression and even suicide attempts are more frequent during estrogen lulls.

WHAT'S SO FUNNY?

Here are some ideas for entertaining your playful spirit.

- Create your own compilation videos of film clips and television episodes that make you laugh. That way, you'll have them on hand when you need to lighten up. You can also rent or buy compilation tapes like *Saturday Night Live* reruns or Monty Python sketches and watch bits of them every night.
- Stock up on silliness. Find joke books and comics that are laugh-out-loud funny, and keep them by your bed, in the bathroom, on the refrigerator—anywhere that you can always see them.
- Take a stand-up artist for a ride. Get cassettes or compact discs of comedians that you can listen to in your car so that long drives actually cheer you up.
- Humor your inner clown. Go to a photo booth with a friend and take whimsical pictures. Or cut and paste photos of you, your family friend, or coworkers onto pictures you find in magazines. Also, make a different goofy face in the mirror with each bathroom visit throughout the day. And get yourself a pair of Groucho glasses or a silly wig as a reminder to not take yourself too seriously.
- Sign up for a free joke-a-day service on the Internet via e-mail. Just type "joke" into your Web browser, or try logging on to Web sites such as www.humorproject.com, www.aath.org, and www.laugh-of-the-day.com.
- Catch the bug. Laughter is not only the best medicine; it's contagious, too! When you read a humorous anecdote, quote, or cartoon, post it on your front door or another place where you'll be able to share others' enjoyment.
- See the comical side of the change. Read a funny book about menopause, like *The Noisy Passage* by Marie Evans and Ann Shakeshaft.
- Instead of the typical dinner and a movie, why not take a friend or your spouse to comedy clubs or social clubs that feature a comic for the night's entertainment?
- When you host or attend parties, suggest funny-bone-tickling interactive games like Pictionary, Cranium, Taboo, Guesstures, and Balderdash. Or play poker for a ridiculous stake like gummy bears.

Conventional treatments for depression include a variety of antidepressant drugs, psychotherapy, and a combination of both. Estrogen replacement therapy also seemed to help women with perimenopausal and postmenopausal depression, according to a study, published in the *Journal of the American Menopause Society*, that was a review of the medical literature on women and depression.

While you should seek help from a qualified mental health expert for any sign of depression, there may be some things you can do to help lift the clouds of mild to moderate depression.

Move for your mood. Just as physical activity helps to balance mood swings, it can also prevent and treat depression. Researchers don't know exactly why exercise helps, but they suggest it may enhance our sense of

ST. JOHN'S WORT TO THE RESCUE

If you've tried Prozac or some other prescription antidepressant, but don't like the side effects (lower sexual desire being one), you might want to consider St. John's wort.

St. John's wort has gotten a lot of publicity as "natural Prozac" over the years. Studies have found that St. John's wort alleviates mild to moderate depression as effectively as prescription antidepressants. Scientists aren't sure how St. John's wort works but speculate that it increases levels of the mood-elevating chemical serotonin. One ingredient, hypericin, is believed to be responsible for the herb's antidepressant effects, but newer research indicates that St. John's wort might contain many other active ingredients.

"It's not just one molecule with one effect, as with synthetic drugs," says Harold Bloomfield, M.D., in Del Mar, California, and author of *Hypericum and Depression*. "St. John's wort has many active ingredients, and they all work together."

Widely used to relieve depression in European countries, St. John's wort has some definite advantages over synthetic drugs. It isn't addictive, causes no withdrawal symptoms, and can be safely mixed with alcohol. Nor does it produce the side effects commonly associated with antidepressant drugs, such as nausea, gastrointestinal distress, and lowered sex drive. "Prescription antidepressants aren't necessary to treat mild depression," says Dr. Bloomfield.

mastery so we feel more mentally and physically in control. Aerobic activity may also help vent pent-up frustration. And mood-enhancing endorphins (runner's high) released during exercise could also be involved. Aim for at least 30 minutes of exercise most days. If you want, you can break it into three sets of 10 minutes each.

Expand your exercise horizons. Yoga is an excellent depression remedy. For one thing, if you take a class, you'll bond with others, says Ellen Kamhi, R.N., Ph.D., author of *Cycles of Life: Herbs and Energy Techniques for Women*. Also, some movements and breathing exercises in yoga can stimulate glands to release mood-enhancing hormones. (For more on yoga, see page 363.)

Illuminate yourself. "Before we use any herbs or supplements, we

"St. John's wort is the first thing I prescribe for depression," says Hyla Cass, M.D., assistant clinical professor of psychiatry at the UCLA School of Medicine. "It may not help every woman, but it's unlikely ever to hurt anyone."

If your doctor has ruled out serious depression, you may want to give St. John's wort a try. Here's what you need to know.

Take just what you need, and no more. Doctors who prescribe St. John's wort usually suggest 300 milligrams three times a day. Look for products with 0.3 percent extract of hypericin.

The best dose, says Dr. Cass, "is the lowest one that produces results." She suggests starting with the recommended dosage, then tapering after a few months to find the optimal dosage. Some people will find they can eventually stop taking the herb completely without a recurrence of symptoms.

Take it with food. Some women experience nausea the first few days, which usually vanishes when the herb is taken with food.

Wear sunscreen, wraparound sunglasses, and a hat if you go outdoors. Evidence suggests that St. John's wort may increase sensitivity to the sun if you're light-skinned.

Don't expect instant results. "Like prescription antidepressants, St. John's wort often takes 3 or 4 weeks before it kicks in," says Dr. Bloomfield.

need to find out what's causing the depression," says Dr. Kamhi. Sometimes it's something relatively simple, like lack of sunlight, which can be treated with a light box. These devices shine full-spectrum light on your face, simulating natural sunlight. Light treatment should be considered even before the use of herbs, she says, because there are no chemicals or toxicities in light, and you can operate a light box at work or at home. Use this treatment only in consultation with your doctor, who can explain proper use of the box and set up an appropriate treatment schedule for you.

Brew a soothing tea. "My favorite antidepressant is a tea made of Siberian ginseng and rosebuds—it immediately lifts your spirits," says Dr. Kamhi. Get Siberian ginseng from a health food store in the form of the whole root, in a tea bag, or in a capsule.

Welcome support. Nourish emotional and physical improvements among other women experiencing menopause. Much research has shown that a support group can be an essential element in enhancing both mental and physical health. In a 10-year Stanford University study of women with advanced stages of breast cancer, researchers found that the women who were in a support group lived twice as long as those who were not in a support group.

"The group process offers wonderful energy to support change," says counselor Louise Hay, an expert in creative power and personal growth and author of 27 bestsellers, including *You Can Heal Your Life*. A menopause support group can be a focused opportunity for women to share their experiences on the sometimes unpredictable path of menopause. But don't use your group to sit around and play "ain't it awful. . . . " Share ideas of ways to cope. Use the group as a stepping-stone in your growth process.

To locate a women's support group in your area, check the local newspaper under "community meetings and services." You can also contact the National Self-Help Clearinghouse, 365 Fifth Avenue, Suite 3300, New York, New York 10016, or visit their Web site at www.selfhelpgroups.org. Another option is to jump online for a menopausal women's chat room.

Read on for more ways to connect socially—not just through menopause, but generally—in "Making New Connections" on the opposite page.

ALLEVIATE ANXIETY WITH ACUPRESSURE

A few minutes of acupressure, the fine art of finger pressure, can help ease your body and mind.

If you are experiencing feelings of anxiety as you approach midlife, or if you find yourself generally feeling stressed-out, acupressure can provide you with calming relief, says David Nickel, O.M.D., L.Ac., a doctor of oriental medicine and a licensed acupuncturist in Santa Monica, California.

How does it work? A practitioner could give you a lengthy explanation about how acupressure restores complex energetic pathways in your body. But in Western terms, pressing your fingers or knuckles in the right places improves circulation throughout your body, including your brain. The resulting flood of minerals, enzymes, oxygen, and pleasure chemicals brings relief from muscular and emotional tension.

A quick way to relieve minor anxiety is to apply pressure to the Spirit Gate point, located on the outside of your wrist, below the first crease and in line with your pinkie finger. Press on this spot until you get an aching sensation similar to when you hit your funny bone.

Maintain this pressure for 15 to 30 seconds, then release. For optimal results, do not work the same spot more than two or three times a day.

For help in getting started, see page 352.

Making New Connections

The shadow of sadness can sneak up on you like a runaway shopping cart barreling toward your brand-new car in the grocery store parking lot. It gains momentum, the sharp metal edges charging at the gleaming paint . . . until some kind bystander dives between car and cart and absorbs the impact. Like that bystander, social support can step in and buffer us against the abrasive effects of gloomy feelings, depression, and mood swings.

And when it comes to making those stress-reducing connections, women have the edge. We give one another more frequent and effective social support, we're quicker to provide help when a friend is depressed or sad, and we're more satisfied overall than men with our personal connections.

In fact, new studies suggest we have our own, unique way to deal with stress, called "tend and befriend," and it's more effective than the fight-or-flight mechanism we'd previously been thought to use.

Reducing Stress with Friendship

"Social support is emotionally nurturing, and if it's emotionally nurturing, it's going to be physically nurturing—the classic mind–body connection," says Patricia McWhorter, Ph.D., a licensed psychologist in Palm Harbor, Florida, and author of *Cry Our Native Soul.*

More specifically, social support has many benefits. Here are a few of the best.

It calms. Stress produces physiological responses, including increased heart rate, breathing, and blood pressure, that over time can harm mental and physical health. "And social support cuts off this dysfunctional cycle," says Judith C. Tingley, Ph.D., a psychologist and public speaker in Phoenix.

A study reported in the *Journal of Behavioral Medicine* found that women experienced high blood pressure and increased heart rates only when they performed stressful tasks alone, compared with those who worked with or were in the presence of a female friend or even a female stranger. In the latter cases, heart rate and blood pressure responses were minimal. Just having another woman in the room, whether she was a stranger or a friend, reduced stress.

This calming power appears to work over the long term, too. People who have social connections bounce back more quickly from surgery and illnesses than those without support.

It takes a load off. When you have solid social connections, you have people who are prepared to help, whether it's a lift to work or someone to care for your children in an emergency. "There are people there to say, 'Don't worry, we've got this covered,' which reduces stress," says David Posen, M.D., a public speaker in Oakville, Ontario, and author of *Always Change a Losing Game.*

Social support might also help stop stress from starting in the first place. For example, if you face work conflict but have sufficient social support from your colleagues, you'll be less likely to view the problem as stressful.

It dissolves distress. We feel much better when we talk things through. "And when we hear ourselves talk, we can often get to the root of what's bothering us without the listener saying a word," says Dr. Posen.

It validates. If someone listens empathetically and says things like "Gee, that must be hard" or "I agree" or "That happened to me, too," it makes us feel better, says Mark Gorkin, a licensed clinical social worker, president of StressDoc Enterprises, and author of *Practice Safe Stress*. "You begin to feel like you're not alone or a freak of nature after all," he says.

It boosts self-esteem. "Anything that threatens our self-esteem (for instance, someone's threatening or criticizing us) produces a stress response," says Dr. Posen. Our social connections help us feel better about ourselves—good friends make us feel good, and we feel as if we're part of a larger whole. "And as self-esteem improves, stress diminishes," he says.

It lingers. "Social support instills a kind of inner foundation—you carry around the beliefs and sharing that you receive from your social connections even when they're not there, like that great teacher you had in high school who remains a role model throughout your life," says Mark Gorkin.

Female Friends: The Ultimate Connection

When they're stressed, female prairie voles prefer to be around other female prairie voles. The same goes for humans. It seems that social support from women, rather than from men, is more stress relieving to both sexes.

A study at the University of California in San Diego recorded the blood pressure responses of men and women who gave a 5-minute impromptu speech to either a male or a female audience. Even though the audiences behaved identically, the speakers had lower blood pressure when they talked before a female audience. "We're not sure why this is," says study researcher Nicholas Christenfeld, Ph.D., associate professor of psychology. "But we suspect it may be because the speakers interpreted the support differently when it came from women. When it came from men, the support was interpreted as 'I understand what you're saying, and you're making good points,' but when it came from a woman, it was interpreted as 'I like you as a person.'"

It seems that females are just more socially wired than males are. "Our connections are more naturally feelings-based," says Dr. McWhorter. A landmark anthropology study illustrated this difference, she says. Researchers watched two opposing tribes of chimpanzees. The males from each tribe waited at the imaginary line of territory, throwing rocks and chasing one another away. Meanwhile, the females sneaked into one another's trees, where they secretly bonded, groomed one another, and played with one another's infants.

Finding Your Own Connections

Although simply being a woman provides an advantage when it comes to making connections, there's more you can do. Here are some ways to build social networks (or strengthen the ones you already have).

Be supportive yourself. "Our mothers told us when we were little: 'To have a friend, you have to be a friend,'" says Karyn Buxman, R.N., president of HUMORx, a company that helps people feel better about themselves and their work through humor and laughter, and author of *This Won't Hurt a Bit!* The amount of social support we give is as important as how much we get. Follow these guidelines to be a good supporter.

- Ask questions, and show interest in what the other person has to say.

- Just listen. "Don't judge or tell the person what she should do— that's the last thing we need when we need social support," says Dr. McWhorter.

- Nurture your friendships with regular phone calls, invitations, and support.

- When something is shared with you in confidence, don't tell your five best friends.

Focus on quality, not quantity. A study at Yale University found that people with just a few friends who felt loved and supported had fewer coronary blockages than those with many friends who felt less loved and supported. Here are five characteristics necessary for high-quality social connections.

Compassion. "To feel supported, you have to feel cared for and understood," says Dr. Tingley.

Unconditional love. "You need to feel safe to be vulnerable, goofy, and free to let it all hang out," says Dr. McWhorter.

AGE GRACEFULLY

Is your attitude about growing older fair, or is it ruled by society's stereotypes?

"It's no wonder so many menopausal women get depressed, living in the context of an 'ageist' culture, which assumes that growing older is an inevitable decline into incapacity, fatigue, and despondency," says Alice D. Domar, Ph.D., director of the women's health programs for the division of behavioral medicine at Harvard Medical School and coauthor of *Self-Nurture.*

Certain changes do tend to occur at midlife. For example, losing weight becomes harder, libido fluctuates, and social and family roles may shift. But none of this should mean menopausal women can't feel attractive, be fully sexual, come into their creativity, develop careers, or redefine relations with loved ones in ways that are profoundly gratifying, says Dr. Domar.

Your distorted ideas about aging might come from someone else's fear or stereotype. "In other words, if your mind is a bus, who is driving it? Is it your boss? Your mother-in-law? Your father? A guy who broke up with you years ago? The media? For people who have negative beliefs running around their heads," says Dr. Domar, "the usual answer to 'who is driving your bus' is anyone but themselves."

Have the courage to question the origins of your negative impressions about menopausal and postmenopausal years. Then you can take the wheel and follow your self-guided directions on the road of maturity that leads to peace of mind and vitality.

Accessibility. Solid social support is there for you whenever you need it, even at 4 o'clock Monday morning.

Trustworthiness. "You want someone who won't ridicule you or let the whole world know about your problem," says Linda Sapadin, Ph.D., a psychologist practicing in Valley Stream, New York, and author of *It's About Time: The Six Styles of Procrastination and How to Overcome Them.*

Honesty. Someone who constantly tells you you're wonderful isn't going to be much help. "Find someone who can listen but also be objective," says Mark Gorkin.

Know what to avoid. When it comes to spilling your guts, it's smart to look out for the red flags. Dr. Posen recommends you zip it up when you notice any of these five traits.

Cattiness. Someone who reveals others' confidences to you is also likely to reveal yours to them.

Lack of empathy. If you're having relationship problems because of your infertility, a happily married woman with three children may not be able to empathize. Choose someone you can relate to on this particular issue.

Self-centeredness. The woman who immediately switches the focus of the conversation from your problem to herself probably won't be much help.

Disinterest. If she seems impatient when you're talking, she probably isn't interested.

Insensitivity. If she's uncaring when she talks about others, she's probably not going to be too caring with you either.

Start with what you have. "You might not have to build a support system—you might just have to start being more open with the people you already know," says Dr. Posen. Your "fun friend" (with whom you've never pondered anything deeper than what kind of martini to order) could turn out to be a great listener.

Talk to strangers. "It's often easier to confide in strangers than friends because you don't have to worry about them telling others you know, and you don't have to worry about damaging their opinion of you," says Dr. Sapadin. Support groups and group therapy provide excellent opportunities for stranger interaction.

Join a group. If you run for exercise, join a running group. If you read, join a book club. If you want to do something for the community, volunteer. "You'll meet people with common interests, and they'll also be doing some things you're not doing, which can challenge you to stretch and grow," says Mark Gorkin.

Go online. The Internet helps build social bridges among diverse groups of people. "In some chat groups, people come together and are honest with one another," says Mark. "They gradually open up and meet people with whom they can create a one-on-one relationship."

The proof: A study reported in the *American Journal of Community Psychology* gave 42 single women computer-mediated social support (CMSS) concerning parenting issues. The online discussions revealed close personal relationships among the women, and the mothers who regularly participated in CMSS experienced less parenting stress.

Online groups are also great if you want to remain anonymous. But as with all Web information, consider the source and be cautious. Visit the site a few times before you decide to join. Good starting points for online support groups include www.liszt.com, www.drkoop.com, and www.psychcentral.com.

With all these mood-enhancing options to choose from, we hope you're starting to feel better already. And once you start feeling better, you might find yourself starting to think about all sorts of pleasurable things again . . . like sex. To find out how to have the best time of your life in bed (or anyplace else you find appealing), turn to chapter 9.

Chapter
9

MAKING SEX GREAT AGAIN

IF YOUR SEX LIFE HAS BECOME COMPROMISED BY MIDLIFE CRISES, painful intercourse, chronic disease, a change in your marital status, or any of the hormonal changes of menopause, don't bottle up your desires. Denying your passionate nature is a sure way to sap one of the most sublime pleasures from your life—not to mention your mate's. Besides, frequent sex in midlife and beyond is actually quite good for you and can even help manage some symptoms of menopause.

According to the results of a University of Chicago study, women who engage in sex once a week have higher estrogen levels. In fact, women with sporadic, rather than weekly, sexual activity had a 50 percent chance of developing severely low estrogen levels. The benefit of consistent indulging might very well translate to fewer hot flashes, less vaginal dryness, better odds of withstanding osteoporosis, and slower aging, says Patricia Love, Ed.D., a marriage and family therapist and relationship consultant in Austin, Texas, and coauthor of *Hot Monogamy*.

The specific reasons that sex is good for keeping aging women youthful are a bit complex, says Dr. Love. It all begins with oxytocin, the chemical that triggers orgasm (also released during breastfeeding) and causes you to bond with your partner, she explains. Bonding encourages more touching, and that in turn releases endorphins, the body's natural "opiates." When this happens often, Dr. Love says that it colors your life with a sense of tranquillity and happiness that ultimately offsets aging, both emotionally and physically.

Dr. Love suggests maintaining weekly sexual relations even if you don't always feel like it. "You might just think of sex as meeting your partner's needs. What you don't realize is that it's also good for you because it sends a signal to your body that says, 'I'm still young, alive, and vibrant.'"

Another dividend: Regular sexual activity stimulates the vaginal lining to produce natural lubricants, keeping vaginal dryness at bay. And if your own lubrication is inadequate, sex encourages you to apply creams and moisturizers, which further maintains vaginal health. To reap that benefit, you don't necessarily need a partner. Masturbating twice a week can produce the same results.

But all of this begs the question if sex at midlife is so good for us, why aren't we having orgasms every day? Surveys show that almost one in three women over 50 hasn't had sex in the past year. The same is true for about one in seven over 40.

If this statistic applies to you, then let this chapter help you open the door to a more vibrant—and fulfilling—sex life.

Make the Most of a Midlife Crisis

For many women, menopause signals the beginning of a whole new stage in life. Midlife affords us time to begin thinking about autonomy and individuality, about expressing who we really are. "I see women becoming more assertive, in a positive way, and more active. We move beyond our traditional roles as nurturers and begin putting ourselves first," says Carol Landau, Ph.D., clinical professor of psychiatry and human behavior at Brown University Medical School in Providence, Rhode Island, and coauthor of *The Complete Book of Menopause*. That could mean speaking up more at home and at work, pursuing a more meaningful career or doing volunteer work, choosing new hobbies, or making new friends— or taking other steps that bring new meaning to your daily life. (See our life-enriching suggestions in chapter 7.)

PUT A SLANT ON GREAT SEX

As women age, their uterine muscles tend to weaken and sag downward, undermining full sensations of intercourse or even causing the embarrassment of leaking urine in the heat of the moment. But you can battle gravity by keeping the supporting muscles in the pubic region toned with daily Kegel exercises, says Helen Healy, N.D., a naturopathic physician and the director of the Wellspring Naturopathic Clinic in St. Paul, Minnesota. For the best results, do them while lying on a slantboard, a padded piece of exercise equipment that allows you to lie down on an adjustable incline.

Kegel exercises consist of contracting and relaxing the pubococcygeal muscle, which is used to stop and start the flow of urine. When this muscle is in good working order, the tissues surrounding it remain healthier and better oxygenated, says Dr. Healy. By strengthening it, menopausal women can maintain better control and even better vaginal lubrication. Better yet, women report improved sex lives and more intense orgasms after doing Kegels routinely.

Dr. Healy suggests lying on a slantboard set at a 25- to 30-degree angle (with one end raised about 2 feet) with your head at the low end. While in that position, squeeze the pubococcygeal muscle hard and hold it for about 5 seconds, then release and relax for 3 seconds. Always do this on an empty stomach to prevent a potential hiatal hernia. For optimal benefits, work up to 100 squeezes per day. (Not all of them need to be done on a slantboard!) The beauty of Kegels is that you can pretty much do them anywhere—even sitting at the dinner table or in front of the TV, and no one will know it.

At the same time, a woman might also look more critically at the quality of intimacy in her relationships with her spouse, her children, and her friends, and feel a need for a deeper connection. This type of inward assessment can bring on a wave of growing pains that can strain not only a good sex life but the marriage itself.

And in truth not all marriages survive midlife changes. The divorce rate among middle-aged people is second only to the rate among younger couples who've been married 7 years or less. If one partner has felt alienated for years and has stayed only to raise the kids or out of economic necessity, then midlife can present an opportunity to leave a bad situation and start over.

But do feelings of discontent necessarily mean that you've made all the wrong choices, or that to be happy you need to file for divorce, lose 20 pounds, or take a handsome lover? Of course not! Instead, a strong sense of discontent is a loud signal that it's time to pay attention to your inner needs, not necessarily a sign that your life needs a complete overhaul. Small or gradual changes may make all the difference.

Midlife Crises: What You Can Do for Yourself

To help you sort out your discontent and decide what to do, experts offer this advice.

Let the big questions simmer. Set aside some time to ask yourself questions about your life, and then let the answers rise to the surface. "I ask myself if I'm doing what I really want to be doing. If I'm still happy with my marriage, my job, my social life," says Janice Levine, Ph.D., a clinical psychologist and director of the Couples Health Program in Lexington, Massachusetts. "The questions just simmer in the back of my mind. I notice that little red flags go up if I find I'm doing things that I really don't want to be doing." In the same way, little green flags may go up when you are doing what pleases you most. If you pay attention to the red and green flags, you could have an "aha" moment, when you recognize choices that are working for or against you.

Select a confidante. For most women, the single most important help at midlife is having a close friend you can confide in. Choose someone who can listen without having her own agenda. For instance, if you are married and need to talk over doubts about your relationship, do not confide in a woman who is in the midst of a separation herself.

Put regret in its place. At midlife, many women feel at least some regrets. Some point you toward important actions, such as making peace with your parents or siblings. But others can take on a life of their own, with no resolution. If you find yourself ruminating about the road not taken, it might be time to forgive yourself for simply being human. (After all, if you decided to raise three children and work part-time instead of becoming a research chemist or a concert pianist, remind yourself that you made a great choice. No one can do everything. Put superwoman to rest.)

KEEP UP WITH CONTRACEPTION

When it comes to birth control, better safe than sorry is a rule not to break when you're approaching menopause.

Sex without risk of pregnancy could make those annoying menopausal symptoms seem worthwhile. But don't toss your contraceptives away after your first hot flash. "Pregnancy is possible during the perimenopausal years," warns Brian Walsh, M.D., assistant professor of obstetrics and gynecology and reproductive biology at Harvard Medical School and the director of the Menopause Clinic at Brigham and Women's Hospital, both in Boston. "Admittedly, the risk is low, but it's not zero."

An unplanned pregnancy on the brink of menopause could prove both physically and emotionally burdensome, so it's essential to use birth control every time you have intercourse. Some women assume that the rhythm method is a good option during perimenopause, especially since irregular ovulation lowers their chances of conceiving; however, the accompanying irregular menstrual cycles also make it difficult to judge "safe" times, so the rhythm method is still unreliable.

Barrier methods, which include diaphragms and condoms, are wise choices, says Dr. Walsh. Spermicidal formulas, however, can irritate sensitive vaginal tissue and should be avoided if vaginal dryness, typical of menopause, is a problem. Women who can safely take estrogen may benefit from low-dose birth control pills, which also offer symptomatic relief from hot flashes and menstrual irregularities.

When do contraceptives become extraneous? After your periods have stopped completely for 1 year, says Dr. Walsh. But since on-again-off-again cycles can make the determination difficult, it's best to consult with your doctor before stopping.

Restoring Intimacy

Trying to hide midlife questioning from your partner won't work—and could be dangerous for your marriage, experts caution. "He will probably see changes in your behavior before you do," says Dr. Levine. You might start acting distant, lose interest in activities you've shared for years, stop seeing old friends as often, even change your wardrobe or your hairstyle. He's bound to notice and wonder what's up. And, if you are avoiding sex, that could very well be misinterpreted as rejection by your lover.

More important, resisting change out of fear that your marriage will be altered shortchanges both you and your relationship. "If you hold back in an effort to keep everything the same, your need for change might express itself in unhealthy ways. You might grow to resent your husband, become depressed, even spend money recklessly or have an affair," notes Dr. Levine.

So speak up. For all you know, he might be experiencing similar feelings. "A lot of couples go through midlife changes at the same time," Dr. Landau explains. How men and women deal with change is different, though. While a man might distract himself, a woman might be more likely to want to talk things out.

Think through your frustrations before starting a conversation. If you feel bored with your sex life or your marriage, don't simply blame your husband. Ask yourself why. Perhaps you always imagined that married life would bring a certain kind of excitement, but that hasn't materialized. And so it may be time to give up an unrealistic expectation. Or perhaps the two of you are stuck in old routines—maybe you've made love the same way for decades, or done the same things every weekend for years. It might be time to try something new.

Once you've thought through what you really want to say, try talking to your spouse in a nonthreatening way about your hopes and frustrations. Pick a time when the two of you are relaxed, not tired or rushed. It's usually best to talk about sex outside the bedroom. And be specific about what you want from him, and ready to suggest some alternative activities.

Once you have opened up the lines of communication, together you can experiment with solutions. Perhaps, for example, he needs to understand that at midlife a woman requires a longer period of foreplay, and you can learn seductive massage techniques together. Maybe he'll finally take you on that romance-revving cruise or lingerie shopping date that he's been procrastinating about for the 30 years of your marriage.

The fact is, for many women, menopause becomes a liberating time to experiment with different sexual behaviors, such as oral sex. Communicate—and you're on the road to joining the ranks of women who report their postmenopausal years as their best sex years.

Overcome Menopausal Symptoms

Many women try to keep certain menopausal symptoms private as long as possible, but that can be difficult to do in the bedroom, where many of the most physically intimate moments of the day occur. Here, then, is the best advice for dealing with the two symptoms most likely to interfere with your sex life: hot flashes and vaginal dryness.

Steamy Sex without Hot Flashes

You want hot sex, but instead you have hot flashes. Don't despair. You have enough stress to manage during menopause without straining your most intimate, supporting relationship. If hot flashes and night sweats leave you less than lustful, consider the following solutions.

Take an herbal chiller. Medical research suggests that black cohosh, a popular herbal remedy, contains estrogen-like substances that help relieve menopausal symptoms, especially hot flashes. Anecdotal reports suggest that black cohosh also can increase menopausal women's sex drives, says Kimberly Windstar, N.D., faculty member at the National College of Naturopathic Medicine and a naturopathic physician at New Health Horizons clinic, both in Portland, Oregon.

But unlike conventional hormone therapy, black cohosh doesn't raise blood levels of estrogen. This makes the herb a boon particularly for women who have experienced breast cancer because black cohosh quells hot flashes without increasing the risk of recurrence, Dr. Windstar says.

Germany's Commission E (similar to the Food and Drug Administration) recommends a daily dose of 40 milligrams, taken for no more than 6 months. Some women find that one 40-milligram capsule is enough, says Dr. Windstar, while others might need to discuss increasing their dosages with their practitioners for best results. Because black cohosh is such a potent herb, it's best to consult your health care provider before taking it, especially if you've had breast cancer.

Make love between flashes. Hot flashes seem to be most frequent from 6:00 A.M. to 8:00 A.M. and from 6:00 P.M. to 10:00 P.M., explains Dr. Landau. So if hot flashes are a big impediment to your sex life, you might try scheduling "sex dates" outside these times. If you and

EAT YOGURT, STARVE YEAST

After menopause, your vagina loses some of its protective lining. That means it becomes more easily abraded and more prone to bacterial and yeast infections, which cause itching, irritation, and, often, pain during intercourse.

The problem is that the oral antibiotics designed to take care of the bacterial infections can also lead to more vaginal yeast infections—at a time when you're already more vulnerable. Why the complications? Oral antibiotics are formulated to fight bacteria throughout the body, and, unfortunately, in the process they also annihilate the beneficial ones in the reproductive tract. As a result, the normally small, harmless population of yeast that reside in the reproductive canals can increase wildly.

To fight off yeast naturally, treat yourself to at least one 8-ounce serving of yogurt a day. Most yogurt contains beneficial bacteria in the form of acidophilus and bifidus (often labeled as "active cultures") that help suppress yeast. (Check the carton to make sure it lists active or live cultures.) Yogurt with the least sugar is best since sugar seems to encourage yeast.

If yogurt doesn't agree with you, try taking acidophilus and bifidus supplements, available as drops or tablets from health food stores. Follow package directions for dosage. Take supplements at least 2 hours after the antibiotic. Otherwise, you'll risk killing off the bacteria in the supplement. If you have any serious gastrointestinal problems that require medical attention, check with your doctor before taking the supplement.

---

your partner both work close to home, consider meeting for a lunchtime rendezvous.

Banish Vaginal Dryness

When a woman reaches menopause and estrogen levels are at an all-time low, the walls of her vagina may become weak, thin, and dry enough to cause discomfort, especially during sex. For some, intercourse may hurt even with ample foreplay. To remedy vaginal dryness, experts offer the following advice.

Use the right lubricant. You might be tempted to use reach for the petroleum jelly. Not a good idea! Petroleum jelly can break down condoms.

Plus, it isn't water-soluble, so it remains in the vagina, where it can harbor yeast and other infection-producing microbes.

Instead, try a vaginal lubricant, such as Astroglide or K-Y Jelly, designed to relieve friction during sex by coating your vaginal walls. Unlike a moisturizer, lubricants tend to evaporate, and often need to be reapplied during intercourse.

Try an estrogen cream. These prescription creams are applied directly into the vagina. They relieve dryness by keeping vaginal tissue moist, healthy, and strong, explains Brian Walsh, M.D., assistant professor of obstetrics and gynecology and reproductive biology at Harvard Medical School and the director of the Menopause Clinic at Brigham and Women's Hospital, both in Boston. Because the hormone stays mostly in the vagina, estrogen creams don't raise blood levels of estrogen, making this an attractive option if you experience breakthrough bleeding or other undesirable side effects from estrogen in pill form.

Use a vaginal ring. The ring—about the size of a diaphragm and inserted by either you or your doctor—is kept in the vagina for up to 3 months, where it releases a steady, low dose of estrogen, says Dr. Walsh. Studies show that it works well to relieve both vaginal dryness and urinary tract complaints. Some women prefer the ring over creams because it's less messy.

Moisturize from the inside out. Vaginal moisturizers won't strengthen or build up weakened vaginal walls—only estrogen can do that—but if you prefer to use over-the-counter remedies instead of prescription medications, products such as Replens can hydrate the vagina and relieve irritation for 2 to 3 days. They're available in suppositories, or single-use applicators for convenience. And they're estrogen-free, pH-balanced, nonirritating, and safe to use with condoms. (Check product labeling.)

Lubricate with licorice. Although licorice is better known for treating coughs and ulcers, natural health care professionals have found that it does wonders for toning the mucous membranes of the reproductive system as well. "When tender vaginal tissue needs to be moistened, licorice is a choice remedy," according to Helen Healy, N.D., a naturopathic physician and the director of the Wellspring Naturopathic Clinic in St. Paul, Minnesota.

Unlike topically applied lubricants, which are quickly absorbed into the vaginal tissue, licorice is believed to imitate the role of estrogen in the body, activating the production of mucus and helping to "plump up" the thinning vaginal wall, says Dr. Healy. For that reason, it's a good remedy for women who forgo hormone therapy (HT, formerly HRT, hormone replacement therapy). She suggests using only deglycyrrhizinated licorice, labeled DGL. Whole licorice can stimulate the adrenal glands, which aggravates hypertension and could create serious risks, especially in aging women. Tablets marked DGL provide the benefits without those risks.

Begin by taking two 380-milligram tablets of the dried herb three times daily to keep the vaginal area moist throughout the day, she says. Once the vaginal tissue is fortified, you might find that fewer tablets are

RECLAIMING YOUR SEXUALITY

It's not unusual for a postmenopausal woman to experience a narrowing of the vagina that prevents penetration, particularly if she has spent years without a partner. Fortunately, a vaginal dilator can retrain her anatomy for a sexual relationship.

A dilator is a smooth glass wand that is inserted manually into the vagina on a daily basis for anywhere from 1 to 6 months, explains Brian Walsh, M.D., assistant professor of obstetrics and gynecology and reproductive biology at Harvard Medical School and the director of the Menopause Clinic at Brigham and Women's Hospital, both in Boston. In cases of severe narrowing, a patient may need to gradually increase the size of the dilator over a period of months. Once the muscles are widened, the condition will not return as long as regular intercourse is resumed.

A long hiatus from sex can also heighten the effects of the vaginal atrophy common among menopausal women. Atrophy is characterized by drying and thinning of tissues in and around the vagina, a situation that makes it prone to infection and easily irritated. To offset those symptoms, dilators are normally used in conjunction with topical estrogen creams, which enable the vagina to produce natural secretions and improve suppleness. Both dilators and estrogen creams are available by prescription only.

necessary. Use it as long as needed. Incidentally, if you're a fan of licorice sticks, don't try them—or any other licorice candy—instead of the licorice tablets. Licorice candy contains no herbal licorice at all. (Sorry!)

Avoid antihistamines. The antihistamines you take to relieve your nose and eyes during the allergy season may stifle sexual comfort. That's because in addition to drying out the mucous membranes in your sinuses, these drugs also rob moisture from the lining of your vagina.

As an alternative to antihistamine drugs, consider using the nutritional supplement quercetin, a bioflavonoid derived from citrus fruits and buckwheat, suggests Tori Hudson, N.D., professor at the National College of Naturopathic Medicine and the medical director of A Woman's Time clinic, both in Portland, Oregon. Rather than drying out your body, quercetin goes to work on the cells that release histamines, stabilizing them and preventing such reactions as watery eyes and runny noses. Dr. Hudson recommends taking 200 to 400 milligrams of quercetin three times per day, between meals, through allergy season. Quercetin is available in tablet form from health food stores and drugstores.

Discover Your Alluring Self

If you've been with the same man for years, you might think it's impossible to get that magic back. The thought might even make you smile. Me? Alluring to the man I've shared a bathroom with for years? Yes and yes. That's because allure isn't just a way to get a partner. It's a way to keep one.

"Making an effort to look attractive to your partner is a sign of respect," says Carol Rinkleib Ellison, Ph.D., a clinical psychologist and sex researcher in Oakland, California. "It says, 'You're important to me.'" That said, the simplest changes are often the most dramatic. You'll find lots of great suggestions for enhancing your looks in chapter 6. Here are some of the experts' favorites.

Apply some lipstick. Lipstick lights up your face. You don't have to go for vixen-red lips (unless you want to). Cool colors, such as cranberry and raspberry, look best on fair or ruddy skin; warm colors, such as brick and coral, on darker skin. Add lip gloss over the lipstick for moist, larger-looking lips.

PAMPER YOURSELF CAREFULLY

Bath oils, bubbles, deodorant soaps, douches, decorative toilet tissue, and even some laundry detergents can trigger discomfort in your delicate vaginal tissues—a particular concern for menopausal women, according to Mary Jane Minkin, M.D., clinical professor of obstetrics and gynecology at Yale University School of Medicine and coauthor of *What Every Woman Needs to Know about Menopause.*

Before the onset of menopause, the hormone estrogen keeps your vagina lubricated, which protects it from potentially irritating substances. But as estrogen levels start to drop, the mucous membranes of your vagina become thinner and less moist. Soaps, which wash away your body's protective oils, only enhance that drying effect, increasing the likelihood of painful intercourse. What's more, once damaged by irritants, thin vaginal tissues are more prone to yeast and bacterial infections, another source of sexual discomfort.

Deodorant soaps, which usually contain perfumes and dyes, can be especially hard on sensitive tissue. Two milder brands that Dr. Minkin recommends are Dove (white only) and Neutrogena. When it comes to baths, soaking in a tub of soapy bubbles or scented oils is an invitation for irritation. Showers are best, but oatmeal baths, or even daily baths without added soaps, are also okay.

As for laundry detergents, it's best to stick to the brand your body's used to. But if you notice irritation, switch to something without scents or bleaching agents. Flush your affection for decorative or colored toilet tissue as well, she says. Always use an undyed or white variety since dyes are potential irritants. And definitely don't douche, Dr. Minkin says. Douching further strips your vagina of natural lubricants.

Update your 'do. Many women wear the same hairstyle for decades, which is a big mistake. But you don't want to entrust just any stylist with your new look. Look for a salon with a well-established clientele and a reputation for being trendy but not bizarre. To find the right stylist, look for someone who's around your age and has an attractive, updated look.

Sexier hairstyles are tousled with lots of volume. But ideally your style should also be low-maintenance and loose enough so that you (or your partner!) can run your fingers through it.

Ignore the scale. Just because you might be carrying a few more pounds than you'd like doesn't necessarily mean you're less alluring. (In fact, your spouse might appreciate your curvy, womanly figure a *lot* more than you do. Ask him!) You just have to flatter your proportions. If you have larger hips, for example, balance your silhouette with shoulder pads. Avoid skirts and pants with pleats, and dress in one color.

Flaunt your assets. The greatest beauty secret of all: Work with what you have—and then work it. If you've always been told that you have beautiful hands, treat yourself to a weekly manicure and call attention to your hands with beautiful rings. If he has always loved your breasts, accentuate them with exquisite brassieres and scoop-neck shirts and sweaters.

(Un)Dress for Success

Sexy lingerie really can add spice to your sex life—and we guarantee that it will get his interest. So . . . are you ready to graduate from "plain vanilla" briefs and a bra? As with blouses or shoes, you may not know what

CHANGE YOUR VIDEO FARE

If you're spending too many nights renting *Star Trek* videos rather than shooting off your own rockets, you and your lover might consider a more arousing form of entertainment. Films with steamy love scenes, particularly those depicting the kind of characters you can relate to, can turn up the heat for menopausal women who experience low libidos, according to Barbara D. Bartlik, M.D., clinical assistant professor in the department of psychiatry at Weill Medical College of Cornell University and assistant attending psychiatrist at the New York Presbyterian Hospital, both in New York City.

Since your estrogen and testosterone levels wane as you age, you may encounter diminished sensitivity in your breasts and genital area, often increasing the time it takes to feel sexually aroused. The bottom line is that many women require more intense forms of stimulation, and that's where erotic films can help. Erotic images actually flood the body with some of the same hormones that sex does. Not only can torrid love scenes excite sexual feelings, but they can also introduce you to new, possibly more enjoyable methods for achieving fulfillment, says Dr. Bartlik.

you want until you try it on. But it always helps to have some idea of what you're looking for. Is it elegant or racy, or somewhere in between? Which features do you want to accentuate? What's your psychological comfort level? Here are some ideas to help you choose your new undercover look.

Go on a lingerie safari. Wander through department and lingerie stores and see what catches your eye. Bright colors or dark jewel tones? Silk and satin, or fishnet and feathers? Styles that cover, or that reveal? Whatever you choose, you should feel emotionally comfortable in it, but it should also give you a feeling of excitement and anticipation.

Accentuate the positives. Lingerie should always accentuate the body part you're most proud of while it downplays flaws. If you're big all over, try a full-length silk or satin gown (perhaps with strategically placed lace, ties, or cutaways). If you have heavy hips and thighs, avoid thongs, and choose a knee-length gown or a baby-doll style that comes to just above the knees. And if you're small-chested, don't think that bustiers are only for the well-endowed—many women with a small bust can look

Unlike pornography, the type of film you might want to seek out, as a mature woman, is from the "erotica" category of adult entertainment. Good erotica films feature respectable characters in sensitive, sexually charged relationships. If you're scanning the video shelves looking for a little sophistication, select films produced by women and those depicting more mature couples on the cover, says Dr. Bartlik. Keep in mind also that films featuring characters with less "model-like" bodies will help you connect to the action better than those targeted to a younger audience.

Videos that have a menopausal woman's needs in mind can be discreetly purchased online or through mail order. The Femme Productions company, for example, uniquely offers films written and produced by women and claims to promote a softer, more sensual approach to erotic film by tapping into a woman's version of sexual fantasy. To purchase a video, contact Candida Royalle's Femme online at www.royalle.com, or call (800) 456-LOVE for a catalog.

great in a bustier (or one of the many new water- and air-filled push-up bras designed to amplify your curves).

Pick the right color. Color sends a message. If you want to play innocent, wear white or soft pink. If you want to be the harlot, wear red or leopard-patterned. If you're not sure, go with classic black or a jewel tone.

Add sexy heels. High-heeled pumps make any woman's legs look longer and thinner.

Indulge in Herbal Aphrodisiacs

Herbalists say that you can recapture that "swept away" feeling with the help of herbal potions, oils, and teas. Here are the details on the passion-producing botanicals that can help the most.

Breathe in a sensual aroma. If you want to subtly perfume the air with sensuality and create a passionate atmosphere, there are several essential oils to consider. Rose and amber have long associations with love and sensuality, and some say the scent of sandalwood can make you feel very centered in your body, very aware of physical sensation. Just add a few droplets of your chosen essential oil to a cup of warm water (the heat will release the aroma). But don't drink it by mistake!

Take massage to new heights. Just a few drops of the same essential oils, when added to an ounce of jojoba oil, can bring new sensual dimensions to a full-body massage before lovemaking. Massage each other from head to toe. Concentrate first on relaxation by working on tense spots such as the upper back, then let your touch become slower, more caressing, even arousing. Include erogenous zones like the backs of the knees and the inner thighs.

Drink some damiana. The Mexican herb damiana has a widely established folk reputation for enlivening the feminine libido, explains David Winston, a founding member of the American Herbalists Guild who works in Washington, New Jersey. Experts don't agree on whether or not it's medically warranted as an aphrodisiac, but the herb is generally accepted for its ability to stabilize your emotions. Because of the herb's mild mood-enhancement abilities, Winston recommends damiana when he hears women complain of low libido. The theory is that since the herb can curb your anxiety levels and lift you out of the doldrums, your lovin' feelings have more chance to flourish. To make a quick damiana tea, pour boiling water over dried damiana leaves in a cup and let them steep for 10 minutes.

For more hints on lifting your libido, see page 281.

Sex and Chronic Disease

Couples living with a major illness, such as heart disease or cancer, often struggle with sexual problems. Sometimes they give up on sex entirely. And that's too bad because our sexual feelings and our need for physical closeness don't end when we get sick. If anything, they become more important.

At the same time, it's not fair to expect that a major health problem will have no effect on a couple's sexuality or level of intimacy. So what follows is a condition-by-condition guide to four major health problems, all of which can be experienced by menopausal and postmenopausal women. It explains how each can affect sexuality and offers practical ways to express sexual feelings that don't necessarily involve intercourse.

Arthritis: Go for a Good Soak

In the most common form of arthritis, known as osteoarthritis, the cartilage that covers the ends of bones degenerates, causing bone to rub against bone. This friction causes pain and swelling of the joints, most commonly in the hips, knees, and back. This pain and swelling also limit flexibility, which can make sex difficult.

Not surprisingly, many women with arthritis lose interest in sex, and it's not hard to see why: Being in physical pain doesn't naturally lead most of us to erotic thoughts.

If possible, treat yourself (and your mate) to a hot tub. Water's soothing warmth and buoyancy can relieve joint pain and stiffness (It's also an ideal place to cuddle, talk, or fool around.) If you have lung or heart disease, diabetes, or high or low blood pressure, or have undergone joint replacement, don't use a hot tub without asking your doctor first.

If you never seem to feel in the mood, talk to your doctor. Common arthritis medications, such as prednisone and muscle relaxants, can affect sex drive and the ability to climax. You may be able to take another medication that works just as well but doesn't dampen your libido.

And finally, don't let a negative body image cheat you out of sex. To feel better about your body, pamper it. Take scented bubble baths. Sleep on satin sheets. Treat yourself to a massage. (Ask your partner if he might serve as your masseur.) And if your doctor says it's okay, get regular exercise. Working out often makes people feel stronger, both physically and mentally.

Cancer: Try a Little Kama Sutra

Being diagnosed with cancer—and living with it—can be emotionally devastating. Understandably, both men and women can experience an emotional shutdown that kills sexual desire. To complicate matters, cancer treatments can affect desire and performance. If a woman's ovaries are surgically removed or are damaged by chemotherapy, for example, the resulting sudden loss of estrogen can cause her vagina to become dry and tight, one symptom of sudden menopause.

If lovemaking in the missionary position hurts, experiment with other positions that let you control the movement. The woman-on-top position, for example, often works well. Or you and your partner can try lying on your sides, either face-to-face or in a "spooning" position. If you have had a mastectomy and aren't ready to expose the scar during intercourse, consider wearing a brief nightgown or a camisole, or a bra with a prosthesis inside.

Above all, it's especially important to be patient and flexible with each other. It seems obvious, but when you feel angry, sad, or vulnerable, share those feelings with your partner. While the things you used to do in bed may no longer be possible or practical, learning to express and respond to negative feelings can strengthen your trust in each other, which can increase intimacy and make it easier to be sexually playful.

Heart Disease: Start Small

When we're aroused, our hearts beat faster and we breathe more rapidly. That's why many people still mistakenly believe that sex is a no-no for anyone with a heart problem. And while studies do suggest that women with heart disease may be more depressed and take longer to resume sexual activity than men, it's really common only in the movies for people to have heart attacks during sex. In fact, if either of you is depressed, tender touching may actually make you feel better

Nonetheless, according to one estimate, between 50 and 75 percent of men and women who have had heart attacks drastically cut down on sex or avoid it completely. In order to reclaim your sex life, start with the small gestures. Take the pressure off intercourse and instead focus on holding, kissing, or caressing each other. Discover other ways to give and receive pleasure, such as mutual massage or oral sex.

If you take the prescription heart drug nitroglycerin for chest pain associated with exertion, your doctor will probably suggest that you take it shortly before sex to stave off the pain of an angina attack. If you take other medications, pay attention to how they may affect your sex drive or performance. If either of you seems impaired by prescriptions, your doctor may be able to switch you to a different, yet still effective, drug.

Osteoporosis: Take It from the Top

Sex can't be gratifying if it means putting painful pressure on frail bones threatened or damaged by osteoporosis. In the advanced stages of the disease, the bones in your spine can become so weak that they break, literally, with a sneeze. These fractures are painful and take a long time to heal. What's more, bones elsewhere in your body are also more fragile and susceptible to breaks, especially the hips and wrists.

Therefore, having sex while lying on your back with the full weight of your partner on top can be both dangerous and painful if you have brittle bones. But just because the missionary position is uncomfortable does not mean that you have to take a vow of celibacy. Rather, taking the lead in sex will ensure your safety and comfort.

Climbing on top could take you back into the pleasure zone. "If you want to avoid pain, the woman-on-top position may help because you have more control," explains Domeena C. Renshaw, M.D., professor and assistant chairperson in the department of psychiatry and the director of the Sexual Dysfunction Clinic at the Loyola University Medical Center in Chicago.

The most basic method is to lie over your partner; this is called a reverse missionary position when the woman is on top. Or you can sit up and straddle his pelvis (unless, of course, you have knee pain). In that case, continue to experiment with positions where you are on top. Dr. Renshaw reminds couples to maintain a sense of humor and adventure about testing new positions, and to communicate about what feels pleasurable for both.

The most important thing to remember about sex and menopause is this: It ain't over yet. If you keep an open mind and make the effort to engage your partner, you may find postmenopausal sex to be the best sex of your life. (After all, there are no periods, no birth control, and no kids in the house!) Enjoy yourself: You deserve it.

Menopause Symptoms and Solutions

The best way to get through menopause is to find out everything you can about it—the symptoms, the treatments, the options. In this section, we'll give you an overview of the symptoms you may experience and all the ways to handle them, as well as the benefits and drawbacks of every treatment option. Armed with the latest information, you can make the right choices for who you are, your unique lifestyle, and your menopause experience.

Chapter

10

THE MENOPAUSE
SYMPTOM SOLVER

Menopause ushers in a host of changes to body and mind, some of which are admittedly difficult to ignore, like hot flashes and weight gain. At the opposite end of the spectrum are the silent changes—such as rising blood pressure—which are frequently undetected despite their serious consequences. Somewhere in the middle lurk the easily overlooked changes that are often chalked up to everyday stress, like insomnia or anxiety.

And while the changes that menopause brings can affect the quality of your life, the extent to which they do is largely up to you—that is, if you're prepared to handle them head-on. To help you do just that, this chapter covers the most common symptoms associated with menopause in an easy-to-use A-to-Z format, beginning with Anxiety and going all the way through to Weight Gain. Just look up the symptom or symptoms that are bothering you, and we'll show you exactly what you can do to keep them from undermining your health and happiness. We've also included "Medical Alert" boxes that give you a heads-up on problems that might require attention from your doctor.

Ready to find some answers to keep you from muddling through menopause? Read on, and take charge of what can be the time of your life.

ANXIETY

Rare is the woman who reaches menopause without having lain awake her fair share of nights worrying over *something*, be it her job, a child's grades, or the gray hairs that sprout in her brush. But don't worry. That's normal.

"When we're confronted with problems and don't have solutions, the emotional response is anxiety," says Susan Heitler, Ph.D., a clinical psychologist in Denver and author of the audiotape *Anxiety: Friend or Foe?* "Women are especially likely to experience anxiety when they're vaguely disturbed about a problem, like having too much to do and too little time in which to do it."

In women, hormonal fluctuations may also play a role in aggravating the anxiety response, though scientists have yet to figure out how or why. They do know that women seem more prone to anxious feelings just prior to their periods as well during puberty and around menopause—times of life when hormone levels change dramatically.

The fact is that millions of us worry too much. We virtually train ourselves to worry, sometimes to the point where it brings on feelings of vulnerability, which of course only reinforces the habit. So how do you reverse the process if you've crossed the worry line?

Give yourself permission to feel anxious. Try to perceive your anxiety as a yellow light, not a red stop sign, advises Dr. Heitler. "Anxiety tells you to look at how you can deal more effectively with a potential problem. It doesn't tell you to give up on doing what you want to do."

SIGNS AND SYMPTOMS

ANXIETY

Anxiety is often confused with fear. The difference is that with fear, you know what's scaring you and can take action. Because anxiety is dread of the not yet known, tracing your feelings to a particular problem can be difficult. Left unchecked, anxiety can lead to sleeplessness, irritability, overeating or loss of appetite, and difficulty concentrating. It may also contribute to high blood pressure and heart disease.

What Can You Do?

If you are living with anxiety that amounts to more than everyday worry, prescription medication and therapy with a trained counselor are probably in order. You can take some natural steps, however, to reduce and eliminate worry and negative stress and to minimize anxiety-related episodes.

Never worry alone. When you talk about your worries with a trusted friend, coworker, or relative, the toxicity dissipates. You find solutions; your concerns aren't so overwhelming. Research shows that the more isolated we feel, the more we tend to worry.

Let the worry go. Chronic worriers have a difficult time doing this because they usually do just the opposite. They hold on as though worrying will fix the problem. It won't.

Devise an action plan. "The very best antidote to anxiety is to gather information," says Dr. Heitler. Pull out a sheet of paper and write down exactly what is bugging you. Then review your list and note what you need to handle the problems. "For example, if you're losing your job, write down your fears of not having enough money to pay bills or whether you'll find another job quickly. Perhaps you can get information from your family about loan possibilities or talk to human resources about other positions within your company," she suggests.

Take a breather. When you feel that you are in the grip of anxious feelings, take a relaxing, cleansing breath. Close your eyes and inhale deeply from your belly. Silently repeat the word "calm," drawing out the *m* and exhaling to a count of 10. Repeat three or four times.

Take the fantasy route. Sit down in a comfortable chair, close your eyes, and picture yourself lying on a beautiful beach on a tropical island. Inhale and exhale deeply as you visualize yourself basking in the sunshine, listening to the ocean waves, and seeing the palm trees rustling in the wind. "Soon enough, your breathing and heart rate will slow down, your stress level will drop, your anxiety will disappear, and your thoughts will clear," says Dr. Heitler.

Avoid the superwoman trap. If you usually have 20 errands to run and household chores to do, decide which are the most important and postpone the rest. "You may have to cut back the number of hours you

Medical Alert

ANXIETY

If your symptoms disrupt your life, making it impossible to work, drive, or simply enjoy the day without a torrent of fears and worries, see your doctor. And if feelings of anxiety are accompanied by physical symptoms, such as heart palpitations, trembling, sweating, headaches, nausea, faintness, or shortness of breath, an underlying anxiety disorder may be at play. But you're not alone—more than 19 million people in the United States live with an anxiety disorder, a type of medical illness that includes panic attacks, phobias, post-traumatic stress disorder, obsessive-compulsive disorder, and generalized anxiety disorder. Many different options for medication and forms of talk therapy exist that may help you regain a sense of normalcy in your day-to-day life.

spend on work, split the chores and errands with your husband, or hire some help," says Dr. Heitler.

Find time to have fun. Make personal time a priority. Schedule fun things on your calendar, and don't let other matters interfere—even if it means leaving your job on time (for a change) or saying no to another obligation.

"At the end of the workday, make it a point to leave your job emotionally as well as physically. When you get home, order out for dinner and relax by lying down and listening to music, reading, or playing with the dog or cat," says Dr. Heitler. It's essential to good health that we make time to relax and unwind.

The good thing about feeling anxious is that it's a barometer, giving you feedback on what's going on in your life. "So listen to your anxious feelings and begin shortening your to-do list to a manageable size," she says. (Find more on moods on page 323.)

BREAST PAIN AND LUMPS

Breast pain is so common that just about every woman will experience it at some point in her life. And because women tend to fear breast cancer more than any other disease, it's understandable that "Is it cancer?" is the first question we typically ask. Fortunately, breast pain is rarely a symptom of breast cancer and often resolves on its own.

Hormonal changes or premenstrual water retention, which tend to occur in both breasts, may be to blame since pain and swelling usually correspond to the menstrual cycle. Sometimes, tender fluid-filled cysts or benign lumps develop in the milk glands, leading to fibrocystic breast disease. This common cyclical condition, which is not really a disease, is caused by accumulated fluid and strands of fibrous tissue. Other, noncyclical causes of breast pain include trauma, infection, and injury.

If you're not sure why you have breast pain, try keeping a daily diary for a month or two and see if the pain comes and goes with your menstrual cycle. Note also the degree to which it interferes with your daily life.

Then see your doctor for a clinical breast exam. Ask to have a mammogram, if needed, to rule out a more serious cause for your pain and inflammation—not to mention for your own peace of mind. For persistent breast pain, ask your doctor about taking the prescription medication danazol (Danocrine). The typical dosage is usually 200 milligrams a day.

For more on reducing breast cancer risk, see page 312.

What Can You Do?

Assuming that your doctor has assured you that you have nothing serious to worry about, here is what experts suggest to relieve breast pain and perhaps even reduce the lumpiness on your own.

Strike oil. Evening primrose oil is an anti-inflammatory that can relieve tenderness and help shrink breast cysts. It is rich in gamma-linolenic acid, an essential fatty acid, and is available over-the-counter. Try taking

SIGNS AND SYMPTOMS

BREAST PAIN AND LUMPS

Breast pain and inflammation are more common in younger women who are still menstruating than in postmenopausal women. Discomfort ranges from mild tenderness in some women to excruciating pain in others.

two 500-milligram capsules a day to start—but no more than six a day. For some women, it can take several months before they experience relief.

Cut the caffeine. Coffee, tea, cola, and chocolate contain methyl-xanthines, naturally occurring substances that may contribute to a fibro-cystic breast problem.

Pop extra E. Some studies have shown that taken in significant doses, vitamin E can prevent breast lumps from returning, though the results are mixed. Nonetheless, many people swear by this remedy, and some experts think it may be because vitamin E encourages your body to get rid of the excess estrogen that seems to aggravate sensitive breast tissue. Take 400 to 600 IU a day. (Get your doctor's go-ahead first.)

Feast on fiber. Build your diet around plant foods such as fruits, vegetables, legumes, and whole grain bread, pasta, and cereals. A low-fat, high-fiber diet lowers estrogen levels, which means less lumpiness and discomfort.

Wrap them in ginger. This pungent herb is a powerful anti-inflam-matory that will relieve the soreness and reduce swelling, says Mindy Green, a founder and professional member of the American Herbalists Guild and director of education services for the Herb Research Founda-tion in Boulder, Colorado. Grate one-quarter cup of the fresh herb. Sprinkle the shavings evenly on a thin cloth. Fold in half. Then wet it with hot water. Apply to each breast for 10 to 20 minutes. Repeat two or three times a day, if possible.

If using powdered ginger (the kind found in your spice rack) is more convenient, add 1 teaspoon of powdered ginger to 2 cups of hot water. Dip a washcloth in the solution and apply it to your skin.

If you have sensitive skin, rub some vegetable oil on your breasts be-fore applying the ginger compress. The oil may help prevent your skin from turning red and overheating.

Soothe with castor oil. Castor oil is great for relieving tenderness and breaking up fibrous tissue, says Mindy.

Dip a dry washcloth in some castor oil and apply it to your breasts. Place a hot-water bottle on top of the washcloth for 20 to 30 minutes. Or rub the castor oil directly onto your breasts. Cover them with plastic wrap and a thin towel. Place a hot-water bottle on top for the same amount of time.

Medical Alert
BREAST PAIN AND LUMPS

See your doctor if your breast pain continues every month despite self-treat-ment. You should also see your doctor if you notice:

- Breast pain that comes on suddenly, especially when you haven't been experiencing monthly pain
- Breast pain that occurs after you start a new medication or hormone therapy
- Bloody or milky discharge from one or both nipples
- Any breast lump or thickening, whether or not it is painful

---

Wear a supportive bra. The mere act of not wearing a bra can contribute to breast pain since the weight of the breasts itself can cause discomfort. So, for many women, wearing a supportive bra is helpful. Be sure you wear a bra that's constructed in a way that won't add to the irritation. Look inside the cups and make sure that there are no seams and that nothing is pushing up against you. If there is an underwire, make sure that it's very well-padded so that it doesn't add to the friction. Sports bras usually fit all of these criteria.

DEPRESSION

Women are three times more likely than men to develop depression. In addition, "women have times in their lives when they seem especially vulnerable to depression," says Laura Epstein Rosen, Ph.D., supervisor of family therapy training for the Special Needs Clinic at Columbia-Presbyterian Medical Center in New York City. Sometimes the risk is biologically driven, as when hormone levels fluctuate just after childbirth and just before menopause. Other times it is externally driven—perhaps by the death of a parent, divorce, job loss, or some other major life event.

Even everyday conflict can brew into mild depression, says Susan Heitler, Ph.D., a clinical psychologist in Denver and author of the audiotape

DEPRESSION

Mild depression often manifests itself as deeply negative feelings of sorrow, guilt, discouragement, and powerlessness. More severe cases may be accompanied by symptoms such as loss of appetite, lack of sleep, and difficulty concentrating. (See page 323 for more on mood disorders.)

Depression: A Disorder of Power. "When you want *x* and your partner wants *y*, you have a problem," she explains. If you repeatedly give up what you want so that your partner gets what he wants, without seeking a mutually satisfying compromise, you may pay an emotional price in the long run.

The good news about depression is that once you recognize that you have it, you can treat it. "By knowing when you are vulnerable to depression and by recognizing its signs and symptoms, you can get the help you need," says Dr. Rosen.

What's more, depression may draw your attention to some aspect of your life that needs evaluation and change, says Margaret Jensvold, M.D., director of the Institute for Research on Women's Health in Rockville, Maryland. "If you find yourself repeatedly getting upset or sad about the same situation, you need to come to terms with that situation, one way or another," she advises.

What Can You Do?

For severe depression, you will need to see a doctor, who may recommend a combination of talk therapy and antidepressant drugs. Mild depression responds well to self-care measures like these.

Illuminate yourself. "Before we use any herbs or supplements, we need to find out what's causing the depression," says Ellen Kamhi, R.N., Ph.D., author of *Cycles of Life: Herbs and Energy Techniques for Women*. Sometimes it's something relatively simple, like lack of sunlight, which can be treated with a light box.

Light treatment should be considered even before using herbs, she says, because there are no chemicals or toxicities in light, and you can operate a light box at work or home. Use this treatment only in consultation with your doctor, who can explain proper use of the box and set up an appropriate treatment schedule.

Eat small meals every 2 or 3 hours. Sticking with a regular mini-meal schedule helps keep your blood sugar on a more even keel. "For some people, low blood sugar can trigger depression," says Dr. Jensvold. Of course, you should make sure that each mini-meal is well-balanced. Choose healthy foods such as whole grains, fruits, vegetables, and fat-free or low-fat dairy products.

Grab your partner. A study published in the *Journal of Nervous and Mental Disease* found that having a supportive spouse and other positive relationships reduced the likelihood of major depression.

Move for your mood. Physical activity is a great way to prevent and treat depression. Researchers don't know exactly why exercise helps, but they suggest it may enhance our sense of mastery so we feel more mentally and physically in control. Aerobic activity may also help vent pent-up frustration. And mood-enhancing endorphins (those brain chemicals responsible for the phenomenon known as "runner's high") released during exercise could also be involved. Aim for at least 30 minutes of exercise most days. If you want, you can break it into three sets of 10 minutes each.

Medical Alert

DEPRESSION

See your doctor if you have suicidal thoughts or have had a distinct period during which you felt down and unhappy or unable to enjoy life and have experienced any of the following symptoms for 2 weeks or longer. You may have severe depression, which requires professional care.

- Appetite or weight changes
- Sleep problems
- Excessive fatigue
- Excessive agitation or lethargy
- Guilty feelings
- Slow thinking or indecisiveness

Expand your exercise horizons. Yoga and tai chi are excellent depression remedies. For one thing, if you take a class, you'll bond with others, says Dr. Kamhi. Also, some movements and breathing exercises in yoga and tai chi can stimulate glands to release mood-enhancing hormones.

FATIGUE

Fatigue is such a broad term that it can mean many different things to different people. To women facing menopause, being tired may mean that they can't lift a finger to wash another dish, while for others it means that they're so cranky that they want to sit in their cars and scream. Still others define it as not being able to get out of bed in the morning.

Understandably, such variety in meaning makes it difficult to use in diagnosing an illness. One way to help measure fatigue, however, is to consider its relation to time. Once you've determined how long your fatigue has been around, start asking other specific questions, such as what activities make you feel most tired, whom are you with when you feel tired, and how does being tired feel. This information is like gold to your doctor, who may be able to help you resolve the problem without any further treatment.

Acute fatigue—that is, lasting less than 1 month—is often easier to diagnose because chances are you know the cause. If you have the flu, for example, you probably wouldn't even mention a concern about fatigue to your doctor because you know why you're so tired. Prolonged fatigue typically lasts 1 to 6 months. Often, women who are depressed will have this

---

SIGNS AND SYMPTOMS

FATIGUE

Fatigue is a feeling of tiredness all too familiar to most people. The problem is so common that doctors estimate about 1 out of every 10 people (many of them women) may be troubled by daytime fatigue. In fact, 8 out of 10 people who are referred to sleep specialists don't have trouble getting to sleep—they have trouble staying awake.

type of fatigue—it develops not overnight but over a couple of months of worry, sadness, stress, or sleepless nights. Another fatiguing condition that can come on gradually is hypothyroidism, in which the thyroid doesn't produce enough of its hormone, resulting in low energy levels. If you don't seek help for these conditions, you may stray into chronic fatigue territory, more than 6 months of exhaustion.

Chronic fatigue is definitely not something you should try to cope with on your own since it could reflect a serious health concern, cautions Dianne Delva, associate professor of family medicine at Queen's University in Kingston, Ontario. For instance, chronic fatigue could be a sign of type 2 diabetes. Left untreated, it could lead to kidney or heart disease, blindness, stroke, or other health problems.

What Can You Do?

Prolonged and chronic fatigue require a doctor's care. But to help reverse short bouts of fatigue, try these natural energy-boosting strategies.

Eat early. The sooner you eat, the better. But if you just can't face food first thing in the morning, make sure you sit down to a nutritious meal within 3 hours. Breakfast helps your body rev up after sleeping and helps prevent you from eating too much lunch, which can sap energy in the afternoon.

At midday, focus on protein. The amino acid tyrosine, supplied by high-protein food, synthesizes more of the brain's alertness chemicals and keeps the brain from manufacturing the neurotransmitter serotonin, which slows you down.

Nix caffeine after 4:30 P.M. Since caffeine keeps you alert for up to 6 hours, it can prevent you from getting to sleep at a regular time if you consume it in the evening. That's *all* sources of caffeine, by the way—including chocolate, cola, and tea.

Drink water. Aim for eight 8-ounce glasses of water every day. Dehydration can cause your performance to flag measurably. Keeping a ready supply of water nearby throughout the day will encourage you to drink as much as you need, when you need it. Try leaving a water bottle on your desk or taking it with you in the car.

Medical Alert

FATIGUE

If you have experienced fatigue for longer than a month, see a doctor.

Treat yourself. Sometimes energy levels slump not because of how much you do but because how much energy you expend on behalf of everyone but yourself. So, give yourself a prescription to do something for yourself today—take a half day off and do something just for you!

Take a walk. Just 20 minutes of walking, ideally after breakfast or lunch, will buoy your energy levels for as much as 8 hours afterward. But don't exercise within several hours of bedtime because you may be too energized to fall asleep.

Don't spend too much time in bed. Sleeping too much can make you feel more, rather than less, fatigued, says Alexander C. Chester, M.D., clinical professor of medicine at the Georgetown University Medical Center in Washington, D.C. Most people need 7 to 8 hours of sleep a night, no more.

Count the hours in your day. If you're like many women, you may have an unrealistic idea of how long it takes to perform your daily chores, and you might be trying to accomplish more than is humanly possible— which only leaves you exhausted.

To take stock, write down everything that you do each day. Next to each task, estimate how much time each task truly takes. Don't leave anything out, from the moment you rise until bedtime. Then add up the hours. If you're trying to do 23 hours' worth of work in 16 waking hours, give yourself a reality check, adjust your efforts, and concentrate on doing just one thing at a time.

FRACTURES

Throughout our lives, our bones break down and rebuild in a carefully balanced process. Because the body needs small amounts of calcium circulating in the blood to help with muscle contraction and blood clotting, it frees up calcium by creating small holes in bones. To keep things in balance, the holes are then quickly repaired. Each year, 10 to 30 percent of your skeleton goes through this bone breakdown and rebuilding—but the process changes as we age, and we no longer rebuild bone as quickly as it is broken down.

The result of this imbalance? On average, we lose one-third of our bone in the first 5 years after menopause, when our ovaries stop producing the estrogen that keeps bone loss to a minimum. And although we still get estrogen from body fat, skin, and muscle after menopause, it's not enough to significantly protect against bone loss.

Unless we take protective measures, this bone loss can advance to osteoporosis, a disease in which the bones become fragile and fracture easily. In fact, one in two women will fracture a bone because of the disease.

What Can You Do?

Bone loss may be inevitable, but osteoporosis isn't. Too often, it is dismissed as a normal part of aging, but it's completely preventable. "Osteoporosis should never happen," says Nancy DiMarco, R.D., Ph.D., professor in the department of nutrition and food sciences at Texas Woman's University in Denton.

Most women know that calcium and weight-bearing exercise lower their risk of osteoporosis, but there's much more you can do to protect your bones. "I'm always surprised when women who say they exercise and take calcium think that's all they have to do," says Jane Lukacs, R.N.,

SIGNS AND SYMPTOMS

FRACTURES

After age 50, half of all American women have bones weak enough to fracture. And unfortunately for many, a fracture may be the first sign that osteoporosis has set in because there are virtually no outward symptoms before then.

Osteoporosis-related fractures commonly occur in the vertebra, hip, or forearm from surprisingly minor activities, such as bending over, lifting, jumping, or tripping. Once the disease progresses, just opening a door can result in broken bones.

Ph.D., a research fellow at the University of Michigan School of Nursing in Ann Arbor.

Don't stop there. Find out other ways to slow bone loss.

Count your calcium. Our bodies need to maintain about 2.2 pounds of calcium to keep bones healthy. But compared with younger women, women ages 65 and older are able to absorb less than half the calcium.

Between ages 19 and 50, you need at least 1,000 milligrams of calcium a day. That's about 3½ glasses of milk, Dr. DiMarco says. After age 50, aim for 1,200 milligrams, just half a glass more.

Eating dairy products, especially milk, is the best way to get calcium, Dr. DiMarco says, because they provide the most concentrated and absorbable form of calcium. Women who are lactose intolerant can usually handle a small amount of milk at a time—½ to 1 cup—without feeling sick, she adds.

If you don't like milk, there are plenty of other ways to get calcium, especially with the number of calcium-fortified foods on the rise. But don't go overboard. Try not to get more than 2,400 milligrams of calcium a day. Any amount over 2,400 milligrams may not be absorbed.

Drink tea. Women, especially postmenopausal ones, who drink 2 or more cups of coffee a day have reduced bone density because coffee increases calcium loss in urine.

Tea, on the other hand, has isoflavonoids, plant compounds that help our bones. A study of postmenopausal women in Great Britain found that drinking at least 1 cup of tea a day increased the drinkers' bone density by about 5 percent, compared with the bone density of women who didn't drink tea. Those who added milk had an even higher bone density.

Researchers think that isoflavonoids' ability to mimic estrogen helps maintain bone density in women after menopause.

Stop smoking. Do this, and you lower your risk of osteoporosis while you get rid of your smoker's cough. Women who smoke may have lower estrogen levels than women who don't, and they go through menopause 2 years earlier.

Drink moderately. Having seven or more alcoholic drinks a week increases your risk of falls and hip fractures. Alcohol also lowers your body's ability to build bone. Further, many women who drink too much

Medical Alert

FRACTURES

Fortunately, bone density tests can reveal signs of osteoporosis before breaks occur. Review the following list of risk factors and talk to your doctor about what type of screening is right for you.

- Thin and small-boned frame
- Irregular menstrual periods or fewer than 10 cycles a year
- History of eating disorders
- Family history of osteoporosis
- Generalized bone pain and tenderness
- Smoking
- History of taking corticosteroids, anticonvulsants such as phenytoin (Dilantin), thyroid medications, or blood thinners.

alcohol have poor nutrition habits, says Robert Marcus, M.D., an endocrinologist at Stanford University.

Fall-proof your house. If you've received a low score on a bone-mass screening, then a short fall for you could lead to a fracture, so take precautions around your home and in daily activities. Wear shoes that are appropriate for the surface you are walking on. Remove slippery throw rugs from your home, and keep electrical cords tucked out of the way. Watch where you walk, especially if the surfaces, such as streets and sidewalks, are uneven.

You'll find medical options for osteoporosis on page 324.

HAIR LOSS

Sure, men fret when they go bald. Some grow their remaining hair longer in the front or on one side and then comb it to cover their bare domes. Some even get toupees. But no matter how they cope, they have millions of other men with whom to share their pain.

Baldness is a different story for women. We're not *supposed* to go bald. "And with all the research that's gone into male-pattern baldness, the issue

---

SIGNS AND SYMPTOMS

HAIR LOSS

It's normal to lose 100 scalp hairs a day, but you have to lose much more, over 50 percent of your scalp hair, before the loss is noticeable. And that's just what happens to about 40 percent of women—they notice that their hair has thinned by the time they reach menopause.

---

in women has been relatively ignored," says Ellen W. Seely, M.D., director of clinical research in the endocrine–hypertension division at Brigham and Women's Hospital in Boston.

Most balding in women is caused by a condition known as androgenic alopecia (AGA)—the same condition that causes the majority of male baldness. Those of us with thinning hair can blame our genes, for one. "Many women with this problem had grandmothers who had it, and great-grandmothers who had it," says Dr. Seely.

But we can also blame our hormones. Testosterone, for one. Too much (in men or women) means that we're more likely to lose the hair on our heads yet *grow* hair on other parts of our bodies. A woman with this problem will go bald in the same places as her husband, such as on her temples and the top of her head, but grow hair on her chin, under her belly button, and on her inner thighs and lower back. This unusual kind of hair growth or loss could also indicate a medical problem other than AGA, so it should be checked out by an endocrinologist, says Dr. Seely.

Estrogen, on the other hand, *prolongs* the hair follicle's growth period. "So with more estrogen, the hair can grow longer, and there's more hair on the scalp," says Dr. Seely. This explains why women experience some hair loss after childbirth and menopause, when estrogen levels are falling. It also explains why we can grow our hair longer than most men.

If you're concerned about baldness, first make sure that there isn't a medical issue. "Tumors can make male hormone, which can cause baldness," Dr. Seely says. Apart from that, hair is dependent on your stress levels and diet. "So avoiding major stresses and getting enough vitamins can help," she says.

What Can You Do?

Given the number of factors that can cause temporary and long-term hair loss, it's tough to know what to do. Treatments that have been reported to work in some studies include exotic herbs, amino acids, and a soft laser scalp massage. Before looking into these more involved therapies, read on. You might find number of solutions that will work for you.

Relax. If you've just gone through a divorce, a move, or some other major stress, your hair loss might be stress-related. Major stress can cause your roots to close down and rest for 3 months.

Think about other changes. If your hair is coming out in patches but you haven't experienced any major life stresses, think about the other changes in your life. Have you started taking a new medication or changed your eating habits? Antithyroid drugs, anticonvulsants, diuretics, and even ibuprofen can trigger hair loss in some people.

Ease up on hair treatments. Don't perm, straighten, or color your hair until it's back to normal. Chemical treatments can inflame and irritate your scalp.

Adopt an easygoing style. Give your hair a break from tight braids and rollers, which can break hair and exaggerate thinning.

Use what the guys use. Apply minoxidil, an over-the-counter hair-restoring treatment, to your scalp twice a day. It has been proven effective, especially for the 25 to 30 percent of women who lose their hair because of heredity factors.

Have patience. Nothing restores hair loss in 6 weeks. Experts say it usually takes 6 months for the process to turn around.

Medical Alert

HAIR LOSS

If you have no idea why you're losing your hair, promptly consult a dermatologist who deals with hair problems. It's better to stop the process as soon as possible instead of waiting for years because it usually becomes more difficult to treat hair loss over time.

HIGH BLOOD PRESSURE

Thanks to estrogen, high blood pressure (or hypertension) hits women later in life than it does men. Not that this female hormone's protection is ironclad. Women can—and do—develop high blood pressure before estrogen production wanes at menopause.

Doctors take two measurements when they check your blood pressure. The first is called the systolic reading. It indicates how hard your heart pumps to push blood through your arteries. The second, called the diastolic reading, shows how much your arteries put up resistance to the bloodflow. Blood pressure is measured in millimeters of mercury, or mm Hg, and a reading of about 120 mm Hg systolic and 80 mm Hg diastolic is considered healthy. We read that simply as 120/80.

Everyone's blood pressure varies widely throughout the day. Generally, it will rise when you're exercising and drop when you're asleep. But when your baseline, or resting, reading creeps up to 140/90, you have borderline high blood pressure. That means your heart is working too hard to pump blood, either because your arteries have narrowed or stiffened with plaque or because you have too much blood in your system on account of water retention or other problems.

"If you're borderline hypertensive, there's a lot you can do to either prevent the need for drugs or reduce the amount of drugs you have to take," says Thomas Pickering, M.D., Ph.D., a cardiologist and professor of medicine at New York Hospital–Cornell Medical Center and author of *Good News about High Blood Pressure.*

SIGNS AND SYMPTOMS

HIGH BLOOD PRESSURE

Blood pressure normally fluctuates from day to day and even from minute to minute, depending upon activity, posture, temperature, diet, drugs, and a person's emotional and physical states. But odds are that you'd never know it unless you took your blood pressure throughout the day. That's one reason high blood pressure is so dangerous—it's a symptomless disease.

What Can You Do?

Uncontrolled high blood pressure increases your risk of heart disease, kidney failure, and stroke. But for most women, elevated blood pressure can be controlled before it has a chance to do any permanent harm. Here's how to get a handle on hypertension.

Have it tested. There's only one way to know for sure if you have high blood pressure: Have your doctor check it. Once a year should be sufficient, unless your doctor orders more tests. It's a quick, painless procedure. The doctor puts an inflatable cuff around your arm and checks your pulse with a stethoscope. If you show a borderline-high reading, the doctor may order several retests over a couple of weeks or months.

Stop smoking. Smoking markedly increases your risk of developing a stroke or blood vessel damage from high blood pressure. It also encourages your body to deposit cholesterol within your coronary arteries. This decreases the size of your vessels and forces your heart to work harder. Anyone with high blood pressure should stop smoking immediately.

Eat more fish and less fat. In a study conducted in Australia, overweight men and women who ate 4 ounces of fish a day dropped 6 blood pressure points in 4 months. But those who ate fish *and* cut back on dietary fat got extra blood pressure–lowering benefits. For women who have elevated blood pressure, Dr. Pickering recommends three to seven fish meals a week—more than the usual, twice-a-week directive.

Cook with garlic and basil. A cornerstone of Mediterranean cuisine, garlic has a documented blood pressure–lowering effect. Try to eat a clove or two each day. Fresh basil leaves also help keep blood pressure in check. Think pesto.

Load up on fiber and shun processed wheat. Dietary fiber has clear cardiovascular benefits. Processed wheat, on the other hand, creates an insulin surge, which triggers a rise in blood pressure for several hours. One study, at Tulane University in New Orleans, found that subjects with the highest blood insulin levels were three times more likely to have high blood pressure. So substitute fiber-rich unprocessed whole grain bread for that white bread to reap the benefits of the former while avoiding the harm of the latter.

Medical Alert

HIGH BLOOD PRESSURE

Your blood pressure readings ideally should be below 120/80 millimeters of mercury (mm Hg), although readings as high as 130/85 are considered normal. If your blood pressure consistently creeps above that mark, you need to start watching it carefully. A reading of 140/90 or higher means that medical treatment is appropriate.

Consume potassium, magnesium, and calcium. All three minerals help keep your blood pressure down. Even better, choose food sources over supplements. "Getting these minerals in combination naturally from food has more of an effect than taking them individually as supplements," says Dr. Pickering. This could mean a difference of 3 to 4 mm Hg.

For potassium, eat four or five daily servings of fruits and vegetables, especially cantaloupe, baked potatoes, bananas, citrus fruits, and tomatoes. You'll find the highest amounts of magnesium in almonds and pumpkin seeds. Low-fat or fat-free dairy products like milk and yogurt provide ample calcium, but so do calcium-fortified orange juice, soy milk, and waffles.

Move it and lose it. Thirty minutes of daily aerobic exercise in the morning will help lower your blood pressure for most of the day. Do it regularly, and the benefits will be permanent. Packing a few extra pounds? Just losing weight will lower your blood pressure. Better yet, the *combination* of losing weight and getting regular exercise can pare your pressure by 20 points.

Reduce stress and add quiet activity. Stress raises blood pressure, so eliminate what you can. For example, ask for more authority on the job; the resulting sense of control reduces stress. Insist on clarity about whom you report to; trying to please too many bosses is stressful.

Then manage the stress that's left by using relaxation techniques. In one 3-month study, 20 minutes a day of meditation lowered study participants' blood pressure by 11 points. Others find success with breathing exercises, nature walks, or even watching tropical fish.

HOT FLASHES

No one knows exactly what triggers hot flashes, but they seem to be linked to the hormonal changes that occur before and during menopause. "These changes somehow stimulate the part of the brain that controls body temperature, throwing off its usually fine-tuned control," explains Robert Freedman, Ph.D., director of the Behavioral Medicine Laboratory at Wayne State University in Detroit. As a result, the brain signals the body to dissipate heat—in other words, to flush and sweat.

If you took your temperature during a hot flash, you wouldn't have a fever. "But hot flashes are synchronized with your core temperature (deep inside your body), which rises and falls in a predictable pattern over a 24-hour period," notes Dr. Freedman. Things start sizzling just about the time your body reaches its peak core temperature for the day—usually late afternoon or early evening. But hot flashes can occur at any time of the day or night.

Though considered physically harmless, hot flashes can make you flustered and self-conscious. The good news about hot flashes is that they actually cool down once menopause finally arrives. For the women in one study, the number of incendiary episodes dropped to 20 percent of their peak frequency within 4 years after the onset of menopause.

What Can You Do?

Hot flashes may take you by surprise the first couple of times they occur. But if you are like many women, you will eventually be able to tell

---

SIGNS AND SYMPTOMS

HOT FLASHES

During a hot flash, blood surges to the surface of the skin on your chest, neck, and head. With this increase in bloodflow comes a rise in skin temperature, a slight acceleration of heart and breathing rates, and perspiration. As the hot flash dissipates heat, your body's core temperature drops (which is why you may feel cold and clammy afterward). The entire episode usually lasts 2 to 5 minutes.

when one is coming on (except when you are asleep, of course). These strategies can help you weather a hot flash and prevent it from becoming too severe.

Practice deep breathing. In one study, women who had been having 20 or more hot flashes a day reduced that number by half with the help of deep breathing, says Dr. Freedman. "This technique seems to short-circuit the arousal of the central nervous system that normally occurs in the initial stages of a hot flash," he explains.

When you feel a hot flash creeping up on you, prepare for deep breathing by sitting up straight and loosening your belt or waistband if it feels tight. Begin by exhaling through your nose longer than you normally would. Then inhale through your nose slowly and deeply, filling your lungs from the bottom up while keeping your belly relaxed. When your chest is fully expanded, exhale slowly and deeply, as if sighing. Continue this pattern of inhaling and exhaling until the hot flash subsides.

Adjust the temperature of the room. Ideally, set the thermostat at 60°F. Simplistic as it may seem, turning down the heat or cranking up the air-conditioning is solid advice, according to Dr. Freedman. "Anything that raises body temperature even a tiny bit, such as being in a room that's too hot, can aggravate a hot flash," he says.

Monitor your reaction to spicy foods. Garlic, ginger, ground red pepper, onions, and highly acidic produce such as citrus fruits and tomatoes may fuel your hot flash fire, according to Judyth Reichenberg-Ullman, N.D., a naturopathic doctor with the Northwest Center for Homeopathic Medicine in Edmonds, Washington, and coauthor of *Homeopathic Self-Care*. If you tend to experience hot flashes after eating one of these foods, eliminate the food from your diet for a week or so and note if your symptoms improve.

Wean yourself off the bean. Hot caffeinated beverages are a common hot flash aggravator. "You can drink soda or hot herbal tea if you'd like," says Mary Jane Minkin, M.D., clinical professor of obstetrics and gynecology at Yale University School of Medicine and coauthor of *What Every Woman Needs to Know about Menopause*. "It's not the heat or the caffeine alone that seems to cause hot flashes. But the combination of the two really seems to bring them on strong."

Medical Alert

HOT FLASHES

See your doctor if your hot flashes become so frequent or severe that they disrupt your daily routine. Also see your doctor if hot flashes at night (called night sweats) continue for several weeks and you are having trouble sleeping as a result.

Avoid alcoholic beverages. Alcohol causes you to flush even when you aren't in a state of hormonal upheaval. It can certainly fan the flame of hot flashes.

In a study at the University of North Carolina at Chapel Hill, women who had at least one alcoholic beverage a week were about 13 percent likelier to experience hot flashes than women who never drank. "Alcohol consumption proved to be one of the strongest lifestyle risk factors for hot flashes," according to Pamela Schwingl, Ph.D., senior epidemiologist at Family Health International in Research Triangle Park, North Carolina, and the study's main author.

INCONTINENCE

It's only when our bodies stop making estrogen that we realize just how much this hormone does. Take the bladder, for instance. Estrogen keeps the linings of the bladder and urethra (the 1-inch-long tube that carries urine from the bladder) supple and healthy. When we stop making estrogen, our bladder control muscles weaken, often to the point where a simple sneeze or chuckle can generate an embarrassing accident.

Researchers believe that urinary incontinence affects 30 to 60 percent of all postmenopausal women. But the good news is that it's easily controlled and, better yet, cured, says Rodney Appell, M.D., Scott Professor of Female Urology at Baylor Medical College in Houston.

Among women ages 55 and younger, stress incontinence is the most common form of urinary incontinence. Women with stress incontinence may dribble urine when they cough, laugh, lift heavy objects, exert

INCONTINENCE

In women, incontinence usually takes one of two forms: If you leak urine during exercise or when you cough, laugh, or sneeze, most likely you have stress incontinence; if you have the urge to go the bathroom but can't get there in time, you probably have what is called urge incontinence. The good news is that doctors say that 8 out of 10 women with incontinence can be helped—if they know what to do.

themselves suddenly, change positions quickly—any action that increases pressure on the bladder.

Stress incontinence results from stretched and weakened pelvic floor muscles, which can result from menopausal changes and abdominal surgery. These muscles, which extend from the pubic bone to the tailbone, provide hammocklike support for the bladder and uterus. Both the vagina and the urethra pass through this muscular sling. When you contract the pelvic floor muscles, you squeeze your vagina and urethra shut.

While stress incontinence gives you no advance warning of a urine leak, urge incontinence sends the signal that you have to go. Unfortunately, it leaves you no time to get to a bathroom. The bladder may release just a bit of urine, or it may spill its whole load.

With urge incontinence, some factor disrupts communication between your brain and your bladder. As a result, your brain gets the message that your bladder is full, but your bladder doesn't receive its instructions to wait until you find a toilet. Weak pelvic floor muscles may contribute to urge incontinence, but other factors—such as menopausal changes, urinary tract infections, and even food irritants—likely play roles as well.

What Can You Do?

To get your bladder back on track, you need to look at a variety of lifestyle factors. Be sure to include these self-care measures in your treatment routine.

Try the Kegel cure. Kegel exercises build strength and endurance in the muscles of the bladder. Most doctors recommend them as the first-line approach in treating most types of incontinence. They can be hard to learn to do correctly, however, so if you don't see any results from the following exercises after about 8 weeks, talk to your doctor about getting some coaching from a health care practitioner.

To do Kegels, you quickly contract your pelvic floor muscles (the ones that you use to control your urine stream) for 1 to 2 seconds, then relax the muscles between contractions to prevent muscle fatigue. Do 10 repetitions three to five times per day. As you repeat the exercise, hold the contractions for 5 seconds, and gradually increase to 15 seconds three to five times daily.

When done correctly, Kegels are just as effective as surgery and medication for mild to moderate stress and urge incontinence, minus the side effects. One study found that women who practiced Kegels three times a week had the most success, even after 5 years.

Retrain your bladder. This technique works especially well for women with urge incontinence. Begin by allowing yourself one bathroom trip every hour for a week or two. Then for another week or two, extend the time between trips by a half hour. Continue this pattern of adding half-hour increments to your routine until you are able to hold your urine for 3 or 4 hours at a time. This exercise teaches your bladder to hold more urine and become less spastic when it is full.

Medical Alert

INCONTINENCE

If home remedies don't help eliminate your incontinence, see your doctor. You should also see your doctor to rule out a more serious contributing condition if you have any of the following symptoms.

- Pain or burning upon urinating
- Voiding more than 2 quarts of urine a day
- Blood in your urine
- Change in bowel habits
- Pain during intercourse
- Numbness or weakness in your arms or legs
- Changes in vision

Quit smoking. Women who smoke cigarettes are more than twice as likely to develop stress incontinence as women who have never smoked, according to a study performed at Virginia Commonwealth University School of Medicine in Richmond. Cigarettes deliver a double whammy to your bladder. Nicotine irritates it, and coughing (as most smokers do) puts pressure on it.

Drink enough fluids each day. Restricting your fluid intake won't prevent leaks. In fact, it can actually aggravate incontinence by producing concentrated urine, which is highly irritating to your bladder. So in addition to cranberry juice, drink lots of water. How do you know that you are well-hydrated? Your urine should appear clear or pale yellow.

INSOMNIA

From decades of research, sleep scientists have determined that, barring unusual circumstances, women naturally sleep between 8 and 8½ hours a day. This is 1 to 1½ hours more sleep per night than the average man requires. The irony is that women very often have less time available for sleep than men, even though they need more sleep than their male counterparts.

Just how does the sleep process work? Scientists point to a biological "clock" that each of us has within us; this internal clock operates on a 24-hour cycle and helps your body know when to do certain things, such as ready itself for sleep. For example, about an hour or two before bedtime, the pineal gland in the brain responds to signals from the biological clock

---

SIGNS AND SYMPTOMS

INSOMNIA

One-third of all adults can't sleep at one time or another. Over time, losing even as little as an hour or so of sleep a night leads to irritability, difficulty performing tasks well, and memory loss, says Virgil Wooten, M.D., associate director of the Sleep Disorders Center at Eastern Virginia Medical School of the Medical College of Hampton Roads in Norfolk.

and secretes a hormone called melatonin that makes you sleepy (among other things). The same clock signals your body to slow your heart rate and lower your body temperature and blood pressure in anticipation of sleep. It then reactivates these vital signs a few hours before you wake up.

Your biological clock works under the assumption that you sleep at night. Therefore, its timing is governed by the cycles of daylight and darkness. This is one reason that some people who are blind experience insomnia. It is also why some people lose sleep if they don't get enough light during the day or wake up too early if light streams in through their bedroom windows. Other factors—like drinking too much coffee or exercising late at night or feeling just plain nervous—can keep you awake, too.

In addition, as women age, they're especially prone to insomnia. Once they turn 40, women are 40 percent more likely to experience some degree of insomnia, thanks to the midlife hormonal changes that precede menopause. A few years before and after menopause, a common cause of insomnia is night sweats. (For practical ideas on how to manage them, see "Night Sweats" on page 287).

What Can You Do?

For most women, occasional insomnia isn't much of a problem. But a wakeful night can leave you less than perky for the day at hand. To prevent future episodes of sleeplessness, follow this advice.

Take a morning walk outside. "Light exposure during the day helps keep your body clock regulated," says Mary A. Carskadon, Ph.D., professor of psychiatry and human behavior at Brown University Medical School and head of the sleep research lab at E. P. Bradley Hospital, both in Providence, Rhode Island. "An early-morning walk in the daylight upon rising will help promote sleep at night."

Resist the urge to nap. Napping during the day after a sleepless night will only throw your body clock further off balance. Instead, experts recommend consolidating your sleep to make sure you get enough of it at night.

De-stress your bedroom. You probably don't sleep in your office. Conversely, experts point out, you shouldn't work in your bedroom. Your

---

Medical Alert

INSOMNIA

If you've tried the advice presented in this section and still can't easily get to sleep or stay asleep throughout the night for a month or so, see your doctor. She may refer you to a sleep disorders clinic for further evaluation.

---

bedroom is for two things only: sleeping and sex. So remove your computer, your office reading pile, your fax machine, and even your phone, if you can. And put your TV back in the den, where it belongs.

Set a bedtime. Adults, just like children, need a regular bedtime, says Dr. Carskadon. "We have body clocks that synchronize our systems. Establish a set sleep and wake time, then stick to it every day. That tells your clock to make you sleepy at night and wakeful in the morning."

Take a hot bath. A hot bath taken early in the evening will cause your temperature to go up and then drop more quickly when you hit the hay, so you can fall asleep more easily.

Wind down before you get into bed. Giving yourself about 45 minutes of "quiet time" before you get into bed helps signal your body clock that the day is done and sleep time is imminent. Listen to soft music, write a letter, read something boring—but don't do anything that jazzes you up (and absolutely nothing work-related).

Turn the clock to the wall. Staring at the clock makes you more tense about getting back to sleep. Instead of checking the time, concentrate on restful thoughts.

Picture some numbers. If you can't sleep, try this technique, recommended by Henry Lahymeyer, M.D., a physician in Northfield, Illinois. Close your eyes and relax. Count backward slowly from 100 to zero. As you do, visualize the numbers in some beautiful way. Maybe you see them being written by a calligrapher. Or try seeing the numbers being drawn on a huge blackboard across a giant sky. Continue until sleep overtakes you.

Don't overcompensate. Don't stay in bed for 10 or 11 hours, trying to make up for lost sleep time. If you usually need 8 hours, you will just have an extra 2 hours to toss and turn. You won't get more sleep, say the experts. And if you extend your sleep time too much, you may begin to wake up too early in the morning. It is more important to get the sleep you need on a regular basis.

IRREGULAR PERIODS AND FLOODING

Your cycles used to be regular, but now they're not. You used to know roughly how many tampons or napkins you'd use during each period, but now you haven't got a clue. Nothing about your period is as it used to be.

If you're like a lot of women, you wonder whether this new irregularity is a normal part of perimenopause—or if it's a sign that something sinister is going on. More than likely, bleeding irregularities that begin in your forties or fifties—or even as early as your thirties—can be traced to the beginnings of menopause, says Susun S. Weed, an herbalist and herbal educator from Woodstock, New York, and author of the *Wise Woman* series of herbal health books. To distinguish normal from abnormal changes, keep records. You may find that there's a certain regularity to your irregularity. If your periods are indeed erratic or profuse, consult your doctor or other expert in women's health.

What Can You Do?

Sometimes natural remedies can even out irregular menses; sometimes they can't. Our experts suggest:

Turn to vitex. Although it's slow to act, vitex tincture (also called chasteberry) is highly recommended for women who are bothered by

---

SIGNS AND SYMPTOMS

IRREGULAR PERIODS AND FLOODING

As they approach menopause, many women report changes to their menstrual cycles that include either lighter or heavier bleeding, and longer, shorter, or skipped periods. In most cases, there is no need for concern.

menopausal irregularities. Susun recommends a dropperful in a small glass of water or juice two or three times a day for 6 to 8 weeks after every irregular period.

Take a hip-swinging stroll. Walking stimulates the pelvic region and gets fluids moving through the area, so it reduces pelvic congestion, says Mary Bove, N.D., a naturopathic doctor and director of the Brattleboro Naturopathic Clinic in Vermont. "I tell women to work on their pelvises, letting their hips lead their stroke as they walk, letting their hips and arms swing freely so that the whole body has a chance to stretch out." A daily 20-minute-or-so walk will decrease the likelihood of cramps, reduce them if you have them, and brighten your mood, she says.

Savor some cinnamon. Cinnamon bark invigorates the blood, helps regulate the menstrual cycle, and checks flooding, says Susun Weed. For heavy bleeding, take 5 to 10 drops of tincture once or twice a day, or chew on a cinnamon stick. You can also simply sprinkle ground cinnamon freely on food, she advises.

Visit a lady. In a clinical study, 5 to 10 drops of lady's mantle tincture controlled menstrual hemorrhage in virtually all of the 300 women who participated, says Susun. When taken after flooding began, lady's mantle took 3 to 5 days to become effective. When taken for 1 to 2 weeks before menstruation, it prevented flooding. She suggests using 5 to 10 drops of the fresh plant tincture three times a day for up to 2 weeks out of every month.

Keep your iron up. Try to consume more iron from herbs and food sources on the days that you bleed heavily, says Susun. You'll feel more energetic and alive within 2 weeks, and your flooding will diminish noticeably by your next period, she adds. Herbal sources of iron include dandelion leaves, milk thistle seed, dang gui, black cohosh, echinacea, and peppermint, according to Susun. Food sources include leafy greens, tofu, raisins, carrots, beets, pumpkin, tomatoes, cauliflower, mushrooms, soybeans, and salmon. Of course, lean red meat is the best source of iron because it contains heme iron, which is readily absorbed by the body.

Reach for yellow dock root. Another iron source, yellow dock root contributes 1 milligram of iron per 20-drop dose of alcohol tincture or per 3-teaspoon dose of vinegar tincture, says Susun. Yellow dock also contains thiamin and vitamin C, which assists absorption of iron, as well as compounds, called anthraquinone glycosides, that stimulate bile production, thereby aiding digestion and nudging a sluggish liver. Either an alcohol or a vinegar tincture is fine, taken daily in tea or water, she advises. Iron is absorbed a little at a time, so she suggests taking it throughout the day. Acids and proteins increase iron absorption, she says, so take your iron with some orange juice or milk.

Limit "iron-eating" foods. Coffee, black tea, soy protein (such as tofu or soy milk), egg yolks, bran, and supplements containing more than 250 milligrams of calcium impair iron absorption, Susun notes. Limit consumption of coffee and tea, and take your calcium at night or with meals that don't include iron-rich foods.

LOW LIBIDO

If hitting an unexpected speed bump with your car equates to the best sex you've had lately, you know your hormones are sending you a signal.

Nearly three out of four women suffer from some kind of sexual difficulty, whether it's decreased sex drive, vaginal dryness, or trouble reaching orgasm. Even if we don't have any severe sexual dysfunction, nearly all of us, according to one survey, have at least one sexual concern.

In the past, the best advice doctors usually offered to improve our sex lives—if we had the nerve to ask—ran from drinking a glass of wine to buying some lingerie. Most likely, they'd claim it was all in our heads.

LOW LIBIDO

Plummeting estrogen levels during menopause can lead to minimized sensation in the labia, interfere with lubrication, and make the tissues in the vagina very delicate and prone to bleeding. In one study, 67 percent of menopausal women experienced low arousal and pain during sex, and 92 percent reported trouble reaching orgasm.

And it's true that emotions and relationship issues are indeed a huge part of desire and sex. But researchers are discovering that quite often the problem lies in our hormones, which become more finicky as we age.

But getting older doesn't have to equate with making love less often. In one study, women over age 65 had almost 10 percent more sex than women ages 39 to 50. Drug companies, inspired by men's reaction to the arousal drug Viagra, are discovering an equally enthusiastic, untapped market in women.

The good news is that the enormous amounts of research resulting from this quest provide numerous ways we can preserve our sexual function *without drugs* and knowledge we can use now to have better sex *tonight*.

What Can You Do?

For women who find themselves less interested in sex at menopause, experts suggest:

Recall pleasurable sensual experiences. Of course, good sex begins long before you even set foot in the bedroom. "Reconnecting to powerful feelings of sensuality—not necessarily sexuality—can go a long way toward helping you feel desire," explains Gina Ogden, Ph.D., a sex therapist in Cambridge, Massachusetts. "Sometimes these playful, sensual memories predate adult sexual experience—like the time you went skinny-dipping when you were 8 years old or you rolled around on the floor with your first puppy. Summoning the energy that infused your joy as a little girl can revitalize your sex life today."

Stay physically active. Regular exercise will relieve stress, improve your mood, and help you feel great about your body, says Yula Ponticas,

Ph.D., a clinical psychologist in the Sexual Behaviors Consultation Unit at Johns Hopkins University School of Medicine in Baltimore. When researchers looked at women 50 years and older, they found that those with the highest levels of physical fitness were also the ones who enjoyed intimacy more often.

Aerobic exercise wakes up your nerves and primes your sympathetic nervous system for sex, says Cindy Meston, Ph.D., a sex researcher and assistant professor of psychology at the University of Texas in Austin. It also improves your cardiovascular system and increases bloodflow, a key part of arousal and orgasm.

Yoga, a more sedate exercise, may also help, says Deborah Moskowitz, N.D., a naturopathic physician in Portland, Oregon.

Get your blood flowing. Stimulating herbs that get blood circulation flowing enhance sexual feelings in women, notes Aviva Romm, a professional member of the American Herbalists Guild in Bloomfield Hills, Michigan. "With more bloodflow to the pelvis, you'll feel more aroused."

Simmer these herbs in 2 cups of water for 20 minutes: 1 tablespoon of grated fresh ginger, 7 to 10 cloves, 2 or 3 cinnamon sticks, 4 or 5 black peppercorns, and 7 to 10 cardamom pods. Strain and add small amounts of milk and honey to taste. If you wish, add ¼ teaspoon of vanilla. "Vanilla comes from the orchid family, and orchids are incredibly sensual flowers," says Aviva. "It's an aphrodisiac."

Use the right lubricant. Vaginal dryness is a prime cause of painful intercourse, so you may be tempted to reach for the petroleum jelly—but that's not a good idea. Petroleum jelly can break down condoms. Plus, it isn't water-soluble, so it remains in the vagina, where it can harbor yeast and other infection-producing microbes.

So what's the better option? Try vaginal lubricants such as Astroglide and K-Y jelly, which are designed to relieve friction during sex by coating your vaginal walls. Unlike moisturizers, they tend to evaporate and often need to be reapplied during intercourse. For more tips on overcoming vaginal dryness, turn to page 237.

If you smoke, quit. Women who smoke complain of vaginal dryness and painful intercourse a lot more than nonsmokers do. The reason? Smoking restricts the bloodflow necessary for a clitoral erection,

---

Medical Alert

LOW LIBIDO

See your gynecologist if your sexual desire continues to wane despite your having tried measures such as those described in this chapter. You may have an underlying health problem, such as chronic fatigue syndrome, depression, Lyme disease, or a thyroid disorder. And if you suspect that an emotional conflict is sapping your sexual desire, consider getting counseling from a psychotherapist or sex therapist. See chapter 9 for some ideas on rekindling your sexual fire.

---

engorgement of the vaginal walls and labia, and lubrication. So much for those sexy cigarette ads.

Consider hormonal help. If the strategies above don't help, you may want to consider testosterone therapy. Several studies have shown that supplementary testosterone (in pill or shot form) can increase sexual arousal in some postmenopausal women, especially in women whose ovaries have been removed. Your doctor can explain the benefits and drawbacks of testosterone therapy.

MEMORY PROBLEMS

You walk into the living room to get something—but what? You drive right past the grocery store and forget to turn in. What's going on?

The connection between memory and menopause has long been an issue of debate. In ongoing research into brain function, scientists are trying to determine whether estrogen receptors or estrogen metabolites (the breakdown products of estrogen) affect memory function. But so far nothing has been proven, says Adelaide Nardone, M.D., a gynecologist in Mount Kisco, New York.

In recent research at Yale University, magnetic resonance imaging (MRI) was used to study the influence of estrogen on the brain patterns of postmenopausal women. Therapeutic doses of estrogen affected brain activity in memory tasks, like remembering a just-looked-up telephone number. This seems to support the theory that estrogen aids short-term information storage.

This small study provides a tantalizing clue to estrogen's role in brain function, but definitive links have not been forged, says Dr. Nardone, who believes that much of menopausal "mental misfiring" can be traced to fatigue.

Women undergoing change of life are prone to insomnia and night sweats, which often leave them exhausted, she says. And increased anxiety about memory lapses may further distort their perception of memory loss.

What Can You Do?

If you want to remember better naturally, work these easy remedies into your daily routine. The first two tips are helpful if your memory problems are sleep-related. The others will help to boost your memory power any time of day.

Practice good "sleep hygiene." Be sure that your bedroom is dark and shielded from noise so you can sleep beyond 6:00 A.M. Eliminate any stimulating input, she says—no watching TV in bed. Take care not to eat any heavy foods after 7:00 P.M. since vigorous digestion tends to inhibit deep sleep. The same goes for caffeine and chocolate, which can keep you awake.

Take a sip of moo juice. If restorative rest still eludes you, Dr. Nardone suggests taking 300 to 500 milligrams of calcium (a glass or two of fat-free milk will do the trick) an hour before bedtime to encourage sleepiness. Calcium may soothe the body into a deep sleep that is interrupted less often, she says.

Get some mental exercise. The more you challenge your brain, the better it'll perform. Any kind of mental exercise, such as working crossword

SIGNS AND SYMPTOMS
MEMORY PROBLEMS

For many women, menopause and forgetfulness seem to arrive hand in hand. Frequent memory lapses, sudden blanks, and forgotten names can be scary and may lead you to believe that you're not as sharp as you used to be.

Medical Alert

MEMORY PROBLEMS

If your memory seems to be failing steadily, don't hesitate to consult your doctor. Many treatable conditions can cause forgetfulness—among them, depression, drug side effects, and thyroid disorders. Your doctor can determine whether or not you have age-related memory impairment or something more serious.

puzzles, can help improve your memory. Just be sure it's something you enjoy; if you don't enjoy the activity, it won't feel as rewarding.

Get physical. In one study, researchers found that volunteers who got an hour of aerobic exercise three times a week performed better on memory tests than those who didn't work out. Exercise, they speculate, may increase oxygen flow to the brain and speed glucose metabolism, improving recall. Exercise can also reduce stress, which can interfere with memory.

Make meaningful connections. To remember things like street addresses or a shopping list, make up a story or a sentence that links that information in a meaningful way. To remember someone's address—for example, 65 South Street—tell yourself, "Sixty-five is retirement age, and many people move to the South after they retire."

Paint a mental image. Concrete visual images can help connect new names. Assume that you meet a prospective boss, Ms. Saucer, at a job interview, and her most striking feature is her green eyes. Envision saucers painted to look like huge green eyes. So, later in the conversation, or the next time you meet her, her eyes will remind you that her last name is Saucer.

Avoid distractions. Make a mental note of what you're going to do before you do it. It will minimize distraction, which makes you forget why, for example, you walked into the living room. You head for a room to find something in particular, but as you enter, something else gets your attention.

So, instead, tell yourself, "I'm going into the living room to get the photo album," for example, and you will be less likely to get distracted by the magazines and papers on the coffee table.

NIGHT SWEATS

It's one thing to feel a hot flash spread from your chest to your neck and your head, leaving you sweaty and flushed midday. Hot flashes are uncomfortable, inconvenient, and sometimes embarrassing, but after your first few hot flashes, you realize, as other women approaching menopause do, that you can deal with them.

Nocturnal flashes—night sweats—are a different story. Waking up in a pool of perspiration disrupts your sleep. So does getting up from a deep sleep to change your soaking wet nightclothes and sheets.

"But night sweats, hot flashes, and the chills that sometimes follow are nothing to worry about and last only 9 to 16 months, on the average," says Lila A. Wallis, M.D., professor of medicine at Weill Medical College at Cornell University in New York City, and past president of the American Medical Women's Association (AMWA). It's believed that the drop in the production of the female hormone estrogen and other hormonal changes interfere with the way the body regulates heat.

Okay, so nightly heat waves are seemingly harmless and temporary. That's no consolation, however, if you can't get the rest you need. In addition, some experts believe that some of the mental symptoms attributed to hormonal changes before and after menopause—foggy thinking, for instance—are more likely a result of sleep deprivation.

What Can You Do?

If your sleep time suddenly becomes hot and steamy for all the wrong reasons, try these simple strategies to help you sleep through your next night sweat (or get back to dreamland in a wink).

SIGNS AND SYMPTOMS

NIGHT SWEATS

Night sweats are hot flashes that occur during sleep. You wake drenched in sweat, sometimes several times a night. Because night sweats disturb sleep, you're often tired during the day.

Medical Alert

NIGHT SWEATS

If you haven't slept well in weeks and generally feel lousy, make an appointment with your doctor, who can give you even more advice on eliminating night sweats.

Have a cup of sage tea before bed. Sage—an ordinary kitchen herb—can help reduce or sometimes even eliminate night sweats, according to herbalists. To make a sage infusion, place 4 heaping tablespoons of dried sage in 1 cup of hot water. Cover tightly and steep for 4 hours or more. Then strain, reheat, and drink. (Used in therapeutic amounts, sage can increase sedative side effects of drugs. Do not use medicinal amounts of sage if you're hypoglycemic or undergoing anticonvulsant therapy.)

Sleep on all-cotton sheets and pillowcases. Cotton is a breathable fabric that wicks moisture away from the skin. Avoid cotton/polyester blends, flannel, and satin—they'll leave you feeling hot and clammy. And keep a light cotton quilt at the foot of your bed to pull over yourself if you get the chills after a hot flash.

Wear cotton. Wear all-cotton underwear and short-sleeved, knee-length nightgowns (long-sleeved gowns will be too hot and uncomfortable). Avoid nylon or polyester blends, which will trap rather than release heat. Keep a dry nightie handy at the foot of your bed or in a chair next to your bed. If you have to change in the middle of the night, you won't have to get out of bed and rummage through your dresser drawers.

Keep the right supplies on hand. Leave a small cotton towel next to your bed to wipe the sweat off your chest, neck, and face, and place a fan next to your bed to cool those heat waves.

Drift back to sleep. Try keeping your eyes closed and letting yourself drift into that semiconscious state between sleep and waking. You will be more likely to fall back asleep, says Sonia Ancoli-Israel, Ph.D., professor in the department of psychiatry at the University of California in San Diego.

Get out of bed. If you can't fall back to sleep within 15 to 30 minutes, get out of bed and do something relaxing for a half-hour, like reading. Then try to go back to bed. Repeat as often as you need to until you fall asleep.

PAINFUL URINATION

To some extent, women get urinary tract infections (UTIs) simply because of their anatomy. Because the rectum, vagina, and urethra are within centimeters of one another, it's easy for infection-causing bacteria such as *Escherichia coli* to enter the urinary tract. And at menopause, normal changes in the vaginal tissues can contribute to UTIs. Most women will experience at least one or two UTIs at some time in their lives.

If the infection is limited to the urethra, it's called urethritis. More often than not, the infection travels farther up the tract and into the bladder and becomes cystitis (or, simply, a bladder infection). Treatment usually consists of a 1-day or 3-day dose of antibiotics. Unless treated promptly, a bladder infection can move to the kidneys, leading to a more serious condition, called pyelonephritis.

Anything that alters the bacterial balance of the genitourinary tract can render women more susceptible to UTIs. Women who use certain birth control methods—for example, spermicides containing nonoxynol-9—are at higher risk for UTIs. This ingredient is found in spermicidal jellies, spermicidal foams or inserts, and condoms with spermicidal lubricant.

What Can You Do?

While UTIs require a doctor's care, you can ease the pain and protect yourself from future infections with this expert advice.

Drink more water, not less. You may be tempted to drink less because urinating afterward is so painful. But if you drink a gallon of water within 24 hours of discovering UTI symptoms, you might be able to flush the bacteria out of your system.

SIGNS AND SYMPTOMS

PAINFUL URINATION

Painful urination is often a sign of a urinary tract infection (UTI). Other symptoms you may experience are a burning sensation when urinating, frequent urination, voiding just a few drops at a time, and passing blood.

Medical Alert

PAINFUL URINATION

If you have more than two UTIs (or what you think are UTIs) in 6 months, or more than three episodes in 12 months, see a doctor and get a urine culture for an accurate diagnosis. Also, see your doctor if your UTI symptoms are accompanied by blood in the urine, chills, nausea, vomiting, or lower-back pain.

If you've received a prescription for your UTI and symptoms don't start clearing up within 2 days, call your doctor promptly.

Fix a baking soda cocktail. At the first sign of symptoms, mix ½ teaspoon of baking soda in an 8-ounce glass of water and drink it. The baking soda raises the pH (acid–base balance) of irritating, acidic urine.

Get juiced. Cranberries contain unique substances called condensed tannins that make it more difficult for bacteria to adhere to the lining of your urinary tract. Accordingly, drinking cranberry juice cocktail can both prevent and treat UTIs. In several published studies, drinking just three 8-ounce glasses of cranberry juice cocktail a day significantly reduced the incidence of UTIs in elderly women.

Doctors caution, however, that in some women with urinary tract sensitivity, cranberry juice may act as an irritant because of its high acid content. If cranberry juice seems to make your symptoms worse, try diluting it before stopping it altogether.

Wear knee–highs and skirts or loose pants. If you have an infection, wearing tight undergarments or jeans forces the bacteria that normally line your vaginal area up into your urethra. If you have irritation, constrictive clothing can worsen pain and discomfort because it presses against the already inflamed urethral opening.

Nix other offenders. Whether you have a simple irritation or an infected urinary tract, the last thing that you need are known bladder irritants. The most notorious bladder irritants are citrus, tomatoes, aged cheeses, chocolate, spicy foods, caffeine, alcohol, and nicotine. For certain people, anything carbonated—especially beer and soft drinks—may irritate the bladder and make you urinate more frequently or urgently.

Ask about estrogen cream. If you suddenly start experiencing more

UTIs as you approach menopause, you may want to ask your doctor about estrogen cream. Applied topically, it helps your body maintain a normal vaginal environment and helps the urethra to produce mucus; both of these protect against bacterial infections such as UTIs.

SNORING

So, you think you don't snore? Think again. Ever awaken with headaches? Morning fatigue? In women, these symptoms can be signs of sleep apnea, interruptions in sleep when you actually stop breathing several times a night. This disorder affects the quality of your sleep, making you restless during the night and tired during the day.

"Snoring is a key sign of sleep apnea in men and women alike, but women are less likely to know they snore," says Joan Shaver, R.N., Ph.D., professor and dean of the College of Nursing at the University of Illinois at Chicago and one of the first researchers to study sleep problems in women. "If a man snores, his wife will complain and prompt him to find a solution. But if a woman snores, often the guy won't notice because he's too busy snoring himself."

But there may be other factors at work as well. When women suddenly start snoring, for example, it's usually a sign that estrogen is plummeting. As this hormone drops, it affects the sensory nerves in the soft palate, causing it to lose muscle tone and become flaccid. As you sleep, the soft palate flaps, creating the lovely sound known as snoring.

SIGNS AND SYMPTOMS
SNORING

Snoring can be a symptom of sleep apnea, a breathing disturbance characterized by explosively loud snoring interspersed with pauses of silence. During those pauses, which can last 10 seconds or longer, the snorer actually stops breathing. Because these episodes typically happen dozens of times each night, the snorer awakens feeling unrefreshed and exhausted.

Medical Alert

SNORING

Apnea is a serious disease that may increase your risk of stroke, high blood pressure, or an enlarged heart. And the longer it goes undetected, the worse it can become because apnea worsens with age. So see your doctor for a complete evaluation if snoring doesn't respond to self-care after a few weeks.

Menopausal weight gain, also known as the Buddha belly, is another culprit. As belly fat crowds the internal organs, pushing them up and putting pressure on the diaphragm, you have to work harder to breathe. Forcing the air in and out causes you to snore.

Hypothyroidism can also be the reason that some women snore. A sluggish thyroid aggravates sinus problems; plus, it contributes to weight gain. Menopause itself triggers hypothyroidism in many women; about 70 percent of all American women have an underactive thyroid by age 70.

What Can You Do?

Short of buying your spouse earplugs, give these tips a try. If you don't see improvement in a couple of weeks, see your doctor to rule out a more serious underlying condition.

Change sleeping positions. Snoring is usually worse when you sleep on your back, so try elevating your head, which may reduce soft palate flapping. Sleeping on your side is another good option for many.

Use a decongestant. Low-dose, over-the-counter decongestants may help keep your sinuses open during the night. Take the smallest dose you can since decongestants can keep some people awake.

Take your estrogen by moonlight. If you're on estrogen replacement therapy, take it at night. This will enhance sleep, too, guiding you to a deeper level faster.

Kick the butts. Smoke may cause swelling and inflammation of the throat tissues, which, when swollen, are more likely to vibrate and produce snoring. Add this to your list of 1,001 reasons that it's a good idea to quit smoking.

Drop that drink. Alcohol relaxes all the muscles in the throat that vibrate. And it's dose-related: The more you drink, the louder you'll snore.

UNWANTED FACIAL HAIR

In up to 90 percent of women with unwanted facial hair, there is no underlying problem. But for the other 10 percent, such problems could be caused by a tumor, polycystic ovary syndrome, or a benign condition called hirsutism, in which hair grows fast and thick on the cheeks, chin, forehead, and chest.

There is no cure for hirsutism. But a new cream on the market called Vaniqa (eflornithine HCl) helps slow hair growth—no matter what the cause. Oral contraceptives, hormone therapy, and a prescription drug called spironolactone (which reduces the amount of male hormones floating around in our bodies) may also help remove unwanted facial hair. Keep the men in your life away from Vaniqa, though. It hasn't been found safe for men, who might be tempted to try it as an alternative to daily shaving.

What Can You Do?

Of course, you can always follow the tried and true: shaving, waxing, depilatories, and electrolysis. Here's what the experts have to say about each method.

Ready, set, shave. Shaving is by far the easiest way to remove unwanted hair; try a double-edged razor for the closest shave. And contrary

---

SIGNS AND SYMPTOMS
UNWANTED FACIAL HAIR

As we age and our estrogen levels drop, problems with unwanted facial hair may worsen. If this scenario applies to you, you're not alone. About 20 million women in America try to conceal or remove facial hair at least once a week. For additional how-tos, see page 152.

UNWANTED FACIAL HAIR

If you experience any sudden change in hair growth—especially in those areas where men typically sprout hair, such as the cheeks—see a doctor to rule out an underlying health condition.

to the old wives' tales, shaving facial hair doesn't cause it to grow back faster or coarser.

Pick up a waxing kit. Waxing pulls hairs out by the roots, which can be painful depending on your tolerance. It's best for light, fuzzy hairs you'd rather live without. As far as the waxing options are concerned, most women find that the prewaxed plastic strips aren't as painful to use as warm wax that hardens as it cools.

With sugaring, a variation of waxing, hair is coated with a paste of sugar and wax—it's easier to pull off than wax and therefore less traumatizing to the skin.

Take the chemical route. Chemical depilatories are creams that contain chemicals to dissolve hair, so they're best for places on the body where the skin is not easily irritated. To ensure best results before using a depilatory for the first time, smear a quarter-size amount on your forearm, let it sit for the amount of time specified on the package, and then wipe it off. Wait 24 hours before proceeding so that you can see if any itching, redness, or irritation develops.

One advantage to depilatories is that some contain hair growth inhibitors and fruit enzymes—ingredients that interfere with the protein that lets hair grow back.

Make an appointment for a permanent solution. Electrolysis is the only permanent hair removal option. But you can't do it yourself— a professional performs it in a salon or a hair removal office by inserting a probe into each individual hair follicle and passing an electric current through it. Removing all of the hair on your upper lip may require several sessions.

Make sure that you choose a highly experienced technician since improper electrolysis can leave permanent scars. Qualifications to look for include membership in a state or national electrolysis association and designation as a certified professional electrolysist (CPE).

WEIGHT GAIN

Even medical experts can't agree whether it's aging or menopause that causes extra pounds to migrate toward the middle. They just know that the average American woman puts on up to 15 pounds during late adulthood, most of it around her waist. One reason is that aging causes your metabolism to slow down and your lean muscle mass to decrease. Since lean muscle cells burn more calories than fat, the less muscle you have, the fewer calories you burn. Add to this the fact that the shape of your body is determined by muscle strength, and it's no surprise that as muscles grow weaker, paunches start.

Now think back to puberty and childbirth, two other major hormonal shifts in your life. Both events triggered changes in body composition and weight. Menopause is no different, except that as your estrogen decreases, a subsequent increase in insulin makes losing weight more difficult.

Even women who don't gain weight can see 10 to 15 pounds shift to the waist, an effect of aging known as central obesity. Osteoporosis

---

SIGNS AND SYMPTOMS
WEIGHT GAIN

If you're even 20 percent overweight (say you should weigh 120 pounds but tip the scale at 144 pounds), health risks soar for high blood pressure and cholesterol, diabetes, and other diseases. Luckily, the news is not all bad. Dropping even 10 excess pounds can lower your cholesterol by 5 to 10 points and your blood pressure by as much as 6 points.

magnifies the problem as it causes the spine to shrink, shortening the waistline.

Besides making you feel unattractive, extra pounds around your middle are sometimes associated with cardiovascular disease, high blood pressure, and an increased risk of breast cancer. What's the best way to combat abdominal spread? Sensible eating and exercise.

Don't deprive yourself of too many calories, or your body will go into starvation mode, which lowers your metabolism even more. Follow a low-fat diet and do some kind of aerobic exercise for at least 30 minutes three times a week to boost your metabolism and burn fat. Weight-bearing exercise, like walking, will also strengthen your bones and prevent osteoporosis.

And don't look to hormone therapy (HT, formerly hormone replacement therapy, HRT) as some kind of magic answer. Research to date is inconclusive. One study found that women on HT gained more weight than those not on HT, while another study found that HT appeared to prevent the increase in abdominal fat. Any decision regarding this type of therapy should be based on your overall health, not on your desire to lose weight.

As you move through menopause, try not to curse your fat cells. They help convert other chemicals in your body into estrogen, which may ease your transition by reducing the incidence and severity of hot flashes, mood swings, and sleep disturbances.

What Can You Do?

If ever there is a time in your life to accept yourself, menopause is it. Concentrate on being fit and healthy rather than squeezing into your jeans from college. The following advice may help.

Keep a food diary. Write down not only what you eat but also how much you eat, when you eat it, and what you're doing at the time. This process helps you shape healthier dietary habits by uncovering hidden sources of calories and fat. It also identifies situations that switch on your appetite—for instance, you may realize that you consistently turn to food when you are bored or stressed-out.

Trim 600 calories a day from your present diet. The simplest way to do this is to eat less. You can also switch from whole milk to fat-free, order foods like fish and potatoes baked instead of fried, switch to fat-free mayo and salad dressing, and take similar small calorie-saving steps.

Eat half as much. Do you usually fill your plate or, if you're eating at a restaurant, eat everything that you're served? Instead, try eating half as much. Chances are, you'll be able to meet your need for nutrition without feeling deprived.

Increase your physical activity level. Find little opportunities to be more active throughout the day, and you'll give yourself a huge boost toward reaching your weight-loss goals. If you walk to work, for example, tack an extra block onto your route. You'll burn 10 more calories per day, or roughly 3,500 more calories per year—the number of calories in 1 pound of fat. Some other strategies are to take the stairs instead of the elevator, go for a brisk walk at lunch, and park your car at the far end of the parking lot when you go to the supermarket.

Create the changes that count. For best results, some experts recommend that you make only one or two minor changes at a time in your eating and exercise habits. For example, look for ways that you can cut your calorie intake by roughly 125 calories a day. You might try putting mustard instead of mayonnaise on your sandwich or using low-fat milk instead of cream in your coffee. Same goes for exercise: Start with a 10-minute workout and gradually build from there. By going slowly and giving yourself time to adjust to the lifestyle changes you make, you set yourself up for lasting weight loss.

Make a date with the weight. If you use a scale to monitor your progress, weigh yourself at the same time every day. Your weight fluctuates over the course of 24 hours. Stepping on the scale in the morning one day and at bedtime the next can leave you with an inaccurate (and discouraging) picture of how you are doing.

Chapter

11

MAKING THE MOST OF YOUR MEDICAL OPTIONS

MODERN WOMEN HAVE THE OPTION TO DO MANY THINGS THAT our grandmothers never dreamed of—ride whitewater rapids, work shoulder to shoulder with men, and postpone or entirely bypass child-bearing. Unlike our foremothers of a century ago, whose average life expectancy was 47, women today can expect to live at least 30 years beyond menopause. And while the very term *postmenopausal* fills many women with anxiety, even dread, we all would probably agree that it sure beats the alternative.

Of course, in order to make the most of those extra years, you'll want to continue in the best possible health. And that means staying informed of the latest health issues and getting the care you need before small problems become serious. This chapter will discuss some of the issues you may encounter as you make your way through the world of conventional medicine: Are there any good reasons to take hormone therapy? Does breast cancer risk decrease—or increase—after menopause? When the doctor suggests a hysterectomy, do any other options exist? What can you expect when facing a disease? But first, read on for advice on choosing—and working with—your doctor.

GETTING THE CARE YOU NEED

To get the medical attention you need during menopause, your first step should be to find a good doctor, and then continue to see her regularly. "If you wait 5 years for a checkup, you'll have a million questions that will never get answered," says Margaret Houston, M.D., a family practice physician with the Mayo Clinic.

Know the specialties. There are several types of doctors most people choose to use as a primary care physician, and understanding the specifics of their practices can help make sure that you choose the one that's right for you.

Family practitioners are trained to cover the whole spectrum of family health, so their study is rather broad and includes general adult medicine as well as pediatrics, gynecology, obstetrics, and in-office surgical procedures. On the other hand, internists receive more in-depth training in the diagnosis and treatment of adult illnesses, such as diabetes and heart disease.

Some women also choose to use their gynecologists as their primary care physicians, which saves time for the generally healthy because they can include a lot of preventive tests in their annual pelvic exams, such as blood pressure and cholesterol monitoring. Gynecology, however, is actually a medical-surgical specialty, so these skills are best used to treat illness of your reproductive organs.

Ask around. One of the best ways to find a competent doctor is to ask around, but don't just ask anyone. If you can, question people who work in the medical field. Emergency room physicians and nurses are often in a good position to judge the abilities of local doctors. If it's a gynecologist you're after, ask midwives and nurse-practitioners.

Find a doctor with time. When choosing a new doctor, call several offices, and ask how much time the doctor allots for new-patient visits, annual physicals, and regular visits. One might allow 10 minutes, while another spends 30.

See other health professionals. Physician's assistants and nurse-practitioners are qualified to treat most common problems and usually spend more time with patients than doctors do.

Maximize Your Doctor Visits

If there's one fact about medical care that doctors and patients whole-heartedly agree on, it's that there isn't enough time in the average visit to cover everything. In fact, research shows that most doctors are so pressed for time that they tend to interrupt a patient, on average, after 23 seconds.

With that in mind, here's how you can beat the time crunch and get the most from every visit.

Be up-front and early. When you make an appointment, briefly tell the scheduling person what your issues are. She can help determine how much time you need with the doctor. And to avoid a long wait when you arrive, try to get the first appointment of the day. Or call just before your appointment to find out if the doctor is behind schedule.

Discuss the biggest issues first. Prepare a list of key points that you want to bring up, and during your visit, start with the most important ones.

Present your complaints chronologically. For instance, if your first symptom of dizziness started 2 months ago, then got worse a month ago, then became a constant problem last week, say so. If you lost your balance and fell in the past 2 days, this type of background information should help your doctor put things in perspective.

Explain your strategy. Let your doctor know what, if anything, you've done to try to remedy your condition. Tell her if you've changed your diet in any way or taken any vitamins, herbs, or over-the-counter remedies. Describe their effects, if any, on your symptoms.

Make Teamwork Count

Every woman should perform monthly skin and breast self-exams. But over age 40, you should also talk to your doctor about the following tests and about adding them to your schedule of routine medical care. Your individual health and history factors will need to be taken into account, but here's a general idea of when you should expect to have each type of test.

After age 40, schedule all of the following:

- Mammogram every other year to spot early signs of breast cancer.

- Pelvic exam once a year, along with a manual breast exam and digital rectal exam.

- Blood pressure screening by a health professional at least once a year. High blood pressure (indicated by readings consistently above 140/90) is a risk factor for heart disease and stroke.

- Cholesterol screening once a year. Make sure you know your total cholesterol, LDL, HDL, and triglycerides.

- Complete annual head-to-toe skin exam by a knowledgeable physician to detect any signs of skin cancer.

After age 45, schedule all of the above, plus:

- Serum estradiol test every 2 years. The results of this test can help gauge the onset of menopause.

- An electrocardiogram (EKG) every year. More than one-third of the women who have heart attacks don't have any warning signals beforehand. An EKG can help spot heart damage from the previous year that you may not be aware of.

After age 50, schedule all of the above, plus:

- A thyroid function test every year, which involves lab analysis of a blood sample.

- Fecal occult blood test every year to reveal any hidden blood in your stool, which can be a warning sign of colon cancer and other diseases.

- Bone density screening to help determine your risk of developing osteoporosis. In many cases, women only need this test once.

MAKING THE HORMONE DECISION

Scared and confused about whether or not to take hormone therapy (HT, formerly replacement therapy, HRT)? You're not alone.

"The doctors are confused, so I can't imagine that women aren't," says Machelle M. Seibel, M.D., clinical professor of gynecology and obstetrics

ETHNIC DIFFERENCES MAY INFLUENCE HT DECISION

While 12 out of every 100 white women are on hormone therapy (HT), only 7 out of 100 non-white women take the hormones. Researchers point to numerous reasons for the difference.

First, and possibly foremost, most studies looking at the risks and benefits of HT were conducted with white women. Doctors may be reluctant to recommend HT to non-white women because there is uncertainty about whether the risks and benefits differ according to ethnicity.

Another reason could be differences in how some groups use the health care system. For instance, some research shows that certain ethnic and racial groups are less apt to have health insurance, making it less likely that these women will have a regular physician. Multiple studies have shown that a doctor's recommendation is the primary factor in influencing women to use HT. Without regular medical care, a woman probably wouldn't be given the option of HT.

Even if women have comparable numbers of medical visits, HT tends to be prescribed more often to white women than to black women. Part of this may be that African-American women don't see their gynecologists as often as white women do. And it's gynecologists more than other physicians who are more likely to prescribe HT.

There may be more than just race and ethnicity at work, however. Traditionally, women who go on HT are more affluent and educated than those who don't. Why? These women have easy access to medical care, tend to be healthy, and may visit physicians more often for preventive care.

Other possibilities: There may be differences in how certain groups of women view menopause. Some research suggests that African-Americans perceive menopause more as a natural transition than a disorder. This outlook might make them more accepting of their symptoms and less likely to seek medical treatment. Also, patients with physicians of the same race may be more inclined to take HT.

at Boston University School of Medicine and a reproductive endocrinologist at the Fertility Center of New England in Reading, Massachusetts.

So what's causing all the confusion? In case you missed the big news, 16,000 participants in the Women's Health Initiative (WHI), a landmark study of hormone therapy, opened their mailboxes to find a letter that said, "Stop taking your pills." The researchers sent the letter after they'd found a higher risk of breast cancer among users of a combination HT (a mixture of estrogen and progestin), plus increased risks for heart attack, stroke, and blood clots. To make matters more frightening, the FDA recently used these findings to declare *all* forms of estrogen to be known carcinogens.

Now, thanks to these alarming headlines, many menopausal and post-menopausal women don't know *what* to think about hormone therapy. And with about 50 million of us heading into menopause, plus greater numbers to come, a lot of us are left scratching our heads.

So, to take HT or not? When you get through all the research and hoopla, it essentially boils down to this: HT is not the source of all women's evils as its critics say, but neither is it the cure-all that others claim.

Basically, you're facing an individual decision as unique as you are. Along with your doctor, you need to consider your health, family medical history, risks, and just plain how you feel about it deep in your gut, says Sharon Youcha, M.D., who is on the clinical faculty at Thomas Jefferson University Hospital in Philadelphia and is a gynecologist with a special interest in menopause.

Making Sense of the Headlines

What troubles most of us isn't what we know about hormone therapy— it's what we don't know, or at least don't know enough about. The real risk of breast cancer in conjunction with HT is still up in the air. Meanwhile, one of the potential benefits of long-term HT—prevention of heart disease—has been called into question. Here's what we know for sure.

The Breast Cancer Connection

Ask any woman considering HT about her greatest concern, and she'll probably tell you: breast cancer. The specter of this dread disease looms large over our decision regarding hormones. In fact, some experts say that it's the number one reason holding most women back.

But in evaluating your individual risks, it's important to recognize that both truth and exaggeration exist in the information that's presented to us. The key is to put it all in perspective. And the first step is to understand the hormone therapy–breast cancer connection.

A cancer cell forms when the DNA that controls cell division is damaged. By stimulating breast cells to divide, estrogen increases the chance that one of those new cells will have damaged DNA and will then multiply out of control, causing cancer.

HOW DO THEY MAKE PREMARIN?

The safety and effectiveness of estrogen aren't the only controversies swirling around hormone therapy. How some forms of estrogen are made has people up in arms as well.

The estrogen that many doctors prescribe today is called conjugated equine estrogen, better known in prescription form as Premarin, one of the most prescribed drugs in the country. The word "equine" gives you a hint—Premarin is derived from the urine of pregnant mares. Mares produce high levels of estrogen in their urine until the middle of their third trimester.

The controversy comes on two fronts. On one side, animal rights activists believe that breeding horses just so the mares can produce estrogen-rich urine is cruel. They also claim that the foals of these pregnant horses are unwanted "by-products."

On the other side are those who feel women shouldn't put a substance such as horse urine into their bodies and that they should be using "natural," or bioidentical, estrogens processed from plants.

"Some women view the estrogen in Premarin as an unacceptable choice because it is derived from pregnant mares. But for the majority of women I see, it is a point of interest but not a point of decision making. Would they rather it came from a plant or some other source? Yes. But I don't think that alone is going to stop women from taking estrogen," says Machelle M. Seibel, M.D., clinical professor of gynecology and obstetrics at Boston University Medical School and a reproductive endocrinologist at the Fertility Center of New England in Reading, Massachusetts.

Studies show that women who take HT for 5 years or less—the usual amount of time required to treat menopausal symptoms—probably have little to worry about, except for a very small risk of blood clots.

Questions arise for women who take HT longer. More than 50 population studies found that the risk of breast cancer increased approximately 30 percent for women who used HT for 5 years or more. And it's possible that progesterone—added to estrogen replacement therapy (ERT) to reduce the risk of endometrial cancer—actually *increases* the risk of breast cancer. In the landmark WHI study, which was suspended after 5 years, researchers saw a 26 percent increase in the number of breast cancer cases among HT users.

But before you flush your Premarin down the toilet, consider what those numbers actually mean, a reality that is often lost in the hysterical headlines. According to the authors of the WHI study, for every 10,000 women taking hormone therapy, 38 cases of invasive breast cancer would occur, 8 more cases than you would expect to see in a group of women not taking HT. So taking HT long-term may increase your *personal* risk of developing breast cancer, but probably only slightly.

Future research seeks to clarify the link between HT and breast cancer. Until then, you and your doctor have to make decisions based on your history and, obviously, your comfort level. If you're lying awake at night worrying about breast cancer, then you shouldn't be taking HT.

Hormone Therapy and Heart Disease

For years, many doctors viewed HT as the ultimate double whammy against osteoporosis and heart disease—two problems that plague women most after menopause.

Years of observational studies backed up this theory by showing that women who took the hormones had fewer heart attacks than those who didn't. Other studies found that women on HT saw their LDL ("bad") cholesterol levels drop by about 10 percent, while their beneficial HDL cholesterol increased by about 9 percent.

But a 4-year study of 2,700 women, part of the Heart and Estrogen/Progestin Replacement Study (HERS), found in 1998 that women who already had heart disease were 50 percent more likely to have a heart attack during their first 2 years on HT than those not taking hormones. The WHI backed up these results, revealing that compared with the group not taking HT, 22 percent more participants developed cardiovascular disease while taking HT.

The bottom line: If you have heart disease and are considering HT for osteoporosis or perimenopausal symptoms, find other treatment options. If you haven't had a heart attack and don't have severe arteriosclerosis, you're probably fine taking HT for short-term relief of menopausal symptoms.

But heart disease prevention shouldn't be the reason you're taking HT, anyway. The cholesterol benefits you get from hormones are about the same you'd get from a low-fat diet. And cholesterol-lowering statins and other medications provide better protection.

The Good and the Bad

Think of the decision to take HT as a scale: You weigh the benefits on one side, the drawbacks on the other. Whichever side tips the scale determines your decision. But before you start weighing, you have to know the facts.

The Pros

Bones. The ads might as well say, "Got estrogen?" Next to calcium, estrogen is probably the biggest ally we have in the quest for strong bones. Basically, it increases factors that stimulate bone to grow. So when we lose estrogen in middle age, we begin losing bone. If you take HT, studies show that bone loss slows. One study found that women who took HT for 5 or more years reduced their risk of back and neck fractures by 50 to 80 percent. Another series of studies found that women taking hormones reduced their risk of hip fractures by 25 percent. Once you go off HT, however, you're likely to lose whatever gains you've made.

Hot flashes. Without question, hormone therapy is the most effective treatment for hot flashes and other perimenopausal symptoms, says Deborah Kwolek, M.D., medical director of the Women's Health Center at the Chandler Medical Center of the University of Kentucky in Lexington. Women who take HT reduce their hot flashes (or power surges, as some of us like to call them) by up to 70 percent.

For many women, Dr. Youcha adds, HT is the only way to get through menopause without investing in a towel company. How does it help? One theory is that as estrogen declines during menopause, a chemical called luteinizing hormone (LH) rises, possibly throwing off the way your body's thermostat works. HT affects the release of that hormone, stabilizing the thermostat.

Sleep. Estrogen helps you get a better night's sleep. A study conducted in Turku, Finland, found that HT eliminated the hot flashes, night sweats, and headaches that kept women up at night. Another study, at Brown University Medical School, found that in menopausal women, HT helped alleviate sleep apnea (in which you stop breathing several times during the night). Somehow, researchers speculate, estrogen helps stimulate breathing during sleep.

Mood. It could be the result of getting a better night's sleep, or it could be that HT actually helps regulate mood, but women on hormone therapy often report feeling less irritable, says Wulf H. Utian, M.D., Ph.D., executive director of the North American Menopause Society in Cleveland.

Memory. The studies aren't completely conclusive yet, but research suggests that estrogen replacement therapy helps improve memory and cognitive function and may even ward off or at least slow the progression of Alzheimer's disease.

Weight. In what may be the greatest incentive to take HT, researchers at Boston University discovered that women on hormone therapy had significantly less body fat than non-HT users. And a study at Johns Hopkins University found that HT increased muscle mass while decreasing body fat. Researchers speculate that it's the estrogen drop that contributes to the all-too-common postmenopausal weight gain.

The Cons

Blood clots. Hormone therapy more than doubles your risk of developing blood clots in your legs, which could dislodge and travel to your lungs (causing a pulmonary embolism) or to your brain (causing a stroke or other serious problems). Oral estrogen elevates blood-clotting factors produced by the liver, which may trigger the formation of blood clots.

Gallstones. HT also slightly increases your risk of developing gall-stones. Estrogen stimulates the liver to remove cholesterol from the blood and divert it into the gallbladder, and gallstones form if too much choles-terol flows into the gallbladder.

Endometrial cancer. Because the additional estrogen stimulates the cells lining your uterus to continue to divide, using estrogen therapy alone can increase your risk of this cancer. But that risk is essentially eliminated when progesterone is added to the hormone mix.

Periods. Just when you thought it was safe to throw out the tampons, you start on HT and begin having periodic vaginal bleeding again. Blame HT. This is the major reason women stop taking hormones. (Hey, 40 years of periods is more than enough!)

Side effects. Like most drugs, HT has a laundry list of possible side effects, including severe stomach pain or swelling, pain or numbness in the chest, shortness of breath, severe headaches, changes in vision, and breast lumps. Other, less serious side effects include bloating, breast pain and ten-derness, nausea, headaches, and mood swings.

Restrictions. You may not be able to take hormone therapy if you've had breast cancer, liver disease, large uterine fibroids, or endometriosis be-cause HT may aggravate these conditions.

Questions to Ask Yourself

Now it's time to put all the pros and cons on the scale. How do you measure it out? Try answering these few simple questions, Dr. Utian sug-gests. Along with your doctor's input and recommendations, your answers will help guide you down the right path.

"Do I have perimenopausal symptoms such as hot flashes?" If the answer is no, you don't need HT.

"Why do I need hormone therapy?" You should not take hor-mones just because you're a menopausal woman. Your doctor should clearly state why she thinks you need HT and what your long-term plan of action should be.

"What does my medical history show?" You'll have to go over this with your doctor, but many women either underestimate or overestimate their own risks of certain diseases. You may fear breast cancer, but your family history and your own bone density may predispose you much, much more to osteoporosis.

"Are there other options?" Obviously, lifestyle changes can make a big difference. And there are other drugs on the market that help treat hot flashes and bone loss. That's not necessarily to say these are better than HT. In fact, you may find that hormone therapy is perfect for you. But look at all your other options before deciding.

"How do I feel about HT?" Gut feelings go a long way, Dr. Youcha says. If taking HT seems right medically, but you're stressing out about it, talk to your doctor about the alternatives.

Customizing Your HT Plan

"Gone are the days of one-size-fits-all hormone therapy, when all menopausal women received a standard dose of estrogen and progestin and either lived with the results or abandoned the therapy altogether," says Andrew M. Kaunitz, M.D., professor of obstetrics and gynecology at the University of Florida Health Science Center in Jacksonville and director of gynecology and menopause services at the University of Florida Medicus Diagnostic Center. Today hormone therapy uses various forms of estrogens (such as conjugated estrogen, estradiol, estropipate, or esterified estrogen) and progestin (such as medroxyprogesterone acetate, norethindrone acetate, or micronized progesterone) in various doses. "If you stopped taking HT—or are worried about starting—because of side effects like headaches or spotting, don't assume it's not for you. Unpleasant side effects can be reduced or, in most cases, eliminated," says Dr. Kaunitz.

To find the hormone mix that's best for you, talk to your doctor about tailoring therapy to your needs. Here are your options.

Continuous combined. Estrogen is taken along with a low dose of progestin every day. The constant dosage of progestin (which signals the uterus to shed its lining) means that you may experience erratic bleeding or spotting, with no pattern or regularity. For some women, this eventually stops.

Sequential/cyclical. Estrogen is taken every day and progestin is taken on a cyclical schedule so that bleeding occurs on a regular, predictable schedule, as if you're having a period.

Quarterly progestin. Another option is to take estrogen every day and progestin every 3 months, or quarterly throughout the year. You'll have just four periods per year.

Low-dose estrogen. Taken in a very low dose with no progestin, estrogen produces none of progestin's PMS-like symptoms, and the dosage of estrogen is low enough that there appears to be no increased risk of endometrial cancer. Your doctor, however, may recommend regular tests of the endometrium if you choose this option.

THE INVENTORS OF HORMONE THERAPY

Maybe we're the first generation openly talking about taking hormones for health, but we sure aren't the first ones who thought about it. There's evidence that more than 5,000 years ago, Chinese emperors ingested the urine of young women to gain the restorative powers of hormones.

In the modern era, we can thank the research team of Edgar Allen and Edward A. Doisy. They got the ball rolling on the hormone revolution in 1923 with their landmark paper in the *Journal of the American Medical Association*, "An Ovarian Hormone: Preliminary Report on Its Localization, Extraction, and Partial Purification and Action in Test Animals."

The two met in their medical school library in the early 1920s and quickly became friends. So when Dr. Allen wanted to make extracts from ovarian tissue, because of previous research that showed removing the ovaries from rats stopped their estrus cycle (basically, an animal's menstrual cycle), he asked his good friend Dr. Doisy to help. The two set about identifying the hormone that turned out to be estrogen.

As for the progesterone part, they got some help from G. W. Corner and Willard Allen, who identified and explained the role of progesterone in 1927. Then in 1929, Dr. Doisy—continuing his previous estrogen research—actually crystallized estrogen, which was originally called theelin. So by the end of the 1920s, scientists understood and could re-create the roles of both estrogen and progesterone in a woman's body.

Ironically, Dr. Edgar Allen was just 31 and Dr. Doisy only 29 when they published the findings that would later change the science of aging.

Pill, Patch, or Cream?

The form in which you take hormone therapy can be as important as the type and dosage that you take. The most common method of administering HT is orally, either with separate pills for each hormone or with a combined pill.

HT is also available in a patch, which is ideal for women who find taking pills unpleasant, who have problems absorbing the oral medication, or who have high triglyceride levels.

Hormone cream, applied topically inside the vagina where it has an immediate effect, works especially well for women who experience sexual discomfort after menopause and tolerate neither pills nor the patch. Topical treatments have such a low dose that progestin may not be necessary, but they don't treat hot flashes or protect your bones the way a pill or patch does.

Interested in natural hormone therapy? See page 327.

WHAT YOU NEED TO KNOW ABOUT BREAST CANCER

With all the races, the pink ribbons, and the celebrities talking about their breast cancer, it's difficult to ignore the disease. And we shouldn't ignore all the hype because close to 183,000 women get breast cancer each year.

Although estrogen is considered a key player in breast cancer—in both its advent and its progress—there are two schools of thought on how much of a role it actually plays.

Some research suggests estrogen may do to our breast cells what too many desserts do to our fat cells—make them grow and divide. And if any of the breast cells are already cancerous, estrogen feeds their growth. The other school disagrees and sees estrogen as more protective than causative in breast cancer development. If you do develop breast cancer while on estrogen, it will typically be a type that is more easily treated.

REDUCE YOUR BREAST CANCER RISK

Worried about breast cancer? You can start reducing your overall risk today with a number of small lifestyle changes.

Load up on colorful foods. Want to lower your risk of cancer three times a day? Then eat at least seven servings of fruits and vegetables in all hues of the rainbow. That's because carotenoids, the plant chemicals that create bright colors in fruits and vegetables, may help prevent cancer. So make it a habit to dine on blueberries, grapes, raisins, plums, dark green lettuce, spinach, kale, collards, carrots, strawberries, tomatoes, beets, and red, green, orange, and yellow peppers.

Try a new fruit or vegetable each week and learn new ways to prepare old favorites. You don't have to give up meat completely; just shift toward a more colorful, plant-based diet. A good tool for expanding your produce menu is a vegetarian starter cookbook, such as *Vegetarian and More!* by Linda Rosensweig.

Slim down. More fat equals more unopposed estrogen (estrogen without a progesterone parent keeping it under control), which increases your risk of breast cancer. So a lean body means less estrogen and a lower risk of breast cancer.

Take your breasts for a walk. A study conducted at the Keck School of Medicine of the University of Southern California showed that women who had exercised at least 4 hours per week for at least 12 years and hadn't gained much weight in adulthood were 29 percent less likely to get breast cancer than women who had never exercised at that level.

Make it a virgin daiquiri. Your arteries may feel pretty good after a few drinks, but your breasts have a low tolerance. A combined report of more than 50 studies found that drinking as few as two alcoholic drinks a day can increase your breast cancer risk by 25 percent, no matter whether you drink cheap vodka or a fine red wine.

Unfortunately, passing the menopause milestone doesn't seem to lower your chances of estrogen-positive breast cancer.

The older you get, the greater your chances of getting breast cancer. One reason may be that although your ovaries no longer make estrogen after menopause, there's still enough estrogen hanging around in your tissues to stimulate breast cancer cells to grow.

Yet despite the theories and recent headlines, steering clear of estrogen replacement therapy (ERT) won't completely remove your breast cancer risk. "In fact, most breast cancer cases occur in women who are postmenopausal and have never been on hormone therapy," says M. Michelle Blackwood, M.D., breast surgeon at the Blackwood Breast Center in Stamford, Connecticut.

Another theory suggests that we get more breast cancer as we age because of the overall deterioration our bodies undergo, not the estrogen. "We're at the highest risk of breast cancer when we have the *least* estrogen in our bodies," says Dr. Blackwood.

Progesterone, too, causes cells in the breasts to divide, says Malcolm Pike, Ph.D., professor in the department of preventive medicine at the University of Southern California in Los Angeles. A study conducted at screening centers throughout the United States and published in the *Journal of the American Medical Association* looked at 46,355 postmenopausal women who had used hormone therapy (HT) in the previous 4 years and found that the breast cancer risk of women who had taken ERT alone increased by 1 percent each year they took the therapy. The risk of women who had taken an estrogen/progesterone combination increased by *8 percent* each year they continued that therapy.

Testosterone may also play a part. Women with breast cancer have 30 to 100 percent more testosterone than do healthy women. It's not known exactly what testosterone does in breast tissue to increase the risk. One theory suggests that it stimulates breast cells to grow and divide, increasing the odds that one of those cells will have the cancer switch turned to "on."

Hormones also play a role once the cancer has developed. Some breast cancers have receptors for estrogen or progesterone, sometimes referred to as ER-positive and PR-positive. On the one hand, it's good to have a hormone-sensitive tumor, because it's more likely to respond to hormone-blocking drugs like tamoxifen (Nolvadex). On the other hand, ER- or PR-positive breast cancer is fueled by estrogen or progesterone, so you have to be extra careful to avoid exposure to those hormones.

Understanding the Tamoxifen Trade-Off

Tamoxifen is a great treatment for the majority of breast cancers, especially estrogen-sensitive ones. But doctors are hesitant to prescribe the drug to *prevent* breast cancer, mainly because it can increase the risk for

SHE FOUND A LUMP

At 48, Helene Kosakowski of Reading, Pennsylvania, felt very tired. Then one day she found a lump in her breast. It turned out to be estrogen-sensitive breast cancer.

"I never did routine checks on my breasts," says Helene. "I was a nurse, and I taught other women to do them, but I never performed them on myself. I didn't think it could happen to me.

"When I did find a lump, I went immediately to my family doctor. He sent me for a mammogram that day.

"When they repeated the mammogram a few times, I knew something was wrong. Being a nurse, I wasn't about to leave without talking to the radiologist, so I was able to look at my film that day. The lump looked like a small sphere. It had fingerlike protrusions, so I knew it had spread. I made an appointment with a surgeon for the following week, and I left for a Disney World vacation.

"Needless to say, I was panicked throughout the weeklong vacation. I still had some hope that it wasn't cancer. When I returned, the surgeon put my hope to rest—it was cancer. And from the biopsy, he could tell that the tumor was estrogen-sensitive, meaning the cancer cells were using estrogen to grow. He scheduled my surgery—a lumpectomy (removal of the tumor) and a partial mastectomy (removal of part of my breast)—for March 7, which was my birthday.

"Then, in April, I had a modified radical mastectomy (removal of my entire

endometrial cancer. So before you decide to take tamoxifen as a preventive measure, you should carefully examine the pros and cons.

It might be worth it to take tamoxifen is if you're genetically at risk for breast cancer. Then your risk of getting breast cancer is higher than your risk of getting endometrial cancer from the drug. If you still have your uterus, doctors will carefully monitor you with ultrasound for any signs of endometrial cancer and any endometrial thickening. They'll do occasional biopsies to look for any tissue changes. If you've had a hysterectomy, you don't have to worry at all about endometrial cancer.

Obesity seems to worsen the effects of tamoxifen on the endometrium. In postmenopausal women, a reaction can occur in body fat that actually creates the most potent form of estrogen—estradiol—which can feed endometrial cancer cells. So if you're overweight, you should give tamoxifen careful thought and talk to your doctor about your options.

breast) and an axillary dissection (removal of some of my lymph nodes) because the cancer had spread. I chose not to have breast reconstruction. Instead, I wear a prosthesis.

"Six months of chemotherapy followed. Emotionally, this was a scary time. Every day, I just got up and tried to make things as normal as possible. I drove myself to chemo. It was still business as usual. If I went on social outings or traveled with my husband, I simply put on a scarf and a hat and dressed myself up.

"After my chemotherapy was complete, I started taking tamoxifen (Nolvadex). Tamoxifen stops estrogen from being produced in my body so the hormone won't feed the cancer. Tamoxifen has its downsides; it brings on hot flashes, weight gain, and the fear of endometrial cancer. My treatment ended in October 2001, and since then I've been able to lose weight and start exercising again.

"Today, at age 54, I'm doing well. I devote a lot of my time to volunteer work for the American Cancer Society, helping women who are going through the same thing I did. And this past year, I traveled to Washington, D.C., to share my experience with legislators to press cancer bills and issues.

"If I can give any advice to women going through a bout of breast cancer, it's that you have choices. You don't have to have a breast reconstruction. I never had one. I look good and have a nice body, except I'm missing a breast and wear a prosthesis. It's your body, and you need to look at all the choices before you make a decision."

Another catalyst for endometrial cancer is estrogen replacement therapy. If you're on ERT, you're already at an increased risk for endometrial cancer. In that case, the tamoxifen may be the straw that breaks the camel's back. Make sure you discuss this with your doctor.

Stay in Touch with Your Breasts

Unless the First Lady invites you to lunch on the day you've scheduled a mammogram, keep your appointment. And frankly, there's no excuse for not making a monthly breast self-exam part of your regular health routine. "Early detection can really make a difference in the long-term outcome," says Donna Sweet, M.D., professor of internal medicine at the University of Kansas School of Medicine in Wichita. Roughly 90 percent of the time, breast lumps are found through self-exams.

So regardless of whether you've gone through menopause or not, the importance of these tests simply cannot be emphasized enough. (See "Why You Still Need Mammograms" on page 388.) Experts recommend that all women perform a monthly self-exam and receive a mammogram every 1 to 2 years after age 40. If you have a mother or sister with breast cancer, get one every year from age 35 on.

As far as the self-exam is concerned, try to do your exam at the same time every month, ideally 5 to 7 days after your period ends. Begin by standing in front of a mirror with your hands at your sides. Raise your hands and hold them together behind your head. Look for any change in the size or shape of your breasts, as well as for nipple discharge, redness, puckering, and dimpling. Next, press your hands on your hips, pull your shoulders and elbows forward, and look for similar changes.

After this visual exam, you need to check your breasts again by touch. Follow a definite pattern, and make sure that you repeat the exam the same way every time—it's the best way to ensure you'll notice anything out of the ordinary. Three common examples that experts recommend are the circle, the wedge, and the vertical patterns.

To use the circle pattern, your fingers travel in small circles, moving from the outer portions of your breast toward the nipple. With the vertical pattern, you slide your hand up and down in vertical lines from one side of the breast to the other. Similarly, with the wedge pattern you start from the nipple and work your fingers out to the edge of your breast and then back toward the nipple again. Whatever pattern you choose, make sure that you cover one breast thoroughly before proceeding to the other one.

Visualize a Pain-Free Mammogram

In order to examine as much of the breast as possible during a mammogram, the breast is compressed between an x-ray plate and a plastic cover. For many women, this image alone is enough to make the prospect of a mammogram unnerving—not to mention fear of a cancer diagnosis.

"Just about every woman experiences a certain degree of apprehension when getting a mammogram," says Laurie Nadel, Ph.D., a doctor of clinical hypnotherapy in New York City who has coached many women in calming mammogram jitters. Her own first mammogram was so painful that she put off scheduling another one for years. "I used mental imagery to pick up the phone and make another appointment." The trick is to give yourself a boost by remembering a positive experience, she adds.

If your mammogram appointment is just around the corner, practice this exercise three times a day, then again just before you step up to the mammography plate. Ball up your hands into fists. Close your eyes and think about a wonderful place where you once felt calm, relaxed, and safe. Remember the sights, sounds, and smells as you relive every moment.

To enhance your sense of peace, add more color to that picture-perfect place in your mind. Make the images larger or sharper, or increase the tightness of your fists, until your calmness reaches its peak.

As your anxiety slowly fades, release your hands, shake them out, and open your eyes. To recapture that warm, fuzzy feeling, make those fists again and say to yourself, "Take me back."

The more you practice this exercise, the faster your brain will make the connection between your fists and total calm, says Dr. Nadel. "The painful part takes 3 seconds, then it's over. If you learn to quickly flood your body with feelings of happiness, you'll reduce the perception of anticipated pain."

To further reduce discomfort, try to schedule your mammogram about 1 week after the last day of your menstrual period, when breast swelling and tenderness are minimal. And a few weeks before your appointment, cut down on caffeine and start taking 200 to 400 IU of vitamin E daily.

HOW TO AVOID
SURGERY-INDUCED MENOPAUSE

If you're one of the 600,000 women a year who are told by their doctors, "You need a hysterectomy," don't panic. Maybe you need surgery, and maybe you don't.

Each year, more than half a million women undergo hysterectomies (removal of the uterus) for fibroids, endometriosis, and abnormal bleeding.

If a woman's ovaries are also removed, her estrogen levels plummet, and she is thrown full-tilt into menopause. And even if the ovaries are preserved, there's some evidence that menopause will occur earlier as a result of a hysterectomy. Overall, it's the second-most-common surgery in America among women in their reproductive years. (For those who've gone through natural menopause, it's far less frequent).

But here's the real kicker: About 90 percent of women who had the surgery could have been offered uterus-sparing treatments instead, says Brian Walsh, M.D., chief of surgical gynecology at Brigham and Women's Hospital in Boston. That's important if you still want to have children or want to avoid an early menopause.

So why aren't we told about other options? "Doctors are either unaware of the alternatives or just not comfortable with performing the procedures that require higher levels of skill," says Mitchell Rein, M.D., an obstetrician-gynecologist, reproductive endocrinologist, and associate professor at Harvard Medical School in Boston. Hysterectomy should be necessary only if a woman's condition doesn't improve after she has explored all other possibilities, or if she has invasive uterine cancer, says Dr. Rein.

Cancer accounts for fewer than 5 percent of all hysterectomies, says Dr. Walsh. Non-life-threatening conditions make up the rest.

Following are three of the most common conditions that normally prompt a hysterectomy and the ways to treat them that don't involve removing your uterus. If your doctor doesn't mention any of these options, ask, especially if you still want to have children.

Fibroids

As many as 4 out of 10 hysterectomies are done to remove fibroids, or uterine leiomyomas, bundles of muscle and connective tissue that can grow inside or outside the uterus. Uterus-saving treatments include:

Ibuprofen. Over-the-counter pain relievers like ibuprofen (such as Motrin and Advil) can sometimes help ease the pain and heavy bleeding of fibroids. For mild symptoms, they should be your doctor's first line of treatment, says Dr. Rein.

Uterine artery embolization. This nonsurgical procedure cuts off the blood supply to the fibroid, causing it to shrink, says Linda D. Bradley,

M.D., director of hysteroscopic services in the department of obstetrics and gynecology at the Cleveland Clinic Foundation in Ohio.

Recovery is quick, and side effects are few, but the impact on fertility is questionable. "After a woman has this procedure, we don't know if her uterus is strong enough to sustain a pregnancy," says Dr. Bradley.

Myomectomy. This surgical technique removes fibroids but leaves the uterus intact. The size of the fibroids and where they occur determine what type of myomectomy your doctor performs. With a hysteroscopic myomectomy, fibroids are removed vaginally. In laparoscopic surgery, the doctor extracts fibroids through a small incision made in the abdomen. The more complex procedures for multiple and large fibroids are done through larger abdominal incisions, says Dr. Rein.

For more information about the new hope for fibroids, turn to page 383.

Endometriosis

About one out of five hysterectomies is done for endometriosis, where fragments of the uterine lining grow outside the uterus in the abdomen and on the ovaries. Fueled by estrogen, the tissue then grows and bleeds on a monthly cycle, causing chronic pain, inflammation, scar tissue, and other problems. Fortunately, because of the estrogen connection, this is one condition that usually slows the closer you get to menopause. Other ways to control endometriosis include:

Oral contraceptives (birth control pills). Most effective for milder cases of endometriosis, oral contraceptives alter the balance of estrogen and progesterone, slowing the progression of the disease, says Dr. Walsh.

Hormonal drugs. GnRH agonists are powerful hormonal drugs that reduce estrogen production and shrink endometrial tissue. The most commonly used are nafarelin (Synarel) and leuprolide (Lupron). Two problems: They send you into early—but reversible—menopause. And they can cause premature bone loss if used long-term, says Dr. Rein.

Laparoscopic surgery. With this surgery, possibly performed when endometriosis is diagnosed, stray endometrial tissue is destroyed with an electrical device or a laser, says Dr. Walsh. Endometriosis has a tendency to recur, but birth control pills can help keep it in check.

Laparotomy. More invasive than laparoscopic surgery but less so than hysterectomy, this procedure destroys the endometriosis tissue and/or associated scar tissue.

Abnormal Bleeding

Persistent or heavy bleeding accounts for another 20 percent of hysterectomies performed. Other options to consider:

Ibuprofen. In mild cases, NSAIDs such as Motrin or Advil can sometimes help slow down the bleeding, says Dr. Walsh.

Hormone treatment. Contraceptives like Depo-Provera, administered by injection, or regular birth control pills are often ideal for women who are not ovulating regularly and who are bleeding throughout the month, says Dr. Walsh.

Endometrial ablation. This destroys the lining of the uterus and the layer under it, and the procedure can be done vaginally. Ablation will usually leave you infertile. And while one-third of all patients will have no more bleeding, one-third will have spotting or a light flow. Twenty-five percent will have average periods. A few—5 to 10 percent—will be no better off than before.

FACING DISEASE

"The stinging shock of cold water . . . "

"An unexpected slap in the face . . . "

"Hearing voices in the room fade as the sound of your pounding heart fills your ears . . . "

DON'T GO IT ALONE

When it comes to facing disease, two heads are definitely better than one. If you're undergoing treatment for a serious health condition, consider asking a relative or close friend to go to your doctor appointments with you. Talk beforehand about the questions you have so that your companion knows what information you need to get from your doctor.

Every woman has different words to describe her first moments after receiving an unexpected diagnosis. And while the reactions may differ, the flood of questions that follow are usually similar. What's next? What should I expect? What are my options?

That's why we've put together this guide to facing the conditions most common to women as they approach menopause. After all, knowledge is power. And if you know the basics of what to expect, you're already a step ahead.

Breast Cancer

If you detect a lump or if anything else seems abnormal during your monthly self-exam, see your gynecologist. Make sure that your doctor checks your breasts in at least two positions, such as lying down with your arms raised over your head and then standing or sitting upright. This will help your doctor get a complete sense of the size, shape, and texture of any suspicious lumps.

Then, if your doctor suspects anything abnormal in your breast, she may order further tests such as a mammogram or an ultrasonogram, which uses high-frequency sound waves to determine if a lump is solid or fluid. If those tests confirm her suspicions, then a biopsy is usually the next step. This can be done with a special needle, or the surgeon may opt to cut out all or part of the lump. Once the lump is removed, a pathologist will examine it to look for cancer cells.

If cancer is confirmed, treatment will depend on several factors, including the size of your tumor and whether it has spread to the lymph nodes or other parts of your body. You will likely receive a combination of surgery, radiation, and/or chemotherapy. Surgery for breast cancer used to mean one thing: mastectomy. A lumpectomy, which removes only the tumor, followed by radiation is far more common now, however.

Radiation therapy uses very sophisticated equipment to direct high-energy rays at cancerous tissue, thereby killing cancer cells in their tracks. Another variation of radiation therapy involves placing radioactive implants into your breast. In some cases, both forms of treatment are warranted. Typical side effects may be limited to a sunburnlike burn on the treated breast, fatigue, and the loss of underarm hair near the treated breast.

GET ANOTHER PROFESSIONAL PERSPECTIVE

If you've been diagnosed with a serious disease that requires difficult treatment, your insurance company may require you to get a second opinion. But even if your insurance company doesn't insist, it may be in your best interests to hear what another doctor has to say, especially if surgery may be required. Second opinions can lend valuable insight into your original diagnosis and may shed new light on your different options.

Chemotherapy, which may involve a variety of anticancer drugs, is a standard treatment for premenopausal women whose breast tumors are greater than 1 centimeter in diameter. Because these drugs travel through the bloodstream, they are often able to destroy cancer cells that other treatments may miss. This treatment is also scarier for many women because of its reputation for nasty side effects, including hair loss, nausea, vomiting, and loss of appetite. But in many cases, these side effects can be controlled or eliminated.

Heart Disease

Heart disease takes many forms, from heart attack to stroke to chronic chest pain, and involves just as many methods to diagnose it. For example, your doctor may begin a physical exam with a blood pressure reading. Blood tests may also be ordered since cholesterol problems help advance heart disease.

From there, further tests may be in order depending on your risk factors, health history, and symptoms. These may include an electrocardiogram, a chest x-ray, an exercise stress test, or a nuclear imaging test. A noninvasive test known as electron beam computed tomography (EBCT) rapidly scans the beating heart with x-trays to examine any potential problems in the arteries. This test is so effective that it can detect heart disease in women who have no outward symptoms.

Depending on your diagnosis, your doctor may prescribe preventive medicines. These commonly include a class of drugs called statins, which reduce cholesterol and consequently lower the risk of having a first heart attack. Low-dose aspirin therapy has also been shown to prevent recurrence of heart attacks among women who've already had them. Long-acting drugs called nitrates and beta-blockers are usually prescribed for chronic chest pain.

If a blockage is detected, there are several surgical procedures that doctors use to restore proper bloodflow through the heart. With balloon angioplasty, a doctor inserts a catheter, or tube, into a narrowed artery and inflates the balloon. This allows him to implant a wire-mesh tube within the walls of the artery to keep it from closing again. Bypass surgery is another option, and in this arena there's good news especially for women—there's now a less invasive type of bypass surgery, in which the incision is made under a breast instead of down the middle of the chest. Of course, it's not an appropriate approach for all cases, but it's definitely worth discussing with your doctor if you need bypass surgery.

Mood Disorders

If you perceive your moods to be especially volatile as you move through menopause, share your concerns with your doctor. You may find that getting an accurate diagnosis can be the first step toward feeling better. For many, it's a relief to be able to put a name and label on what they are experiencing.

As far as treatment is concerned, there are many antidepressant drugs available to help correct chemical imbalances in the brain. Your doctor should ask a lot of questions about your symptoms and general health to determine which medication would be best for you. In most cases, it may be several weeks before you notice its effect.

About 60 to 70 percent of people who can tolerate the side effects of antidepressants get better with the first drug they take. If after 8 to 12 weeks you feel that the particular prescription isn't working for you, talk to your doctor about trying another antidepressant.

In part, your medical history will determine how long you need to take these drugs. Previous episodes of depression usually indicate that a longer time frame is in order.

Women who combine talk therapy with prescription medicines often do better in the long run. Two short-term and highly effective methods to consider are cognitive behavior therapy and interpersonal therapy.

In a cognitive behavior session, your therapist will help you focus on changing behavior and improving mood by identifying which situations make you happy and which lead you to feel depressed. You'll then examine your behavior and thought patterns and find ways to change them. Interpersonal therapy, on the other hand, focuses on your personal and social interactions with others and how they affect your mood. Basically, you'll work on improving your relationships so that you feel better about yourself.

Osteoporosis

If you are at or beyond menopause, have experienced a fracture, or have one or more risk factors for osteoporosis, experts strongly recommend that you have the appropriate medical tests to determine your bone mineral density. Knowing your bone density is really the only way to detect the disease before a fracture occurs or to predict your chances of another break, as well as to monitor the rate of bone loss.

Presently, the best test for determining your bone mineral density is called DEXA (dual-energy x-ray absorptiometry). Don't let the name unnerve you—the test is painless, noninvasive, and brief (usually about 15 minutes). With very low dose radiation, the DEXA machine will scan your hips and spine, two areas where osteoporosis can have the gravest consequences, and compare your bone density with that of the average woman. A reading between −1 and −2.5 standard deviations from normal indicates low bone mass. A standard deviation of +1 or +2 is great news, showing you have good bone density.

If you've been diagnosed with osteoporosis, you should repeat this test every 2 years to make sure that your treatment is working. If your initial score was very low—more than 2.5 standard deviations below normal—have it rechecked annually.

As far as treatment is concerned, osteoporosis is a unique disease in that it doesn't "belong" to a particular medical specialty. Most likely, you would talk to your gynecologist first; however, there are three other types of experts who may be called upon as needed: an endocrinologist, who treats hormone-related conditions; or a rheumatologist, who specializes in diseases of the joints and connective tissues; or an orthopedist, who deals with skeletal problems.

There are also some new drugs available to prevent and treat osteoporosis. One of the most recent contenders, teriparatide (Forteo), takes a new approach in treating osteoporosis because it helps restore the body's ability to build new bone, rather than slowing bone loss. Other drugs include raloxifene (Evista), which is a drug that imitates estrogen without the same potentially harmful effects, such as raising the risk of breast cancer. Raloxifene has been shown to increase bone mass in the spine and hips and to reduce the risk of fractures in the spine by up to 50 percent. Other drugs making a difference include alendronate (Fosamax), which is especially effective for reducing spine and hip fractures, and a companion drug called risedronate (Actonel). Calcitonin, a hormone that slows bone loss and modestly builds spinal bone density, is a common treatment for women at least 5 years beyond menopause.

Reproductive Cancer

Endometrial cancer can occur before or after menopause; but since the number one symptom is abnormal bleeding, it's easy to detect, fortunately. For this reason, any bleeding after menopause, even simple spotting, warrants a trip to the gynecologist right away. Ovarian cancer, on the other hand, is more difficult to diagnose because its symptoms mimic everyday womanly complaints—cramping, bloating, and swelling in the abdomen. What's more, a family history of ovarian cancer is the biggest risk factor for the disease, so there aren't a lot of hands-on things you can do to reduce your risk. Any symptoms that persist for longer than a month should be evaluated by your doctor.

Most endometrial cancer is caught fairly early and treated with a hysterectomy. More advanced cases may require removing the ovaries, fallopian tubes, nearby lymph nodes, and upper part of the vagina. Sometimes follow-up includes radiation treatments, hormone therapy, or chemotherapy.

The primary treatment for ovarian cancer is surgical removal of the tumor. If the case is more severe, one or both ovaries, nearby organs, and lymph nodes may be removed as well. Unfortunately, because surgery rarely cures ovarian cancer, chemotherapy is usually prescribed.

Chapter

12

THE WIDE WORLD OF ALTERNATIVE TREATMENTS

IF YOU'VE BEEN WATCHING THE NEWS, YOU'VE PROBABLY HEARD plenty about alternative treatments for menopause. With the sudden drop-off in the number of women using conventional hormone therapy, our news media are filled with headlines about the latest options. Ironically, much of this "late-breaking news" comes from healing traditions that are thousands of years old! But what you might not have heard about natural healing is this: Alternative medicine offers a lot of satisfaction beyond healing. Because many alternative treatments help integrate the healing of mind and body and put *you* in control of your treatment options, they can also help restore vital balance, perspective, and meaning to life in the menopausal years.

Consider this chapter your tour guide to alternative options. You'll learn about the natural plant-based hormone alternative your doctor can prescribe for you, as well as the wide range of supplements you can pick up on your own at your health food store. Plus, we'll cover all of the other great healing methods, such as acupuncture and yoga, used by women around the world to treat menopausal symptoms.

But first, let's talk about what you should do before you make any changes that could affect your long-term health.

Coordinate Your Care

If you decide to add an herb or supplement to your diet, or if you're interested in trying out an alternative therapy, tell your family physician about your plans. She may need to monitor your progress or adjust your medication. In some cases, an herb or supplement may have a dangerous interaction with a drug you're already taking, so make sure to review "Using Herbs and Supplements Safely" on page 402.

And be patient. Don't expect natural healing methods to work in quite the same way that Western medicine does.

"We're used to quick-fix treatments that work almost immediately," says Adrian Fugh-Berman, M.D., former head of field investigations for the Office of Alternative Medicine at the National Institutes of Health in Bethesda, Maryland. "Natural medicine tends to be slower, gentler, and often easier on your system." So listen to your body, find what works for you, and give it time.

TRAVELING DOWN A DIFFERENT ROAD: HT ALTERNATIVES

For some women, the answer to the hormone therapy (HT) question is a clear no. Whether it's because you can't take HT—or you just won't—there are plenty of other options that can help you deal with the symptoms of perimenopause and safeguard your health.

Natural Hormone Therapies

If you are interested in hormone therapy but concerned about the side effects, you might want to try "natural" hormones that are derived from plant compounds and are identical to the progesterone and estrogen your body produces. Though plant-derived hormones have actually been in use for a long time, the natural hormone therapies, when compared with conventional HT, offer similar relief from symptoms without the number or severity of commonly reported side effects, such as depression, breast tenderness, and bloating.

Bear in mind, however, that another point of contrast concerns the research. Hands down, there have been many more studies conducted to determine the effects (and risks) of conventional hormone therapy—but natural hormone proponents are quick to point out that you simply can't take conclusions drawn from the studies of conventional HT and apply them to the use of natural hormones. They are quite different medicines. To explain more, here's an overview about your options and what we know about how natural hormones can help.

Why Do I Need Hormones Again?

Your body is designed to produce just the right amounts of estrogen and progesterone to keep the rhythm of your menstrual cycle balanced and regular throughout your reproductive years. Estrogen is the hormone that revs up at the beginning of each cycle and makes sure that ovulation occurs every month. And then progesterone steps in to help regulate your cycle and nourish the lining of your uterus in preparation for pregnancy, should this occur. But its job is also to prevent estrogen from causing the lining to thicken too much. So when an egg is not fertilized, progesterone levels drop, causing the lining to be shed in a menstrual period. This is important because it is the monthly shedding that helps lower the risk of endometrial cancer.

As you approach menopause, your ovaries slow down and stop producing progesterone, and you ovulate less frequently or not at all. By the time you reach menopause, the drop in progesterone is almost 100 percent. Estrogen, in contrast, drops by about 90 percent since there are other sources of estrogen in the body.

Decreased estrogen levels are to blame for virtually all menopausal symptoms. So if you're given estrogen to counter them, you're also typically prescribed a progestin (the synthetic version of progesterone) to prevent the estrogen from causing a buildup of tissue in your uterus that can lead to cancer.

Though a progestin acts like your body's own progesterone in its ability to counter the potentially cancer-causing effects of estrogen, your body may well be able to tell the difference. Progestins appear to be the culprit behind many of the unpleasant side effects some women experience with HT. By comparison, side effects are rarely reported among those using natural progesterone, which is derived wild yams, soybeans, and other plant sources.

But Do Natural Hormones Really Work?

Unfortunately, there have been few scientific studies on natural progesterone. In fact, scientists know little about the progesterone you make in your body, let alone the kind made in a lab. But this much we do know: Natural progesterone—which, despite its name, is also created in a lab—is chemically identical to the hormone secreted during the luteal phase of your menstrual cycle, which is the 2 weeks after you ovulate.

The reason you need a lab to intervene is that wild yams and soybeans do not contain progesterone but rather another chemical—a plant compound called diosgenin—that can be turned into a facsimile of your own progesterone, but only in a lab. Until recently, natural progesterone was too quickly absorbed to do the body any good. That's another important difference between synthetic and natural—progestins are easily absorbed. The latest breakthrough, however, is micronized progesterone. In its formulation, the particles are broken into tiny pieces so that when taken in pill form they are steadily absorbed by your body. Prometrium is one brand of micronized progesterone that has received FDA approval.

If you hate pills and are wondering about the natural progesterone creams, it's true that progesterone in this form is more readily absorbed through your skin. Studies have found, however, that it's difficult for a woman to achieve normal levels of circulating hormone by applying it to the skin.

As far as estrogen is concerned, when a woman chooses natural hormone therapy as an alternative to conventional treatment, she uses different combinations of either two or three types of estrogen (identical to the two or three estrogens that her body makes on its own). The working names for these combinations are Bi-est and Tri-est. The exact combinations and the estrogens used to mix them are prescription items prepared by a compounding pharmacist—that is, they are mixed in much the same way that old-fashioned pharmacists once formulated medications, so you get the individualized dosage ordered by your doctor. (If you can't locate a compounding pharmacist in your area, a doctor or practitioner can call in a prescription to one of several mail-order pharmacies.)

If you decide to talk to your doctor about a prescription for natural hormones, know that in general natural hormones are not as strong as the hormones used in HT, so the dosages prescribed will usually be higher. Also, as with any custom-designed product, natural hormone prescriptions can vary slightly from pharmacy to pharmacy. And finally, be prepared to work closely with your doctor for the first few months, making adjustments as necessary until you find the dosage that's right for you.

Herbs

If your menopausal symptoms are limited to a few unpleasant problems that you'd rather do without, perhaps an herbal product can help. But there are so many different herbs. A knowledgeable herbalist, for example, may draw on thousands of different healing plants, and your average health food store or pharmacy may stock dozens upon dozens of herbal products. Which ones do you need? To answer just that question, we've compiled detailed profiles of the 10 safe, easy-to-find herbs that top American and British practitioners consider to be among the best choices for problems that concern women the most in the years before and after menopause. So they're a great place to begin your journey into the ancient and nurturing world of botanical home remedies.

In this section, you'll also learn what makes each herb valuable and unique. Each profile highlights useful information about the herb as well as the botanical name and other common names. Knowing a plant's Latin name is important to help ensure that you gather or purchase the right herbal remedy because it's the name by which it will be known no matter where you are. An herb's common name can vary from region to region or from country to country, making it difficult to be sure what you're using.

You'll also discover how people throughout history—from the ancient

Greeks to Native Americans, from Europeans of the Renaissance to early-20th-century practitioners—used each herb, tracing the link between ancient healing arts and the ways women use herbal remedies today. Most important, you'll learn the specifics of what's available and how different types of herbs and herbal products can help you.

Use these handy profiles to get acquainted with herbs before you explore their use. And refer to them often to refamiliarize yourself with the herbs' potential benefits. Safe use guidelines begin on page 402.

Black Cohosh

Botanical Name: *Actea racemosa*

Also known as black snakeroot, bugbane, and rattleroot, black cohosh was introduced to early settlers by Native Americans and comes from the Algonquin word *cohosh*, meaning "knobby, rough roots." Native American women traditionally relied on black cohosh for "women's diseases."

By the 1800s, herbal healers became convinced that black cohosh was a panacea and used it to treat everything from snakebite to smallpox to hypochondria. By 1912, black cohosh was one of the medicinal herbs most frequently prescribed by American physicians.

Black cohosh supplies estrogenic sterols and glycosides (chemicals that help the body produce and use a variety of hormones) and a host of micronutrients. According to Commission E, the expert panel that judges the safety and effectiveness of herbal medicines for the German government, black cohosh is effective for treating PMS, painful menstruation, and problems associated with menopause. In fact, studies indicate that it can be as effective as hormone therapy for relieving hot flashes and other menopausal difficulties.

Black cohosh can be taken in the form of a decoction or a tincture (sometimes called an extract) or in capsules. Commission E recommends that black cohosh not be used for more than 6 months.

Cramp Bark

Botanical Name: *Viburnum opulus*

Although the bright red berries of the cramp bark bush are so bitter that birds won't touch them, humans have found a number of ingenious uses for them. Siberians distill cramp bark berries into a soul-warming brew, and Canadians substitute them for cranberries in jelly.

For women, the bark of the cramp bark has another, far more useful purpose: For 700 years, this herb has been prescribed as a remedy for menstrual cramps, threatened miscarriage, and pelvic pain, among other problems.

Also known as guelder rose, high cranberry, and red, rose, or water elder, cramp bark is closely related to black haw (*V. prunifolium*). Even under a microscope, the two plants appear identical. (For muscle spasm pain, however, cramp bark seems to be stronger than black haw.)

Cramp bark contains chemicals called hydroquinones, which have various medicinal actions, including one that combats heavy menstrual bleeding. It also contains scopoletin, which fights pain and muscle spasms and relaxes the uterus. Cramp bark is rich in valerianic acid, which has a relaxing effect on the reproductive organs.

Modern herbalists still consider cramp bark one of the best treatments for menstrual cramps. They also recommend it for heavy menstrual bleeding and menopausal flooding, as well as for tension headaches. The dried bark, which is generally regarded as safe, is usually decocted into a tea or made into a tincture (sometimes called an extract).

Dang Gui

Botanical Name: *Angelica sinensis*

One of the first Chinese drugs mentioned in ancient medical books, dang gui (also known as dong quai) dates back to 400 B.C. and is the most popular of all Chinese herbs, especially for women.

In traditional Chinese medicine, doctors treat allergies, arthritis, nervousness, and high blood pressure with dang gui, and they believe the herb has the power to prevent cancer. Because it's also believed that dang gui helps a woman retain her youthful glow long past her youth, dang gui is an ingredient in Chinese beauty creams.

Dang gui contains vitamins B_{12} and E and other active components, including ferulic acid, which eases menstrual cramps, muscle spasms, and other types of pain. Its B_{12} content, along with folate and biotin, stimulates the formation and development of red blood cells in the bone marrow, effectively remedying a type of anemia that commonly accompanies menstrual problems.

Herbalists report that dang gui regulates menstruation, eases cramps, relaxes the uterus, clears up psoriasis and eczema, reduces hot flashes, and eases vaginal dryness. Dang gui root can be taken in the form of tea or a tincture (sometimes called an extract) or in capsules. If you are still menstruating, herbalists recommend that you stop taking this herb 1 week before your period and resume at the end of your period.

Ginseng

Botanical Names: *Panax ginseng* (Korean ginseng); *P. quinquefolium* (American ginseng)

Given that its common names also include "root of life" and "a dose of immortality," it's little surprise that ginseng has enjoyed a near-mythical reputation for thousands of years. This sweet and faintly aromatic root occupied a place of honor in China's 2,000-year-old medical manual *The Herbal Classic of the Divine Plowman*. Today ginseng is still widely employed by Asians to rejuvenate themselves, increase sexual desire, and ease difficult childbirth, among other uses. Native Americans relied on American ginseng for menstrual problems, headaches, exhaustion, fever, colic, vomiting, and earaches.

Growing in popularity in both the United States and China is Siberian ginseng, which is not a true form of ginseng but the root of a plant called *Eleutherococcus senticosus*, which shares certain properties with true ginseng.

Ginseng root contains a banquet of active ingredients, including at least 18 different hormonelike saponins called ginsenosides, which botanists say fight stress and fatigue, protect the liver, and guard against memory loss. Proponents say this herb can be of special help to women by relieving stress-related hot flashes at menopause and easing exhaustion during childbirth.

The age-old methods of using ginseng were to chew the root and to make it into a tea. Ginseng, however, is now also commonly taken in the form of capsules, tablets, and liquid extracts. Experts recommend that to avoid irritability, you avoid consuming caffeine and other stimulants while using ginseng.

Lady's Mantle

Botanical Name: *Alchemilla vulgaris*

With its gray-green leaves and lacy blooms, lady's mantle has a long history of use as a "women's herb" in Europe. The plant may have first been associated with women because the leaves resemble a woman's old-fashioned cloak. Other common names include ladies mantle, lion's foot, and bear's foot.

In any case, as early as the 1600s, lady's mantle was used as an aid to conception, a miscarriage preventive, and—of all things—a folk remedy for sagging breasts. The herb was also used to heal wounds and stop vomiting, diarrhea, and excess bleeding—uses that continue to this day.

Evidence suggests that plant compounds known as tannins, which are found in the leaves and flowers, make lady's mantle an effective, astringent remedy for closing and healing wounds and, when taken internally, for bleeding and diarrhea. In its review of scientific literature on lady's mantle, Commission E, the expert panel that judges the safety and effectiveness of herbal medicines for the German government, recommended it for mild diarrhea that lasts only a few days.

Herbalists believe the astringent properties of lady's mantle work internally, making it an excellent choice for normalizing heavy periods and bleeding due to fibroid tumors. Herbalists say that lady's mantle also improves poor uterine tone, eases menopausal hot flashes, and soothes mild menstrual aches and pains. It may also be used during pregnancy to allay morning sickness.

Generally regarded as safe to use, this herb is usually taken as a tea or tincture (sometimes called an extract). It's also sometimes applied externally as an herbal wash or poultice.

Licorice

Botanical Name: *Glycyrrhiza glabra*

Licorice is a grand old herb. Favored in China for more than 5,000 years, its intensely sweet, fibrous root is still prescribed by herbalists for respiratory and digestive problems, and it is frequently used to heighten the effects of other herbs. In 17th-century England, licorice was boiled with figs to quiet coughs and chest pains, and steeped in teas to relieve constipation and fevers. In fact, licorice has been found in women's herbal formulas for hundreds of years, perhaps because it contains estrogen-like compounds.

If you suck on a slice of dried licorice root, your taste buds will quickly encounter this plant's most active compound: glycyrrhizin, a saponin that's 50 times sweeter than sugar. (Little wonder, then, that one of its other common names is sweet wood.) Structured like your body's hormones, glycyrrhizin may have a mild estrogen-like effect, making it valuable for regulating hormones at menopause, according to herbalists and scientists. Researchers also have found that compounds in licorice have anti-inflammatory, anti-allergic, and anti-arthritic actions. It is also used to ease coughs, clear respiratory congestion, soothe the digestive system, and promote elimination.

While licorice is usually taken medicinally as tea, experts advise against using it daily for more than 4 to 6 weeks. Overuse can lead to water retention, high blood pressure caused by potassium loss, or impaired heart and kidney function. You should also use this herb with caution if you are *at risk for* high blood pressure or water retention. If you have been diagnosed with diabetes, high blood pressure, liver or kidney disorders, or low potassium levels, avoid using licorice altogether.

Motherwort

Botanical Name: *Leonurus cardiaca*

One old herbal text describes motherwort as powerful protection against wicked spirits—and indeed it has been used for thousands of years to dispel doldrums and anxiety. With its dull green leaves and purplish blooms, this ancient herb "makes mothers joyful and settles the womb, therefore it is called Motherwort," according to 17th-century British apothecary Thomas Culpeper. Other common names include mother herb, heart heal, lion's tail, and lion's ear.

A heart remedy throughout Europe and Asia, bitter-tasting motherwort was used in China to lengthen life. (Legend has it that a daily cup of motherwort tea helped one wise man live to see his 300th birthday.) The

Greeks and Romans relied on it to cure all manner of physical and emotional problems.

Motherwort's leaves and flowers contain leonurine and stachydrine, alkaloids (or plant compounds) that herbalists say promote menstrual bleeding and the uterine contractions that lead to childbirth. The herb also contains bitter glycosides, mild sedatives and relaxants that may temporarily lower blood pressure.

Herbalists today use motherwort for a wide variety of "women's conditions." It soothes the stress of premenstrual tension and menopausal hot flashes. Evidence shows that it can also restore cardiac health and regulate a rapid heartbeat brought on by anxiety.

Motherwort is taken as a tea or tincture (sometimes called an extract). If you use it for tension relief, it may take about 15 minutes before you feel the effects.

Oatstraw

Botanical Name: *Avena sativa*

A traditional staple of northern European diets, oats have been cultivated since at least 100 B.C. While oats were prized as a stomach-satisfying grain, tea brewed from the herb's dried, pale green stems, leaves, and grain husks (or straw) was and still is a common folk remedy for nervous exhaustion and sleeplessness. Historically, a good soak in an oatstraw bath was said to relieve arthritis and rheumatism, among other problems.

In 19th-century and early-20th-century America, the plant ranked among the best restoratives for exhaustion brought on by a fever and for headaches associated with overwork or depression.

Herbalists report that tension headaches, insomnia, nervous exhaustion, and that "frazzled" feeling respond well to oatstraw, which is regarded as a tonic that can relieve both physical and emotional fatigue as well as depression. Oatstraw contains calcium and silicic acid (a component of silica), reportedly making this herb a good tonic for hair, nails, and bones.

Herbalists say that drinking a few cups of oatstraw tea every day can increase strength and energy and foster a feeling of calm. It's also believed that oatstraw may encourage sweating and help remedy colds. In addition, it sometimes may be used to fight yeast infections.

This herb is taken as a tea or tincture (sometimes called an extract) or used as a healing wash for skin conditions. Because oatstraw contains gluten, however, you shouldn't ingest it if you have gluten intolerance (celiac disease).

Red Clover

Botanical Name: *Trifolium pratense*

Less than a century ago, red clover was the star ingredient in home-made spring tonics and commercial health tonics alike (including a concoction called Compound Number 7), thanks to its reputation as an all-around wellness herb and blood purifier.

The Chinese revered red clover sap as a remedy for colds and influenza. A popular healing plant in England and Germany, it traveled across the Atlantic with colonists and settlers in North and South America, where it grows wild today. The red, sweet-scented flower heads were "adopted" by Iroquois women, who took the herb at menopause, and by the Cherokee and Rappahannock. At the turn of the century, the herb was typically brewed into a strong tea to halt spasmodic coughing. Mennonite communities still rely on it to ease whooping cough and croup. This herb is also known as purple clover and meadow trefoil.

Herbalists report that red clover brings on a normal menstrual cycle, promotes fertility, balances hormones at menopause when menstrual periods are irregular, calms restlessness, soothes coughing, and eases eczema and psoriasis. Apparently, the blossoms contain hormonelike substances called estrogenic plant sterols. In addition, red clover has important vitamins and minerals, including calcium, magnesium, potassium, and vitamins B and C. To make a red clover tea, soak the flowers in cool water overnight to extract the most minerals.

Vitex

Botanical Name: *Vitex agnus-castus*

To understand the history of vitex, it may help to know that its Latin name means pure, innocent, or chaste—not surprisingly, in ancient Athens women used vitex to quell sexual passion and sacrificed it to the goddess Ceres as a symbol of chastity. The medieval herbalist Gerard called vitex the perfect herb for celibates. In 19th-century France, vitex syrup was given to "suppress the desires of Venus." It's little wonder, then, that some of the other names for vitex include chasteberry and monk's pepper.

Modern herbalists don't buy the notion that vitex dampens a woman's desire; some say, in fact, that it might have precisely the opposite effect. A well-studied herb, vitex appears to work by evening out hormone imbalances that occur during the menstrual cycle. Specifically, it influences the pituitary gland to stem secretion of the hormone prolactin. When prolactin is reduced, an irregular menstrual cycle usually normalizes. This makes vitex useful for women who, month after month, experience premenstrual syndrome, menstrual cramps, and menstrual irregularities.

During menopause, vitex is recommended for flooding, spotting, severe hot flashes, and dizziness. Acne caused by menopausal changes might also be relieved with vitex.

Taken as a tea or tincture (sometimes called an extract), vitex is a slow-acting herb, so use it regularly for several months to reap its benefits. While it is generally regarded as safe, you should know that vitex may counteract the effectiveness of birth control pills.

Vitamins and Other Supplements

Vitamins and supplements are not magic pills. But let's face it: It's really tempting to think of them that way. Anything that can help you ease menopausal symptoms *and* live longer, look younger, boost your energy levels, and stave off cancer, depression, and heart disease certainly sounds miraculous or magical.

Of course, they can't cure everything. But they can do a lot. And while the reasons for taking vitamins and other nutritional supplements are now based on solid science, shopping for them is still nothing less than overwhelming—letters and numbers, capsules and tablets, row upon row of bottles in different sizes and colors covered with enticing claims that compete for your attention and precious consumer dollar.

To sort through the confusion, we've put together this simple guide of seven nutritional supplements you should consider having on hand.

Calcium

By now, it's common knowledge that calcium plays an important role in the prevention of osteoporosis. What is less commonly known is that calcium plays an important role in treating high blood pressure, insomnia, and menstrual and muscle cramps.

Yet calcium comes in so many forms, even as a supplement, that choosing among the varieties may be confusing. Here's a clue: When you're reading labels, look for the "elemental calcium" listing to tell you how much you're really getting, says Robert E. C. Wildman, Ph.D., professor of nutrition at the University of Delaware in Newark. Most labels include this listing, he adds.

If the label does not indicate how much elemental calcium is in each tablet, you can use the table below. If you're taking a 500-milligram tablet of calcium carbonate, for example, you can see that it contains 40 percent elemental calcium—which translates into 200 milligrams of calcium from each tablet. Here are the typical percentages of actual calcium in supplement products.

SUPPLEMENT	ELEMENTAL CALCIUM (%)
Calcium carbonate	40
Dicalcium phosphate	38
Bonemeal	31
Oyster shell	28
Dolomite	22
Calcium citrate	21
Calcium lactate	13
Calcium gluconate	9

You don't absorb all of the elemental calcium that's in a tablet, Dr. Wildman points out—only 30 to 40 percent (in fact, calcium citrate-malate, which is available mostly in fortified orange juice, is perhaps the best-absorbed form). If you take a supplement with food, a tablet of calcium carbonate is the most efficient way to get what you need. With supplements like calcium citrate, lactate, or gluconate, you'll need to take more tablets to equal the amount of calcium in a single dose of calcium carbonate.

All told, aim for between 1,200 and 1,500 milligrams a day if you are over age 50 (1,000 milligrams if you're not quite there). And to get the most calcium from your supplements, divide your daily dose into two smaller doses, no more than 500 milligrams each. If you use calcium citrate, lactate, or gluconate, you can take it between meals without absorption problems, and it also won't interfere with absorption of iron and other trace minerals. All other forms of supplemental calcium are best absorbed when taken with food. Avoid taking supplements at the same time as large amounts of wheat bran. Bran will move the supplements through your system before they can be absorbed.

To further aid absorption, get 400 IU of vitamin D daily from sunlight, fortified foods, or supplements; it's not necessary to take the calcium and vitamin D together.

Good food sources of calcium include milk and other low-fat dairy products, sardines (with bones), kale, and calcium-fortified juices.

Fiber

Worried about gaining weight as you go through menopause? Then pay attention to your fiber intake. Fiber is the indigestible part of all plant foods, including fruits, vegetables, grains, and beans. It is not found in meat or any other animal foods.

Most fiber-rich foods contain both soluble and insoluble fiber. Soluble fiber dissolves in water in your intestinal tract, forming a gluelike gel. It softens stools and slows down stomach emptying, allowing for better digestion and helping you feel fuller longer, an effect that may aid weight loss.

But if you're like most Americans, you're probably not getting enough. The typical diet includes only 10 to 15 grams of dietary fiber a day, but the Daily Value is 25 grams. For many of us, that means we need to double our current intake.

As far as the other health benefits that fiber provides, some studies have shown a link between high-fiber diets and a decreased risk of colon and breast cancers. Studies also have shown that people who get the most fiber in their diets are less likely to have heart disease.

To boost your fiber intake, health experts generally recommend that you get your fiber from food, not supplements. Switch from processed and fast foods to whole foods, including whole grains, fresh vegetables, fruits, and beans, and you get not only a healthy dose of fiber but also a host of other nutrients that supplements don't provide.

Sometimes, though, we can't or won't get all the fiber we need. And that's when supplements can help. Whether you're adding more fiber-rich foods to your diet or taking fiber supplements, you need to increase your intake gradually. Since fiber isn't absorbed, it can ferment in the intestine, causing gas, bloating, cramps, and diarrhea.

And if you choose to use fiber supplements, always drink at least 8 ounces of water with every dose. Fiber acts like a sponge, and if you don't drink plenty of fluids, it can swell and block part of the gastrointestinal tract.

Too much fiber can also block the absorption of vital minerals such as iron, calcium, and zinc. And in some situations, it could also cause calcium losses.

If you supplement, try to get your fiber from a variety of sources in addition to a high-fiber diet. Look for products like psyllium, apple and grapefruit pectin, guar gum, methylcellulose, and calcium polycarbophil. At your local health food store, you may also find wheat and oat bran tablets and multifiber tablets with ingredients such as beet and carrot fibers.

Psyllium is a popular and inexpensive fiber supplement that can act as a laxative and lower cholesterol, says William D. Nelson, N.D., a naturopathic doctor at the Docere Naturopathic Centre in Colorado Springs. This supplement is available in pill, capsule, and powder forms. All are equally effective, but fiber capsules and tablets are more expensive than powders.

Psyllium causes gas and bloating in some people. If that happens to you, try flaxseed, which is easiest to take in capsules or in powdered form. In addition to fiber, flaxseed contains lignans, compounds that may have anticancer, antibacterial, antifungal, and antiviral effects, says Dr. Nelson.

Be leery, however, of marketing claims that fiber supplements containing chitosan (a form of chitin, which is a component of the shells of shellfish) promote weight loss, says Jennifer Brett, N.D., a naturopathic doctor at the Wilton Naturopathic Center in Stratford, Connecticut. "I've never seen any evidence that it works for weight loss," she says. Even if chitosan did remove fat from the body as its proponents claim, it would also bind with and remove fat-soluble vitamins that your body needs, she says.

Animal studies have shown that chitosan can absorb LDL cholesterol (the bad type) and reduce lipid concentrations, but further studies are needed to confirm any cholesterol-lowering action. As for a weight-loss effect, some animals in the studies actually gained weight when they were fed chitosan, while others lost.

Flaxseed

If you're living with hot flashes, you may have been steadily filling your closet with linen clothes, that cool staple of summer wardrobes that is made from flax. According to researchers, you'd be wise, too, to add some flax to your plate. Recent studies have turned up some pretty convincing evidence that in addition to cooling hot flashes, flaxseed and flaxseed oil may improve heart health, fight breast and colon cancers, and boost the immune system.

Flaxseed is the richest source of alpha-linolenic acid (ALA), a plant source of omega-3 fatty acids, which are one of two families of essential fatty acids that the body needs but cannot make on its own. Omega-3s are the building blocks of eicosanoids, hormonelike compounds that regulate blood pressure, clotting, and other body functions.

Plus, these small brown seeds hold some big promise for combating breast and colon cancers. In animal studies, flaxseed has significantly reduced existing breast and colon tumors while stopping new ones from getting started. In one study, researchers at the University of Toronto were able to reduce tumor size by more than half in animals that were fed flaxseed over a 7-week period. Flaxseed and flaxseed oil reduced the growth of existing tumors, but a component of flaxseed, called lignans, appeared to help prevent the development of new ones.

Lignans are plant-based compounds that can block estrogen activity in cells, reducing the risk of certain cancers. Many plants have some lignans, but flaxseed has at least 75 times more than almost any other plant.

Lignans are phytoestrogens, meaning that they are similar to but weaker than the estrogen that a woman's body produces naturally. Therefore, they may also help alleviate menopausal discomforts such as hot flashes and vaginal dryness. They are also antibacterial, antifungal, and antiviral.

Flaxseed also appears to reduce the risk of heart disease and stroke. One way that ALA helps the heart is by decreasing the ability of platelets to clump together, a reaction involved in the development of atherosclerosis (hardening of the arteries). ALA also lowers levels of dangerous, LDL cholesterol and helps the body rid itself of blood fats called triglycerides, which at high levels can also be harmful to heart health.

Flaxseed oil comes in liquid and gelatin capsules, but you may want to skip the oil and just add flaxseed to your diet. The oil contains only trace amounts of the cancer-protective lignans because they are removed during processing.

Flaxseed is also an excellent source of fiber, whereas the oil has virtually none. As little as ¼ cup of ground flaxseed contains 6 grams of fiber—as much as 1½ cups of cooked oatmeal. Grind whole seeds in your electric coffee grinder and sprinkle them on cereal, add them to smoothies, or mix them with yogurt or oatmeal. You can store whole seeds in a cool, dry pantry for up to a year. Use any ground flaxseed immediately or keep it in the freezer, says Diane Morris, R.D., Ph.D., a nutritionist in Winnipeg, Manitoba.

If you choose to use flaxseed oil, try substituting it for salad dressings instead of vegetable, olive, or other oils. Never cook with flaxseed oil because it degrades quickly when exposed to heat and light. And remember to refrigerate it between uses.

To avoid weight gain, be sure to take the high calorie content of oil into account when figuring your daily calorie intake.

SAM-e

Because estrogen levels seem to affect levels of serotonin, the feel-good hormone that helps make us feel mellower and more flexible in how we react to life's curveballs, the sudden drop in estrogen at menopause can have a profound effect on some women. So imagine a natural supplement that could relieve that depression faster than prescription medications, as well as the pain of osteoarthritis.

Sound too good to be true? A nutritional supplement that has been used in Europe for years to treat depression has found its way to U.S. markets, and its benefits look promising. S-adenosylmethionine—or SAM-e (pronounced "sammy") for short—promises to work faster than most prescription antidepressants, without the side effects.

SAM-e occurs naturally in your body and helps in the production of mood-lifting serotonin. Usually, your body can produce all the SAM-e it needs—but depressed women seem to make less SAM-e, so the theory goes that by taking supplements to raise levels to normal, your body follows suit by restoring its serotonin levels as well.

While no large U.S.-based studies have been done to confirm its safety and effectiveness, experts say that you can use SAM-e with antidepressant drugs, or alone for mild to moderate depression, under your doctor's supervision. The usual dosage is 400 milligrams a day, but dosages up to 1,600 milligrams are safe. People who have bipolar disorder should be especially careful about using SAM-e because any kind of antidepressant can tip them over into a state of mania.

Look for enteric-coated capsules to protect your stomach from irritation; they keep the medicine from dissolving before it reaches your small intestine. Also, SAM-e has a better chance of working if you're getting adequate amounts of folate and vitamins B_{12} and B_6 to help the SAM-e along.

Vitamin C

In addition to abating menopausal discomforts such as heavy menstrual bleeding, vitamin C plays an important role in helping your body fight off a host of other conditions, including colds, angina, depression, heart disease, and chronic inflammatory diseases such as lupus and rheumatoid arthritis.

While the Daily Value, the amount you need to take to stave off disease, is a modest 60 milligrams a day (100 milligrams for smokers), some doctors recommend so-called megadoses of vitamin C, amounts far higher than the Daily Value, to flood the body with the vitamin during certain illnesses.

The thinking is this: Many illnesses, including heart disease, involve damage from free radicals, unstable molecules that affect healthy cells. Once it gets started, the damage can cause a chain reaction that quickly depletes inflamed tissue of vitamin C and allows the damage to spread even more.

While there is some research to indicate that taking additional vitamin C can help shorten the duration of a cold, there is little evidence to support the use of large amounts for illnesses such as mononucleosis, hepatitis, cancer, or AIDS, says Balz Frei, Ph.D., professor of biochemistry and biophysics and director of the Linus Pauling Institute at Oregon State University in Corvallis. "I'm not saying that it doesn't work or that the theory behind this isn't sound. I'm saying that there is currently not enough scientific evidence to conclude that megadoses of vitamin C provide health benefits beyond those of more moderate doses of the vitamin," he says.

While vitamin C is considered generally safe at a wide range of dosages, getting more than 1,000 milligrams a day can cause diarrhea; if this occurs, cut back until the diarrhea stops. And if you're taking a high dosage, cut back to 100 milligrams at least 3 days before a physical exam or medical tests, as high amounts can interfere with some tests, including those for blood in the stool and for sugar in the urine. Large dosages may also affect anticoagulants (blood thinners).

If you'd rather stick to the vitamins you can get from food, good sources of vitamin C include broccoli, brussels sprouts, cabbage, chile peppers, citrus fruits, collard and turnip greens, guavas, kale, parsley, red and green bell peppers, and strawberries.

Vitamin D

Open just about any nutrition textbook to the pages on vitamin D, and you'll see haunting photographs of children with rickets, a deficiency condition. Their heads are large because their skull bones haven't fused properly, and their legs are bowed because their bones are too soft to support their weight.

Rickets is no longer common in the United States, but vitamin D deficiency may play a contributing role in the development of osteoporosis, a condition of vital importance to women approaching menopause. The body needs a sufficient amount of vitamin D to make calcium and phosphorus available in the blood that bathes the bones. As these essential minerals are deposited, the bones mineralize, or harden. When blood levels of vitamin D are low, the rate of bone loss accelerates.

Bones aren't the only parts of our bodies that vitamin D befriends. Researchers are finding more and more places where it's active. Forms of vitamin D are being studied in the laboratory for the treatment of breast, prostate, and colon cancers, plus a deadly skin cancer, melanoma. One form of vitamin D, as a topical cream named calcipotriene (Dovonex), showed marked improvement of psoriasis for up to 70 percent of the people who used it.

The irony is that vitamin D is an essential nutrient that our bodies can make on any reasonably sunny day. In fact, it's called the sunshine vitamin because we can make all we need if we have enough sunlight hitting our skin.

Nonetheless, vitamin D deficiency remains a real problem in the United States, and it becomes increasingly likely in people ages 50 and older. As we age, our bodies don't manufacture the vitamin as easily. Plus, people just don't get enough of the few foods that contain vitamin D: milk and fatty fish such as mackerel and salmon.

"Most older people, especially those who use sunscreen, probably don't get enough sun to meet their vitamin D requirements," says Michael Holick, M.D., Ph.D., chief of the section on endocrinology, nutrition, and diabetes at Boston University Medical Center. Nevertheless, it is possible to get an adequate amount of vitamin D from sunlight, he says. Dr. Holick recommends that you expose your hands, face, and arms to sunlight in the midmorning or afternoon. If you live in the north—about the latitude of Boston—you'll have enough exposure if you get 5 to 15 minutes of sunlight three times a week in spring, summer, and fall. Winter sun isn't strong enough to meet your needs for vitamin D unless you live in Florida or a similar clime.

Fortunately, supplements are another reliable way to get what you need if you're not getting enough vitamin D from dairy sources or sunlight. You can take a multivitamin/mineral supplement that offers the Daily Value of 400 IU of vitamin D.

The National Research Council, which sets standard, official guidelines for U.S. health agencies, recommends a daily dosage of 600 IU for people over 70. Some studies show that people over 65 benefit from getting up to 800 IU a day, especially during the winter months.

Vitamin E

Vitamin E apparently has only one major role in the body, but that one is a whopper. "It functions as our bodies' major fat-soluble antioxidant," says Maret Traber, Ph.D., principal investigator at the Linus Pauling Institute and associate professor of nutrition at Oregon State University in Corvallis. Vitamin E is found throughout our bodies in the tissues that contain fat, including in the protective membranes surrounding cells and in their nuclei, which contain the genetic material.

Vitamin E helps neutralize molecular particles called free radicals that are produced as a normal part of reactions that involve oxygen. "A free radical is a molecule that has an unpaired electron, making it unstable," Dr. Traber says. Because the imbalance makes it "hungry" for an electron, it steals one from some other molecule.

Unfortunately, that means that another molecule is short an electron, so it becomes a free radical, which in turn strives to pluck an electron from some other unlucky molecule nearby. The effect is a chain reaction of free radical damage, kind of like a game of tag that's gotten out of control.

This game leads to trouble. When free radicals attack, cell membranes are damaged, sometimes beyond repair. If the cell contents leak out, the cell dies. Or, if the damage occurs in the membranes inside a cell, the cell's genetic material is harmed. If the membrane of the cell's power plant, the mitochondria, is damaged, trouble multiplies like a breakout fight at a hockey game. Free radicals normally generated inside the mitochondria leak out into the cell, and the resulting unrest spreads like wildfire.

Vitamin E can stop all this by donating one of its own electrons to a free radical. When that happens, there's no chain reaction. Vitamin E stops the outbreak of electron grabbing dead in its tracks. You could think of it as a referee for that rowdy game of hockey.

If you go by the research, even an exemplary diet can't give us the amounts of vitamin E that studies suggest provide protection from heart disease or enhance immunity. The Daily Value for vitamin E is 30 IU, but estimates of an optimal dosage really start at around 100 IU. You'd have to ingest 58 cups of boiled spinach, 6 cups of peanuts, 1½ cups of corn oil, or 3 tablespoons of wheat germ oil to get close to that amount.

If you are watching your weight and reducing the amount of fat in your diet, you are even less likely to get close to the DV for vitamin E. In one study of people who had cut their fat intake below 30 percent of calories, daily vitamin E intake dropped from 14.5 to 9.5 IU.

While some researchers recommend getting 100 to 400 IU a day, a number of clinicians recommend even higher amounts for people ages 45 and older and for those with chronic diseases. One study, from researchers at the University of Texas Southwestern Medical Center in Dallas, found that 400 IU a day was the minimum dosage of vitamin E required to significantly reduce LDL oxidation—a process that may contribute to heart disease by thickening and stiffening artery walls. Dosages up to 1,200 IU—which is 40 times the DV—provided additional benefits. Taking 200 IU a day did not significantly reduce LDL oxidation, researchers found. Given this wide range of results, many experts are involved in ongoing discussions about new guidelines for recommending vitamin E.

THE ALTERNATIVE ROUTE: HEALING MODALITIES

The attraction of alternative practitioners is that they typically offer compassionate attention to your overall well-being. And because, according to its proponents, the focus of alternative medicine is preventive, it can help you avoid menopausal health problems altogether. But should the need arise, you can also expect an alternative practitioner to offer a unique array of gentle, nondrug methods to try to relieve your symptoms.

Unlike the approach of conventional medicine, you can expect your prescription from an alternative health practitioner to be a highly personalized program based on your individual symptoms, history, and desires. Practitioners typically include their patients in decisions about what treatments fit since they traditionally value the roles that both mind and spirit play in the healing process.

Be alert when reading this section as to which particular methods appeal to you. Are you drawn to breath work to ease hot flashes? Are you interested in visiting a doctor of oriental medicine to ease heavy menstrual bleeding? Or are you intrigued by the idea of a yoga instructor's teaching you ancient poses that lessen depression and anxiety? If you are still unsure of where to start, your best bet is to visit a naturopathic physician (see "Naturopathy" on page 364) or a holistic gynecologist. These practitioners are skilled in the widest variety of natural therapy options. And for more information on these and other healing alternatives, visit the National Center for Complementary and Alternative Medicine at the National Institutes of Health at its Web site, nccam.nih.gov.

Acupuncture and Acupressure: Find Pain Relief and Fight Hot Flashes

Acupuncture and acupressure are two facets of traditional Chinese medicine that, according to ancient Chinese precepts, can help maintain good health by restoring the body's harmonious balance of chi (pronounced "chee"), or vital energy.

Normally, chi flows freely along invisible internal channels, or "meridians," that traverse the body. Stress, poor nutrition, injuries, or lack of exercise, however, can create obstructions in the meridians that keep chi from flowing freely. Like a stream that's been dammed, chi overflows in certain parts of the body but barely trickles into others. Such imbalance leads to weakness, and weakness can lead to disorder and render the body more susceptible to disease.

Acupuncture needles, inserted at certain "acupoints" along the meridians, trigger healing because they break up obstructions, stimulate energy, or drain energy in a meridian, bringing the body back into balance and allowing chi to flow freely again. Of course, the needles need to be in the right spots in the correct meridians to do the trick. The right acupoint can be a distance from the ailing area.

The needles are so small that there usually isn't any bleeding, except in some areas with a lot of blood vessels, like the hands. (If you see an acupuncturist, make sure disposable needles are used to prevent transmission of blood-borne illnesses. Most acupuncturists use them.)

Acupressure is an offshoot of acupuncture. According to legend, acupuncture originated with China's Yellow Emperor and his ministers in 2500 B.C. Historians, however, suspect that it evolved gradually. When the

CHINESE MEDICINE

What prompts women to give traditional Chinese medicine a try? Usually, some kind of chronic pain, says Barbara Bernie, a licensed acupuncturist and president of the American Foundation of traditional Chinese medicine (TCM) in San Francisco. "Although we don't have statistics on how many people visit TCM practitioners, experience tells me that many people first try acupuncture, one of TCM's therapeutic treatments, for chronic pain that hasn't responded to traditional Western medicine."

But traditional Chinese medicine is much more than the practice of acupuncture. It is a medical system that combines acupuncture with the use of medicinal herbs, massage, and dietary therapy. Practitioners also often recommend exercise, breathing disciplines, and meditation in the form of qigong and tai chi as part of an ongoing, holistic wellness program.

And when it comes to women's health concerns, practitioners say that TCM can't be beat. Though some of the TCM concepts seem decidedly exotic to Westerners, the fact is that they have withstood the test of time, says David Molony, Ph.D., a licensed acupuncturist and executive director of the American Association of Acupuncture and Oriental Medicine, who practices in the northern suburbs of Philadelphia.

If you choose to look further into what this ancient system can do for you, your first traditional Chinese medicine visit is likely to be quite different from the

Chinese healers realized that they could achieve similar results simply by pressing on—rather than inserting needles into—specific points on the body, acupressure emerged as another way to stimulate healing.

Like acupuncture, acupressure is virtually free of side effects. And though it isn't generally regarded as being as potent as acupuncture, it's something that patients can learn to use on their own.

What Acupuncture and Acupressure Can Do for You

While researchers have yet to explain in Western terms why acupuncture and acupressure work, the most widely accepted benefit of these treatments is pain relief. Controlled clinical studies have found acupunc-

doctor visits that you're used to. First of all, TCM uses methods of diagnosis completely different from those of Western medicine. The practitioner will do nothing more invasive than examine your tongue and take your pulse. And before she does anything else, the TCM practitioner will interview you (unlike a Western doctor, who may question you while you're up on the examining table). But be prepared to answer a lot more questions than you're used to being asked—some more personal and graphic than those that your family doctor usually asks.

"Overall, the advantages of traditional Chinese medicine fit nicely with the disadvantages of Western medicine," says Glenn S. Rothfeld, M.D., a clinical instructor in the department of community health at Tufts University School of Medicine in Boston and a practitioner in Arlington, Massachusetts. TCM excels when you have diverse symptoms that don't form a coherent picture, he says. "Western medicine will have you going to specialists who treat your symptoms independently. For example, you might see an ear, nose, and throat specialist for your sinus problems and a gastroenterologist for your stomach problems. A TCM practitioner would see all those symptoms as part of an overall pattern and would treat you accordingly." In fact, he adds, stomach disorders are especially well-suited to TCM.

ture considerably more effective than placebo, or dummy, treatment in relieving pain. Many studies have divided patients into two groups: those who have had actual treatment (needles inserted at appropriate acupoints) and those who have had "sham" acupuncture (needles inserted at the wrong places).

According to Bruce Pomeranz, M.D., Ph.D., a neurophysiologist, professor at the University of Toronto School of Medicine, and one of the world's foremost acupuncture researchers, who has reviewed more than a dozen such studies, 55 to 85 percent of patients who got the real thing reported relief from chronic pain, compared with just 35 percent of those who received the placebo treatment.

Studies show that acupuncture can also help relieve nausea, whether it's the result of a turbulent car ride, chemotherapy, or pregnancy. And other research suggests that acupuncture may help treat arthritis, asthma, bronchitis, cold symptoms, migraines, premenstrual syndrome, and tennis elbow. It may also speed recovery from stroke, partially reverse nerve damage caused by diabetes, ease bladder problems, lessen depression, lower blood pressure, speed labor, and relieve hot flashes during menopause.

Acupressure's tension-relieving potential may also explain its effect on pain and other symptoms. Numerous studies find that the body's physiological response to stress—increased blood pressure and an outpouring of adrenaline—can contribute to heart disease, depression, irritability, insomnia, headaches, difficulty concentrating, dampened immunity, and other problems that often coincide with menopause.

Getting Started:
Self-Acupressure for Good Health

You can learn simple self-acupressure techniques from a trained acupressurist or a licensed or certified acupuncturist, or from tapes or books.

Before you give it a try, here are a few pointers on proper technique and some caveats to keep in mind.

Get trim. Trim your nails before you start so that you don't dig into your skin.

Stick to the middle. Your middle finger is the longest and strongest and the best suited for self-acupressure. If it's not strong enough, try using your knuckles, your fist, or a pencil eraser, suggests Michael Reed Gach, Ph.D., founder and director of the Acupressure Institute in Berkeley, California.

Tread carefully. Avoid applying acupressure to areas with scars, infections, ulcers, or recent burns. Don't apply pressure directly over an artery or over the genitals. And go easy on the abdominal area. Touch, don't press, sensitive areas on the throat, below the ear, or on the outer breast near the armpit, according to Dr. Gach. Also, if you have a serious or chronic illness, such as heart disease, cancer, or high blood pressure, talk to your physician and a professional acupressurist before using self-acupressure.

Don't eat and press. If you've just eaten a heavy meal, wait an hour before beginning an all-body regimen, says Dr. Gach. "Many of the meridians cross the stomach, and if there's a lot of food in the stomach, the energy can get blocked, causing nausea."

Zero in. Search for acupoints by carefully probing with your thumb. Acupoints are usually much more sensitive than the surrounding area, so be on alert for sensitivity.

Make it "hurt good." One of the most common mistakes that novices make is to press too lightly. "You have to press hard enough," says Dr. Pomeranz. "Press until you get an aching sensation. A lot of people don't do that. They're too timid."

Press your fingertips in firmly—at a 90-degree angle to the skin—exploring until you find the sensitive spot. Push hard but not to the point that you puncture the skin. Often you'll feel the same sensation that you get when you hit your funny bone—part pain, part numbness, part tingle. If you have well-developed muscles, you'll need to use deeper pressure. Women often need less pressure than men. Don't press any point that's excruciatingly painful. Acupressure should "hurt good," according to Dr. Gach.

Make it last. Maintain pressure for 15 to 30 seconds per spot. Use a stopwatch or count "one thousand one, one thousand two" to pace yourself. If you're working a spot that has been injured or is painful or tense, hold it until the hurt lessens, but no more than 5 minutes, Dr. Gach says. If you're just starting to use self-acupressure, don't work the same spot more than two or three times a day. "If you do more than that, you could release too much energy in that area, and this could create blockages in other places," he says.

Do it daily. Make sure that you apply acupressure often enough to get results. Dr. Pomeranz recommends doing your regimen every day.

Alexander Technique: Improve Your Posture and Become More Aware of Yourself

Long before menopause, most of us start out with picture-perfect posture; as toddlers, we arrive with our heads up and our limbs loose. But as our bodies develop, we may slouch if we feel "too tall" or hunch our

AYURVEDA

Ayurveda is an approach to physical health, mental clarity, and spiritual ful-fillment that traces its roots to the essential religious texts of Hinduism. Imagine that one of the books of the Old Testament were a treatise on every practical de-tail of achieving physical, mental, and emotional balance in order to perfect the individual's relationship with the Divine Power, and you'll have a sense of the breadth and depth of Ayurveda.

"The most important thing to know about Ayurveda is that it treats the whole person, not just the person's health problems," says Robert E. Svoboda, B.A.M.S., an American who graduated from the Tilak Ayurveda Mahavidyalaya, an Ayurvedic school in Pune, India, and who now works with the Ayurvedic In-stitute, a training center in Albuquerque, New Mexico. "It isn't just about clearing up symptoms or even curing disease. It's also about restructuring the content of a person's consciousness so that he can be aware of the essential na-ture and meaning of life."

One of the core ideas of Ayurveda is that the fundamental energy of life ex-presses itself through the three doshas—vata, pitta, and kapha—which are ba-sically three different types of constitutions. According to Ayurveda, your doshas are determined at the moment of conception, so every person has a different mixture of doshas; usually, one dosha is predominant, and another is secondary.

shoulders to hide our chests. Later, we may succumb to fashion and wear high heels and carry heavy purses that further distort our posture.

And it's precisely these types of poor posture habits that *can* affect your life—and your health, according to teachers of the Alexander Technique, a movement-training program in which an instructor studies how you sit, stand, walk, and bend in order to correct postural and tension-related mis-takes and help you increase your awareness of how you might move more naturally.

Developed in the late 1800s by F. M. Alexander, a Shakespearean actor, the Alexander Technique helps you restore the effortless way of carrying yourself without compressing your spine, says Vivien Schapera, director of the training course at the Alexander Technique of Cincinnati.

"The hallmark of the Alexander Technique is if a movement takes ef-fort, it's wrong. What's causing you to slouch is the excessive unconscious

Of course, the constitution you were born with is affected by day-to-day factors such as your work, the people you spend time with, and the foods you eat. Ultimately, the way to a healthy constitution is to keep your doshas balanced so that no single one becomes too active or too inactive.

In the United States, there are few properly trained Ayurvedic practitioners as there are neither licensing procedures nor an accrediting board. If you're interested in exploring Ayurvedic therapies, your best bet is to choose a practitioner who combines Western medical training with Ayurvedic training or to coordinate Ayurvedic consultations with your regular physician.

If you're not in the care of an Ayurvedic practitioner but would like to try out Ayurveda's health care philosophy, you can start your path toward mind–body healing with these simple lifestyle changes, which are part of the optimal Ayurvedic routine.

- Rise early—by 6:00 A.M., if possible.
- Meditate for at least 20 minutes once or twice each day.
- Keep your diet simple. A vegetarian or modified vegetarian diet is best. Make lunch the major meal of the day, and eat a light dinner early in the evening, preferably between 5:00 and 6:00.
- Take short walks after meals to aid digestion.
- Get to bed early—ideally, by 10:00 P.M.

contraction of muscles—in the stomach, the back, the shoulders—throughout your body," she says. "The Alexander Technique shows you how to free up your body so that you stop pulling on your skeleton with your habitually tense muscles."

By taking stress off the body, the technique can help ease backaches, neck pains, joint problems, headaches, temporomandibular disorder, repetitive strain injuries, and voice strain.

People commonly walk with the head pulled back and down on the neck. This compresses the joints and disks of the neck and back disks and can lead to physical woes such as headaches, says Deborah Caplan, a physical therapist and teacher of the Alexander Technique in New York City. "The head weighs about 12 pounds, and the vertebrae at the top of the spine are very delicate," she says. "People should ask themselves, 'Could I have less tension in my neck and shoulders?'"

What the Alexander Technique Can Do for You

An Alexander Technique instructor can teach you to be more fully aware of yourself when you're walking, standing, sitting, and working. Your teacher will combine manual guidance and verbal instruction, and you will be able to apply what you learn in your lesson to your daily life. "The technique is virtually impossible to learn to do on your own," says Vivien Schapera.

The learning takes place in two ways, says Deborah Caplan. "You learn as the principles are taught to you verbally by a teacher, and you learn on a kinesthetic level by the teacher gently guiding you with her hands into applying the correct use."

Usually, the teacher puts her hand near your head and spine while you sit, stand, or move. This helps remind you to keep your head easefully balanced on your spine and helps you maintain a noncompressing posture, says Judith Stern, a physical therapist on the faculty at the American Center for the Alexander Technique in New York City.

Practitioners use mirrors to show you the difference between what you feel you're doing with your body and what you're really doing. It can be an eye-opening experience. For example, when your shoulder muscles relax, you might feel like you're slouching, but the mirror shows you standing effortlessly upright, says Vivien.

"The teacher guides you through everyday activities, such as sitting, bending, breathing, and talking," she says. "If you were a musician, for example, I would ask you to bring in your instrument so that I could see what you do while you play."

You'll also learn what Alexander Technique teachers call constructive rest, says Judith. You lie down on your back on the floor or a table, knees bent and feet flat on the surface, and learn to release excess muscle tension in your body.

"Allow your neck to release so that your head balances delicately on top of your spine, then allow your torso to release in length and width," she says. "Then you allow your legs to release from your torso and allow your arms to release from your torso."

How many lessons will you need? While this varies from person to person, it usually takes at least 30 visits to make a lasting difference on your postural habits, and most experts recommend scheduling at least one lesson a week.

Getting Started: Balance Your Body

Here are a few hints from top Alexander Technique instructors about how to put your posture into tip-top form.

Kick off your heels. High-heeled shoes are an enemy to good posture because of the way they slant the foot and throw the body out of alignment, notes Deborah Caplan. Flats with cushioned soles give the best support. "Walking in high heels jars the whole body," she says. "The foot is designed to absorb the shock of walking, but with heels the result is a tremendous amount of stress on the back."

Unlock those legs. Perhaps more than men, women commonly cross their legs and hold the inner thighs together, which can lead to back problems because of a twist it creates in the lower spine and pelvis, notes Don Krim, chairman of the North American Society of Teachers of the Alexander Technique and an instructor in Beverly Hills, California. "They're often told to keep their legs together. But keeping your legs together as you move can distort the balance between the hip, knee, and ankle joints, causing strain."

Rather than pulling your knees together after you sit down, keep each knee lined up with your feet. If you wear miniskirts and want to maintain decorum in dress, you may have to trade in your miniskirts for long dresses and slacks in order to sit correctly.

Sit up tall. Many working women spend their days slouched behind a computer, says Deborah. For good sitting posture, it's most important to have a chair that supports the lower back—one that's not so deep or high that your feet can't rest comfortably on the floor. "Slouching undermines support of the spine and weakens the muscles, stretches the ligaments, and strains the facet joints in the back of the spine and the disks," she says. "Plus, the shoulders slip forward and put strain on the neck."

Try to avoid sitting in peculiar positions. Tucking one leg under the other might give you a sense of support, for instance, but it actually causes the body to twist and contort, notes Vivien Schapera. It is ideal to sit with your feet apart and have them resting on an adjustable footrest or flat on the floor, which gives more support to the back.

Bend with care. When you reach down to pick something up, make sure that you're not just bending at the waist, says Judith. "You should be bending over so that the hips, knees, and ankles are doing the work," she

HOMEOPATHY

Developed during the late 1700s by the German physician Samuel Hahnemann, homeopathy (from the Greek words *homeo*, meaning "like," and *pathos*, meaning "suffering") is based on the principle of similars: A substance that causes certain symptoms in a healthy person will *cure* those symptoms in a sick person.

Dr. Hahnemann found that administering medicines that produced symptoms similar to those his sick patients were experiencing relieved his patients' suffering. However, the patients sometimes suffered ill effects from the full-strength medicines. He therefore set about developing a method of making the medicines safer. After much experimenting, he found that diluting and shaking the medicines could enhance their healing effects while reducing their harmful effects. In fact, the more he diluted and shook, or succussed, the medicines, the more potent they became.

Modern homeopathic remedies are *potentized*, meaning that a substance will be added to water, and then succussed 60 or more times. The mixture is then diluted again with water. The process can be repeated up to hundreds of times, until not a molecule of the original substance remains in the remedy.

The principle of potentized remedies gives even experienced homeopaths pause when it comes to explaining how their healing art works. But on one thing they all agree: It does.

"The bottom line is that no one really knows how homeopathic remedies work," says Linda Johnston, M.D., a diplomate in homeopathic therapeutics and founder of the Academy for Classical Homeopathy in Van Nuys, California. "What I do know is that my patients get better. Unlike conventional medicine, homeopathy doesn't treat symptoms—it corrects whatever is disturbing your system and producing those symptoms."

For her female patients, some of homeopathy's benefits include relief from menstrual and menopause difficulties. "I think the fact that homeopathy is non-

says. "When you bend at your waist, the spine has no hinge joints at that point. It's a real strain because the back muscles aren't designed for that kind of work."

Stand up for yourself. Long hours of sitting without a break are sure to aggravate posture problems, notes Vivien. "All you need to do is stand

---

toxic and has no side effects makes it very helpful for women's health problems," says Dr. Johnston.

According to other experts, the real benefit of applying homeopathy to the problems of menopause or PMS is that instead of taking a powerful drug on a regular basis, you can be given a remedy that you might take only a few times to regulate your system. The right remedy can end PMS symptoms entirely.

"Another plus is that unlike other approaches that have you stick to special regimens or keep journals of your symptoms, homeopathy doesn't require that women change their lifestyles to eliminate PMS," says Dr. Johnston. "Instead, homeopathy will correct the physiological problem that causes PMS in the first place."

That doesn't necessarily mean that homeopathy is the answer to everything. Homeopathy might not be the appropriate solution for all the problems many women face around the time of menopause. Vaginal dryness, for example, doesn't usually respond well to homeopathy. Plus, because each woman's menopausal problems present themselves differently, each woman needs a homeopathic remedy individualized just for her.

Homeopathic remedies may not look like any medicine that you've ever taken before. Don't be surprised, for instance, if yours is a couple of dozen of pinhead-size sugar drops, to be downed all at once, one time only. Remedies come in various concentrations, marked with a number and either a "C," for the centesimal scale, which means potencies are diluted 100 times each time that they are shaken, or an "X," for the decimal scale, which means that potencies are diluted 10 times each time that they are shaken. The higher the number, the more dilute the substance, yet the more powerful it is. Of the two units, C is more common.

And with your medicine might come instructions to avoid coffee and strong-smelling substances such as camphor, eucalyptus, and peppermint.

up every 20 minutes or so and then sit back down again. Otherwise, your muscles get fatigued and have no choice but to tighten and collapse into themselves."

Do some heady running. Most people jog with their heads back and down, says Judith. The result is that you end up pulling your head back rather than keeping it aligned with your torso and legs. "Don't move your head in the opposite direction of your legs," she says. "Keep your head balanced and your spine lengthened."

Don't hold the phone. If you're on the phone all day—especially if you're typing while talking—you harm your body by pressing the receiver to your shoulder, says Judith. Use a headset, to avoid spine compression and body contortion, she says.

Cue yourself to remember. Post notes reminding yourself to be aware of your posture, Judith suggests. "You could stick a note on your computer that says, 'Think.' You'll start paying attention to how you're holding yourself: Are your legs relaxed? How are you breathing? Things like that," she says.

Breath Work: Ease Hot Flashes and Restore Your Natural Calm

Truth be told, most of us have forgotten how to breathe correctly. Proper breathing not only helps alleviate psychological problems but also helps soothe physical ones, like hot flashes, PMS, asthma, and insomnia, according to advocates of the therapy known as breath work.

We're born breathing the right way, says C. Shaffia Laue, M.D., a holistic psychiatrist who practices in Lawrence, Kansas. The right way to breathe is deep down in the abdomen. Watch a newborn's tummy slowly rise and fall with each inhalation and exhalation, and you'll see how it's done. Unfortunately, over time most of us unwittingly switch from deep abdominal breathing to "chest breathing," in which we hold our stomachs tight and breathe shallowly.

Shallow breathing spells trouble because it delivers less air per breath to our lungs. Less air per breath means that we take more frequent breaths, but this only makes matters worse, triggering a series of physiological changes that constrict our blood vessels.

"The end result of the whole process is that less oxygen reaches the brain, the heart, and the rest of the body," says Robert Fried, Ph.D., professor of psychology at Hunter College of the City University of New York, director of the Stress and Biofeedback Clinic at the Institute for Rational Emotive Therapy in Manhattan, and author of *The Breath Connection*.

This undersupply of oxygen can leave us feeling dizzy, shaky, groggy, and ill-equipped to make decisions. A chronic undersupply of oxygen can contribute to fatigue, depression, stress, anxiety, and even panic attacks and phobias, explains Dr. Laue.

Shallow chest breathing can also contribute to stress-related disorders such as PMS, menstrual cramps, headaches, migraines, insomnia, high blood pressure, asthma, back pain, and allergies. And since rapid shallow breathing leads to the constriction of blood vessels, it can boost blood pressure and even trigger arterial spasms, says Dr. Fried.

What Breath Work Can Do for You

What makes us switch from deep, satisfying abdominal breathing to shallow chest breathing in the first place? Stress, among other things, Dr. Laue says.

When you're under stress, your diaphragm—the internal muscle between your chest and abdomen—contracts partway. This shrinks the space in your chest into which your lungs can expand, Dr. Fried explains. Your breathing becomes shallow and rapid, your blood vessels contract, and you start selling yourself short on oxygen. Since rapid shallow breathing also contributes to stress, it creates a vicious circle. Stress leads to shallow breathing, which leads to stress, and so on.

Respiratory problems such as asthma can also trigger rapid shallow breathing, says Dr. Fried. Since shallow breathing also exacerbates asthma, this, too, can start a cycle of asthma attacks, shallow breathing, and more asthma attacks.

Getting Started: Breathing Lessons

Fortunately, most of us can relearn deep abdominal breathing by practicing simple relaxation and breathing techniques.

"After people start abdominal breathing, they're less anxious, less depressed, and less stressed, and they sleep better and have more energy," says

Dr. Laue. Women approaching menopause may suffer less severe symptoms, too, once they start breathing abdominally.

The best way to learn how to breathe properly is to find a physical therapist or psychotherapist who does breath work or a doctor who can teach you breathing exercises, watch you do them, and correct any mistakes, says Dr. Laue. Unfortunately, physicians and psychotherapists who use therapeutic breath work are few and far between. If you can't find one, a yoga, qigong, or martial arts teacher may be able to help you since abdominal breathing is an important part of those disciplines. Failing that, look for a good video, Dr. Laue suggests.

If you have diabetes, low blood sugar, or kidney disease, says Dr. Fried, you should not practice breath work without your physician's approval.

First, relax. Relax before practicing abdominal breathing, and you'll find the job easier, Dr. Laue says. She suggests the following progressive relaxation exercise. Though some therapists teach a progressive relaxation exercise that actually has you tense your muscles first, Dr. Laue says that some people have a hard time relaxing their muscles after doing that. She prefers this version, in which you *imagine* tensing your muscles. Wear comfortable clothes for this exercise.

- Lie down.

- Starting at your feet and working up to your head, imagine tensing and then relaxing each part of your body.

- Imagine tensing your feet for 4 or 5 seconds; then imagine releasing the tension for 4 or 5 seconds.

- Moving up to your calf muscles, imagine tensing and relaxing those muscles. Imagine the wind blowing leaves along the gutter on a windy day. In your mind's eye, feel your breath moving the tension down your body and out the bottoms of your feet.

- Continue moving upward through your hips, abdomen, arms, and chest. While you are focusing on your heart, imagine the sun melting the snow on an early-spring day. Feel the energy of the sun melting the tension in your body and then the tension running off your body like the spring melt.

- Continue with your shoulder, neck, and head muscles, and end with your forehead. Finish by imagining yourself tensing and relaxing in a quiet place in nature where you feel very safe and peaceful.

Breathe by the book. Once you're relaxed, remain lying down and place a book on your abdomen. When you inhale, push the book upward, using your stomach muscles. When you exhale, pull the book downward with your stomach muscles. Make sure that your inhalations and exhalations are of equal duration, Dr. Laue says. "If you breathe out to a slow count of three, breathe in to a slow count of three." Practice for 10 to 20 minutes twice a day, and eventually you'll be breathing from your abdomen automatically—even when you sleep, Dr. Laue says.

Imagine. Imagery can also help you breathe correctly, says Nancy Zi, a classical opera singer, voice teacher, practitioner of qigong, and innovator of chi yi, a system of breathing exercises. Chi yi, she explains, is a cross between traditional Chinese qigong breathing exercises and the breath training that professional singers get. Author and executive producer of the book and videotape *The Art of Breathing*, Nancy suggests this simple exercise as a starter.

Imagine that your body is a giant upside-down eyedropper. Your mouth and nose are the dropper's opening, and your stomach is its bulb. With your hands on your stomach, breathe in deeply, imagining the air filling the bulb. Your stomach should expand when you do this. Then exhale, tightening your abdominal muscles as if squeezing the eyedropper bulb.

Yoga: Stretch Your Body and Ease Your Spirit

Started as a spiritual discipline 6,000 years ago in India, the practice of yoga has newly emerged as a powerful remedy for ailments such as menstrual cramps, rashes, mood swings, and varicose veins, making it a valuable healing tool for women.

The term *yoga* comes from the Sanskrit word meaning "to yoke"— that is, to join the mind and body together, says Richard C. Miller, Ph.D., a yoga instructor and psychologist in San Rafael, California, cofounder of the International Association of Yoga Therapists, and founder of the

NATUROPATHY

Naturopathy, also called naturopathic medicine, incorporates a wide range of alternative treatments—Ayurvedic medicine (a traditional form of Indian healing), botanical medicine, exercise therapy, homeopathy, hydrotherapy, massage, meditation, nutritional therapy, and traditional Chinese medicine. Doctors of naturopathy mix and match different treatments, customizing therapy for each individual woman and her particular health condition.

The way naturopaths see it, their job is to teach you how to *stay* healthy. Should you become ill, they're there to bolster your body's defenses with the best that natural medicine has to offer.

"The conventional medical approach is basically: Kill disease, kill disease, kill disease," explains Joseph Pizzorno Jr., N.D., founding president of Bastyr University of Naturopathic Medicine in Kenmore, Washington.

"The natural medicine approach is to help the person live healthier," he says. "While we may use therapies that have a direct impact on disease, we're much more interested in utilizing therapies that help support the body's natural healing processes, rather than those that take over the healing process of the body."

Naturopaths don't reject conventional medicine out of hand, however. For acute health problems such as pneumonia and for life-threatening illnesses such as cancer, conventional medicine is still your best bet, says Dr. Pizzorno. Naturopathic doctors, who use blood, urine, and other standard medical tests in diagnosis, will refer patients with such problems to M.D.'s or D.O.'s. But naturo-

Marin School of Yoga. "Some people interpret yoga as the union of different forces or energies," he says.

The physical, spiritual, and psychological aspects of yoga make it a useful therapy for health ailments, says Carrie Angus, M.D., medical director for the Center for Health and Healing at the Himalayan International Institute of Yoga Science and Philosophy in Honesdale, Pennsylvania. Physically, yoga can build strength and improve flexibility because it stretches and strengthens the muscles, she says. It's good for the spine because it loosens the back and aids good posture, such as correcting slumped, rounded shoulders. Correcting posture misalignment helps free the rib cage, allowing you to breathe more deeply. And in addition to strengthening the body's ability to heal itself, yoga can counteract negative emotions such as anger, anxiety, and depression, she adds.

pathic medicine is the ticket for chronic or less severe conditions that aren't life-threatening, he says.

Unfortunately, there aren't any scientific studies comparing naturopathy with conventional care. Even the best researchers would be hard-pressed to design such a study: Naturopathy includes so many therapies that controlling for all the variables would be virtually impossible.

The diversity in training results in a greater number of options, which is one of the big advantages of the naturopathic approach, N.D.'s say. In naturopathic medical school, students study anatomy, physiology, biochemistry, neurology, pathology, and diagnostic techniques. In addition, they take courses in homeopathy, therapeutic nutrition, hydrotherapy, botanical medicine, spinal manipulation, and other therapeutic modalities rarely taught in conventional medical schools.

Disparate as they are, all naturopathic treatments share the same philosophy: Help the body heal itself. And from the naturopathic perspective, symptoms of illness are also signs that the body is trying to heal itself. A rash, for instance, is a sign that the body is trying to protect itself from an irritant. So according to the naturopathic approach, rather than override the body's attempts at healing—as when a person treats the rash by applying an anti-inflammatory cream—your best efforts should aim to gently enhance the body's own, natural healing efforts.

"Doing yoga postures and concentrating on breathing is soothing and relaxing. And it gives you something else to focus on," says John Orr, an instructor of physical education at Duke University in Durham, North Carolina, and formerly an ordained Theravadin Buddhist monk who practiced in Thailand and India.

After people start doing yoga to relieve stress or physical problems, they gradually discover the deeper psychological benefits, says John. "In spending quiet time alone, you get to know yourself better. So yoga keeps you in touch with your physical, mental, and spiritual self."

The calm and well-being that yoga creates has been shown to counter that stress reaction, says Lee Lipsenthal, M.D., medical director at the Preventive Medicine Research Institute in Sausalito, California. "What we find is that with yoga, heart disease begins to regress and blockages in the arteries shrink," he notes. "The goal is to get people to slow down, which in turn lowers their blood pressure and their heart rate."

What Yoga Can Do for You

Women especially can benefit from yoga. It's claimed to ease the pain of PMS as well as help ease the discomforts of pregnancy, childbirth, and certain changes associated with menopause, such as hot flashes. "It is believed that breathing through your left nostril, for example, creates a cooling breath. This can be used to cool the system down and ease hot flashes," says Dr. Lipsenthal.

Also, evidence suggests that women who practice yoga are better off emotionally—less irritable and more congenial—than others. One study compared two groups: 12 women between ages 27 and 55 who did yoga postures, meditation, and breathing exercises, and 13 women who had no experience with relaxation exercises and who didn't do yoga exercises. The women who practiced yoga scored much better on self-tests designed to measure both positive emotions (such as euphoria) and negative emotions (such as excitability).

Although yoga has hundreds of poses, most routines contain about 20 different ones, with specific poses used to help specific ailments. Poses that emphasize sitting on the floor with your legs spread or lying on your back with your open legs up against a wall can ease cramps and PMS, for example, says Dr. Angus. Poses that focus on your pelvis help direct energy to the area and ease menstrual problems, she adds. Bloating, for example, is said to be caused by stagnation of bodily fluids in the pelvic cavity. When you stretch that area, you get fresh blood pumping to the underlying muscles and tissues.

Getting Started: An At-Home Yoga Routine

Which routine of poses should you choose? It all depends on your physical problems, says Dr. Miller. "There would be a different one for women with back pain than for women with bladder problems," he says. "When teaching yoga, I always individualize the postures to each person in the class." So the best strategy is to sign up for a class with an instructor you feel comfortable with.

Once you start practicing yoga at home, follow these directives from expert instructors.

Get an early start. You can do yoga at any time of the day, but Dr. Miller recommends doing it in the morning. "The effect lasts 8 to 10 hours, so you can enjoy it for the rest of the day."

Get comfortable. Using a mat, blanket, rug, cushion, or chair, sit with your upper body erect but relaxed. Take a minute to check in mentally and put aside all the things that you've been thinking about.

Quiet your mind. Each yoga class begins and ends with a few minutes of meditation to quiet your mind, Dr. Angus says. "It's about focusing the mind on one thing, like your breath or a word such as *peace* or *love*. In that stillness, you can have all kinds of revelations about what you need in life and what's true for you."

A quiet mind can help ease anxiety and depression. You come to realize that lots of things are uncontrollable and that you have to let go of what you can't control.

When clearing your mind for yoga, you should sit up either on the floor or in a chair, with your head, neck, and trunk in a straight line, and take 10 to 15 deep breaths, says Dr. Angus.

Focus. Once your body starts to relax, focus on one sound or one object. "For example, think 'so' while you're breathing in and 'hum' as you breathe out. It takes patience, so if you can do it for 1 minute, you're doing great," says Dr. Angus. With practice, you will be able to focus your mind for longer and longer periods.

Don't make it difficult. Although classes usually run 60 to 90 minutes, a home yoga routine could be effective at 20 to 30 minutes, notes Dr. Miller.

After doing deep breathing for 2 to 3 minutes, do varying yoga poses, synchronized with deep breathing, for about 15 minutes. Repeat this 3 days a week.

Don't push yourself. In yoga, the philosophy of "no pain, no gain" just doesn't apply, says Dr. Miller. "Trying to do more than your body can handle is the way that people injure themselves," he says. "You should be listening to your body the whole time."

Chapter

13

STRAIGHT TALK ABOUT MENOPAUSE

Menopause—and the years before and after—can be a confusing time, between the seemingly endless changes and the health worries that surround it. By now, you may be bursting with questions, or you may be so dazed from information overload you can't start to prioritize what you'd like to ask about. You're not alone! Readers of *Prevention* magazine—women with concerns just like yours—often write in with questions for the experts.

So here are the most commonly asked questions, with complete, detailed, up-to-the-minute answers from specialists like Mary Jane Minkin, M.D., a board-certified obstetrician-gynecologist in New Haven, Connecticut, clinical professor at Yale University School of Medicine, and coauthor of *What Every Woman Needs to Know about Menopause*; Pamela M. Peeke, M.D., assistant clinical professor of medicine at the University of Maryland School of Medicine in Baltimore, *Prevention* magazine advisor, and author of *Fight Fat after Forty*; and Toby Hanlon, Ed.D., women's health editor for *Prevention* magazine.

Predicting Menopause

Q: "Is there a test that tells me if I'm menopausal and should be taking estrogen replacement therapy?"

A: *Dr. Minkin replies:* Tests measuring blood levels of estradiol and follicle-stimulating hormone (FSH) are often used to gauge a woman's menopausal status. But neither test tells you absolutely whether you are menopausal or how far along in the process you are.

Why Tests Fall Short

The only sure way to confirm menopause is by determining when you've gone 12 consecutive months without a menstrual period. If you've reached that point and are also having hot flashes, night sweats, and sleep disturbances, you've probably reached menopause. I don't need a test to confirm that.

But what about a woman in her forties who is having irregular periods and hot flashes and suspects she's headed in the direction of menopause? I don't recommend testing estradiol and FSH levels in this case. They are so variable from day to day and week to week in women approaching menopause that whatever levels you get on a particular day aren't necessarily conclusive. You'd have to repeat the test over time to get any valid results. And neither of these tests can tell you whether you're finished forever with your periods. (*A word of caution:* An elevated FSH and skipped periods for 3 or 4 months doesn't mean you can stop using birth control.)

So although the tests themselves (including the new at-home menopause test) give you legitimate values, I don't think they tell you what you want to know any better than I can from your history and the symptoms you're having.

Making the ERT Decision

Neither the estradiol test nor the FSH test will tell you whether you should take estrogen replacement therapy (ERT). Only you and your health care provider can decide that, depending on symptoms you may be having, such as hot flashes, night sweats, or vaginal dryness, as well as other health concerns, such as your risk for osteoporosis.

Time to Get off the Pill

Q: "I'm almost 50 years old and thinking of stopping birth control pills. I want to see what my periods are like and determine if I'm nearing menopause. How long do I have to stay off the Pill to tell?"

A: *Dr. Minkin replies*: You'll have to wait several weeks to see whether or not you get a period and monitor any symptoms, such as hot flashes. However, the best sign that you've officially reached menopause is when 12 consecutive months have passed without a period.

After you've been off the Pill for several weeks, ask your doctor to do a blood test of your follicle-stimulating hormone (FSH) level to get some idea of where you stand. Keep in mind that your FSH level can fluctuate from day to day as you approach menopause, so one test is not going to give you a sure answer to how close you are to menopause.

HOT FLASH: Don't go off birth control pills in the summer. "If you get hot, you won't know if it's due to the weather or hot flashes," says Dr. Minkin. It's best to go off the Pill during the winter months.

Am I There Yet?

Q: "Since I'm on the Pill and my periods are regular, is there another way to tell whether I'm nearing menopause?"

A: *Dr. Minkin replies*: The first clue for most women that they're peri-menopausal (in the transition to menopause) is that their menstrual cycles become irregular. Their periods may occur more often, the flow may be lighter or heavier, or they may begin to skip periods altogether. But in your case, because birth control pills are so good at regulating the menstrual cycle, you won't have the benefit of these changes to help guide you. Watch for these signs instead.

Look for Other Clues

During the week you're off the Pill and taking the placebo pills, you may begin to experience symptoms such as hot flashes, night sweats, or insomnia. These signs of estrogen withdrawal occur because you're not getting estrogen this week, and your body's own estrogen levels are fluctuating. Those women who are especially sensitive to changing hormone levels may report headaches during this week as well because without the relaxation effect of estrogen, blood vessels constrict.

A second way to gauge where you are hormonally is your age. The average age of menopause in the United States is 51, so you could simply stop taking the Pill and see what happens. Be sure to use another form of birth control in the meantime. (Note that smoking can accelerate menopause by about 2 years due to its toxic effect on the ovaries.)

Another test is your mother's age at the time she began menopause. This can be a reliable predictor of when you will go through it, provided that hers was a natural menopause and not the result of a hysterectomy.

Confirming Menopause

The true sign that you've officially reached menopause is when you've gone without a period for 12 consecutive months. The only way to know this for certain is to stop taking birth control pills.

Some women will request that I check their follicle-stimulating hormone (FSH) level with a blood test. (As your ovaries taper off the production of estrogen, your pituitary gland sends a message to them in the form of a burst of FSH to increase estrogen production.) A woman's FSH levels can fluctuate enormously during perimenopause, so just a single reading isn't conclusive. But it may give you some indication of where you are. Just make sure you've stopped taking the Pill for at least 3 to 4 weeks before the test because it can affect FSH levels and the accuracy of the reading.

But multiple FSH readings over a period of several months are needed for the most accurate results. (This can get pricey if your insurance does not cover the cost of the tests.) This means you need to stop taking birth control pills during this time.

A high FSH—one that falls in the range of 40 to 50 mIU/ml (micro international units per milliliter)—especially if you're having hot flashes or night sweats, could mean you're headed in the direction of menopause.

Too Old for Birth Control Pills?

Q: "I'm in my fifties and have been experiencing irregular periods, menstrual cramping, and other symptoms of perimenopause. My gynecologist prescribed birth control pills. But I'm wondering, am I too old to start taking them?"

A: *Dr. Minkin replies*: Today's superlow-dose pills, containing just 20 micrograms of estrogen, are very safe for healthy, nonsmoking women to use into their early fifties. They ease PMS and menstrual cramps and regulate menstrual changes due to perimenopause. Many women start using the Pill in their forties just to ease irregular bleeding, hot flashes, and sleep disturbances.

However, birth control pills don't prevent sexually transmitted diseases and should not be taken if you smoke, have a personal or strong family history of strokes or blood clots, have active liver disease or hepatitis, or have a personal history of breast cancer.

6 Symptoms You Shouldn't Ignore

Q: "How do I know if my symptoms are caused by menopause, or if I may have a serious disease?"

A: *Toby Hanlon replies:* If you're troubled by hot flashes, skipped periods, achy joints, and mood swings, don't let your doc send you home with a flip "It's only menopause." It could be something more serious.

When I'm out to dinner with my friends Jill and Rande, "I don't remember" or "What's his name?" is a normal part of our conversation. Not surprising for a trio of 50-something women, all of who can claim to be "menopausal." We joke about these "memory adventures," our "mature" skin, and "power surges," as we affectionately call hot flashes.

Tempting as it is to assume that every subtle and not-so-subtle change in your body is just one more thing along for the ride in this host of menopausal symptoms, in fact they could be signs of something more serious.

"When a woman is of the right age for menopause, there's almost a knee-jerk reaction on the part of doctors to attribute any symptom to menopause and not investigate other causes," says James A. Simon, M.D., clinical professor of obstetrics and gynecology at George Washington University School of Medicine and Health Sciences in Washington, D.C.

This "go home, it's just menopause" response is all too common when it comes to women 40 to 60, according to Marianne J. Legato, M.D., founder and director of the Partnership for Women's Health at Columbia University in New York City. "Dismissing or minimizing women's complaints as menopause or 'it's all in your head' puts them at risk for a serious underlying condition going undiagnosed," explains Dr. Legato.

Here's a look at six well-known symptoms associated with menopause, and how to know when you or your doctor shouldn't write them off as menopause.

Changes in Periods

Irregular menstrual periods, one of the most common and predictable signs of menopause, most often occur because of the erratic levels of estrogen and progesterone and because of less frequent ovulation. Every woman has a unique pattern to her periods and knows what's normal for her. But as you approach menopause, what's normal can seem to take on a whole new definition.

"We expect periods to become irregular and differ from a woman's usual pattern," says menopause specialist Jennifer L. Prouty of Fall River, Massachusetts, a registered nurse and chairperson of the consumer education committee for the North American Menopause Society. "But if something isn't familiar to you and represents a change, you need to see a health provider to check it out," she warns.

Irregular means periods with bleeding that is lighter or heavier than usual, periods that are closer together, bleeding for fewer or more days than usual, or missed periods altogether.

Keeping a diary to track changes in your menstrual pattern is a good idea so you can see when and where changes occur and tell your health provider, she says.

It May Be Menopause, But . . .

Menstrual changes that are considered abnormal and need to be checked out include:

- Periods that are very heavy and gushing (flooding), or bleeding with clots

- Periods that last more than 7 days, or 2 or more days longer than usual

- Spotting between periods
- Bleeding after intercourse
- Fewer than 21 days between periods

"Frequently, these symptoms are left unquestioned and untreated for an inordinate amount of time," says Dr. Simon, when in fact they could signal a hormonal imbalance, thyroid disease, uterine fibroids (enlarged by the surge of estrogen as you approach menopause), uterine polyps (noncancerous growths in the endometrium), or even cervical or uterine cancer.

Getting the right diagnosis is crucial if you want to avoid unnecessary procedures such as a hysterectomy, says Michelle Warren, M.D., medical director of the Center for Menopause, Hormonal Disorders, and Women's Health at Columbia University in New York City.

Your doctor will want to know what triggers the bleeding and what makes it stop. Tests used to help determine the cause of abnormal bleeding include a Pap test; a transvaginal ultrasound, which uses sound waves to visualize the uterus and other pelvic organs with a probe inserted into the vagina; endometrial biopsy, in which a small sample of the uterine lining is removed and examined; and hysteroscopy, where a tiny telescope is inserted into the vagina and through the cervix to look directly at the uterine lining.

Hot Flashes

Hot flashes or flushes are the second-most-frequent symptom associated with menopause. When they occur with often drenching perspiration during the night, they're called night sweats.

Hot flashes are the body's way of cooling itself down. Abrupt changes in the body's "thermostat" in the brain can cause it to mistakenly sense that you're too warm. So blood vessels dilate and blood rushes to the surface of the skin to cool the body. That's why you get the red, flushed look on your face and neck. Sweating, which sometimes accompanies a hot flash, also cools the body as the perspiration evaporates.

It May Be Menopause, But . . .

"What I see most frequently misdiagnosed as menopause is hyperthyroidism," says Dr. Warren. That's because its symptoms, which can include flushing, sweating, heat intolerance, heart palpitations, and sleeplessness, can easily be confused with those of menopause.

In hyperthyroidism, the thyroid produces excess amounts of the thyroid hormone thyroxine, overstimulating organs as a result and speeding up many of the body's functions. If left untreated, an overactive thyroid can cause a loss of bone mineral density, which, over time, can lead to osteoporosis. Hyperthyroidism can also result in an irregular heartbeat, which can lead to stroke or heart failure.

Unintended weight loss almost always accompanies an overactive thyroid. So if you're losing weight but not dieting, your heart frequently beats rapidly, or you're always hot even when people around you are cold, don't just blame menopause. "There's a difference between the intermittent flushing and sweating associated with menopause and being hot and sweating all the time that is not menopause," cautions Dr. Simon.

A simple blood test that measures TSH (thyroid-stimulating hormone) will diagnose hyperthyroidism. (It is more accurate than older tests.) TSH, which is made by the pituitary gland, regulates the amount of thyroid hormone that is released into the blood. When the thyroid gland produces too much thyroid hormone, the pituitary compensates by pumping out less TSH. So a TSH level below normal could be a warning sign.

In some cases, hot flashes and sweating can be indicative of an infectious disease such as tuberculosis, Lyme disease, or AIDS. If you also feel sick, your doctor should suspect an infection. "When you're having menopausal hot flashes, you may feel tired because you haven't had a good night's sleep, but you shouldn't feel sick," says Dr. Simon.

Sweating along with a fever could also be caused by cancer such as leukemia or lymphomas. A rare tumor of the adrenal gland called a pheochromocytoma and one that usually occurs in the intestine, called a carcinoid tumor, can cause flushing and feelings of warmth, too, which could be mistaken for menopause symptoms.

Hair Loss

"Once a day, I hear 'I'm losing my hair. Is it menopause?'" says Dr. Minkin. There may well be a connection between dwindling estrogen levels at menopause and thinning hair, but there's no conclusive data.

It May Be Menopause, But . . .

"I'm more concerned that it could be a sign of an underactive thyroid, or hypothyroidism," Dr. Minkin explains. The symptoms are caused by the low levels of thyroxine being produced by the thyroid and circulating through the body. Even subtle changes in thyroid function can affect hair. Complaints of dry skin or brittle nails are also common when the culprit is hypothyroidism.

Women are five times likelier than men to have a thyroid disorder, and it's particularly common as we age. Women between ages 30 and 50 are most typically affected with hypothyroidism, and it's estimated that 10 percent of women 40 and older with the condition go undiagnosed. That's one reason that the American Association of Clinical Endocrinologists recommends that all women over age 40 have a screening TSH test.

Other symptoms of an underactive thyroid also can be easily mistaken for signs of menopause: heavy menstrual bleeding, fatigue, painful joints, mood swings, and weight gain. "Don't let your doctor dismiss these types of symptoms with 'What do you expect at your age?'" warns Dr. Legato. Ask for a TSH test. That way, you can avoid being given a prescription for estrogen therapy when you really need a prescription for thyroid hormone.

If hypothyroidism is not treated, it can raise your cholesterol and increase your risk of heart disease. It can also lead to a decline in memory and concentration.

Achy Joints

The Japanese don't have a word for hot flashes, but they have one for sore shoulders. Joint pain and stiffness are common but not well-recognized symptoms of menopause, says Dr. Warren, because studies have not found a direct link between achy joints and the "change of life." "I see women who have joint pain when they begin having irregular menstrual cycles," says Jennifer Prouty, "and I have to wonder if there is a connection."

We know that a lack of estrogen affects bone and probably cartilage, too, according to John Klippel, M.D., medical director of the Arthritis Foundation in Atlanta. That could explain why osteoarthritis affects mostly women and typically begins when they're in their mid to late forties.

It May Be Menopause, But . . .

Usually joint pain or stiffness associated with menopause isn't localized to a specific joint but is described more as an overall achiness. The pain and stiffness also don't "migrate," or show up in your elbow one day and your knee the next.

But pain in key joints such as the hips, knees, lower back, or end joints of the fingers is most likely not menopause but osteoarthritis. "Osteoarthritis has a pattern to it, so you'll have pain or stiffness when you get up in the morning or after using a joint for a long period of time," explains Dr. Klippel.

See a doctor if the joint pain persists or is accompanied by swelling, or if you have difficulty using the joint. Other causes of joint pain should be ruled out, such as rheumatoid arthritis, fibromyalgia, lupus, and Lyme disease.

Depression

"I'm very depressed, and I know it's menopause" is a complaint that Dr. Minkin hears several times a day from her patients.

We know from studies that giving estrogen to women during perimenopause (the transition to menopause during which menstrual periods become irregular and hot flashes may start) helps reduce their depression. Other studies have suggested that estrogen improves mood in postmenopausal women who feel depressed.

But researchers are still trying to figure out the relationship between estrogen and mood. "There's a growing body of evidence suggesting that neurotransmitters or chemicals in the brain that are associated with mood work better with ample estrogen and may even require estrogen to work properly," explains Dr. Simon.

This doesn't mean that depression is inevitable at menopause, but when it does occur, it should be taken seriously and investigated.

It May Be Menopause, But . . .

The most obvious culprits are untreated hot flashes and night sweats. They can leave you feeling irritable and sleep-deprived, which may result in depression and loss of your overall sense of well-being.

Depression can also be a symptom of hypothyroidism. Make sure you've ruled out this condition with a TSH test.

Don't overlook midlife stresses either. Caring for aging parents, raising teenagers, career changes, or financial problems often hit at this time and can affect anyone's ability to cope. "There's a tendency for women having other symptoms of estrogen deficiency, such as hot flashes, night sweats, and vaginal dryness, to make the snap judgment that their depression is hormonal and maybe they just need a little estrogen," cautions Dr. Simon. But a good assessment by your physician and some soul-searching on your part may reveal that speaking with a mental health professional would be much more beneficial.

Symptoms that go beyond normal feelings of sadness, such as significant changes in weight, social withdrawal, disinterest in life, insomnia, inability to concentrate, and anxiety should never be dismissed as "it's just menopause, and you'll get over it." You could be experiencing clinical depression, which is best treated with a combination of medication and psychotherapy.

Women with a history of depression seem to be more vulnerable to depression at menopause. So it's especially important for a physician to recognize the signs so treatment isn't delayed.

Palpitations

Palpitations can feel like the heart is beating erratically or fast, or skipping a beat, or as if there were butterflies in your chest. Usually they occur with hot flashes and night sweats, but they can appear on their own.

"Levels of estrogen during perimenopause alternate between very high and very low," says Dr. Legato. "This causes a destabilization of the cardiac rhythm, which can lead to palpitations."

It May Be Menopause, But . . .

While palpitations are usually harmless, they could be signs of a serious heart rhythm abnormality or heart disease until proven otherwise.

A revved-up thyroid (hyperthyroidism) can increase the effects of adrenaline, a stress hormone in the body, which can cause a rapid heart rhythm or arrhythmia. It's diagnosed with a TSH test.

Palpitations that occur on a recurring basis in the absence of hot flashes or that are associated with light-headedness or shortness of breath warrant a cardiac evaluation. One test that can be done is an electrocardiogram, called an EKG or ECG, which measures the electrical impulses of the heart and can show an irregularity in the heartbeat. (Your doctor may have you wear a portable ECG device called a Holter monitor for 24 hours to record how your heart responds to normal, everyday activities and to determine whether the sensation of palpitations corresponds to a heart rhythm abnormality.)

A stress echocardiogram is a very accurate method of diagnosing heart disease in women. It's an imaging technique that combines a treadmill stress test with cardiac ultrasound to check your heart's size, movement, shape, and pumping ability.

There's a danger to ascribing palpitations to changing hormone levels. "When a perimenopausal or menopausal woman says to me, 'I'm beginning to experience palpitations,' I don't want to blow it off as 'just that time of her life' and miss coronary disease," says Dr. Legato.

If it turns out that your palpitations are related to menopause, they can usually be relieved with estrogen replacement therapy.

Will Herbs Help You Ease Menopause Symptoms?

Q: "At the health food store, how do I choose the menopause products that work?"

A: *Dr. Minkin replies:* I, too, visited my local health food store recently. The women's nutrition section was filled with various herbal products, all claiming to give your body nutritional and hormonal support for menopause.

I know that many women—including my patients—are experimenting on their own with these herbal supplements as an alternative to prescription hormone replacement therapy (HRT, now known as hormone therapy, or HT) in an effort to eliminate bothersome hot flashes, mood changes, and sleep disturbances. But do they really work?

I spoke with *Prevention* advisor Douglas Schar, DipPhyt, MCPP, MNIMH, a European-trained clinical herbalist who has a sensible two-step approach for managing symptoms. His advice: Come up with a plan, then take only what you need and only those herbs that we know work. "Herbal medicine is medicine, and should never be used in a willy-nilly manner," he cautions.

He prescribes only herbs that have passed his three-part screening process. "For me to work with an herb," he explains, "it must have a substantial history of use, scientific validation that it's effective, and consensus among herbal practitioners that it works." I asked Doug to share his plan.

Step 1: Hormone Balancing

At menopause, the usual orderly ebb and flow of estrogen and progesterone becomes erratic, which underlies the symptoms many women experience. Doug recommends that you choose one of the following hormone-balancing herbs. Although we don't understand exactly how they work, we do know they act on the pituitary gland, ovaries, and estrogen-dependent cells in a way that has been shown in clinical trials to reduce menopausal symptoms. "I've never had a patient fail to respond to one or the other of these herbs," he says.

Black Cohosh *(Cimicifuga racemosa)*

Black cohosh is traditionally known as the menopause herb and is one that Doug considers a hormonal treasure chest. It's been shown to be effective at reducing the severity of hot flashes, memory loss, depression, and mood swings and improving the thickness and elasticity of vaginal tissues. Even the American College of Obstetricians and Gynecologists (ACOG) in Washington, D.C., agrees that black cohosh may be an alternative for women who choose not to take HT.

How much to take: Dried root: two 500-milligram tablets/capsules. Dry standardized extract: Follow package instructions for each dose equivalent to 1.5 milligrams of 27-deoxyacteine. Tincture 1:5, 1 teaspoon; tincture 1:1, 20 drops.

How often: Three times a day.

How long: Take it for at least 3 months to determine if it's working for you. It can be taken as long as you need it.

Cautions: Occasionally causes mild digestive complaints when first taken. Do not use black cohosh in combination with HT. Women with estrogen-dependent cancer, including breast, cervical, uterine, and ovarian, should consult their physician before taking it.

Chasteberry *(Vitex agnus-castus)*

Chasteberry, also called vitex, is probably better known as an herb for smoothing out the hormonal ups and downs of the menstrual cycle and premenstrual syndrome (PMS). In Europe, however, it is widely used at menopause.

How much to take: Fruit: two 500-milligram tablets. Dry standardized extract: Follow package instructions for each dose equivalent to 250 milligrams of 4:1 chasteberry extract. Tincture 1:5, 60 drops; tincture 1:1, 12 drops.

How often: Two times a day.

How long: Take the herb for at least 3 months to determine if it's working for you; it can take several months to have the full effect.

HOT FLASH: If you experience an unpleasant reaction to an herb, stop taking it immediately.

Step 2: Specific Symptom Relief

Despite taking black cohosh or chasteberry, some women may still have hot flashes, insomnia, mood swings, or even heart palpitations. "It's appropriate to take the next step, which is to choose an herb that specifically targets a breakthrough symptom," says Doug.

Sage for Hot Flashes

Add common, garden-variety sage to your program if hot flashes and night sweats persist. It's traditionally used to dry up secretions, including excessive perspiration.

How much to take: As a tea: ½ teaspoon of dried leaf in 1 cup boiling water. Tincture 1:1, 20 drops.

How often: Three times a day.

How long: Sage works right away, so use it as needed.

Valerian for Insomnia

Interrupted sleep patterns are very common at menopause. Some women have a hard time falling asleep, wake frequently, or have difficulty falling back to sleep once awakened. Douglas Schar's favorite all-purpose sleep remedy is valerian, which has been shown to help you drift into a deep sleep and stay there.

How much to take: Tincture 1:5, 1 teaspoon in water or juice.

How often: ½ hour before bed.

How long: Valerian works immediately. It can be used for as long as is required to improve sleep patterns.

Cautions: Do not drive after taking valerian because it causes drowsiness. Valerian should not be used while taking sleep medications or tranquilizers.

St. John's Wort for Depression and Mood Swings

If the blues or mood swings persist, try St. John's wort, suggests Doug. It's recognized by the American College of Obstetricians and Gynecologists as helpful for treating mild to moderate depression.

How much to take: Dried herb: two 500-milligram tablets. Dry standardized extract: one 300-milligram tablet standardized to 0.3 percent hypericin. Tincture 1:5, 1 teaspoon; tincture 1:1, 20 drops.

How often: Three times a day.

How long: You must use this herb continually for 4 to 8 weeks for it to take effect. It can be used long-term.

Cautions: Do not use St. John's wort with prescription antidepressants. It can cause sensitivity to the sun, so use the strongest sunblock available, and reapply often. If your depression worsens, see your health care provider.

Motherwort for Heart Palpitations

Some women experience fluttering or racing sensations of the heart, or palpitations. While benign, they can be alarming the first time you experience them. (Check with your health care practitioner to be sure it's nothing more serious.) A classic European women's herb called motherwort has been used for centuries. It acts on the nervous system to calm palpitations.

How much to take: Tincture 1:1, 20 drops in water or juice.

How often: Three times a day.

How long: Motherwort is safe to use long-term.

Caution: If you're using any kind of cardiac medication, consult your physician before taking motherwort.

HT AND BLACK COHOSH TOGETHER?

Using prescription hormone therapy and black cohosh together is not recommended. "Both of them work on your endocrine system, so it's best to err on the side of caution. Choose one or the other, but not both," recommends *Prevention* magazine advisor Douglas Schar, DipPhyt, MCPP, MNIMH, a European-trained clinical herbalist. "Think of it as double-dipping, using Tums and Rolaids together for indigestion or Motrin and Tylenol together for a headache."

New Hope for Fibroids?

Q: "There's a new procedure for fibroids called uterine artery embolization. What is it, and is it safe?"

A: *Dr. Minkin replies:* There's a lot of buzz these days about uterine artery embolization, or UAE, because it's "minimally invasive" and shrinks a fibroid so it doesn't have to be surgically removed. It's being promoted to women as the way to avoid a hysterectomy or myomectomy (surgical removal of the fibroid alone) to relieve bothersome symptoms such as pelvic pain and heavy menstrual bleeding. This makes it an attractive alternative since the majority of hysterectomies are done to treat fibroids. But that argument doesn't automatically mean that UAE is better. Here's a look at what we know and don't know about this procedure.

HOT FLASH: A fibroid should be checked by a physician every 6 months after it first appears, to make sure it's not growing rapidly.

How UAE Works

UAE is performed by physicians called interventional radiologists, specially trained doctors who use x-rays and imaging techniques to see inside the body while they guide narrow catheters or tubes through blood vessels.

UAE shrinks the fibroid by cutting off its blood supply. An incision is made in the groin, and a thin tube called a catheter is inserted into the main artery of the leg. The catheter is guided to each of the uterine arteries, the main source of blood supply to the fibroid. Then polyvinyl alcohol (plastic) particles are injected into the arteries to permanently plug them and prevent blood from "feeding" the fibroid. All of this is done with the assistance of x-ray images.

Hysterectomy is the only treatment that provides a cure and eliminates the chances that a fibroid will grow back. But the desire to spare the uterus, cut down on hospitalization time, and speed recovery has led to the development of other surgical treatments such as myomectomy, which removes just the fibroid, and hysteroscopic resection, which uses electric current to shave off the fibroid inside the uterus and break it into small pieces so it can be removed through the vagina. UAE was developed to provide women with another option and one that did not require surgery.

Effectiveness. Numerous studies conducted since 1997 have shown UAE to be an effective treatment for improving the heavy menstrual bleeding and pelvic pain associated with fibroids. It has rare serious complications. The most recently published study showed a 58 percent reduction in fibroid size 1 year after the procedure, with an improvement in heavy menstrual bleeding and pelvic pressure in 90 percent of the cases.

Recovery. Expect to stay overnight in the hospital, with total recovery taking 1 to 2 weeks. Recovery can be quite painful, and you'll need medication. (The fibroid is dying due to lack of bloodflow, which is similar to what happens to the heart muscle during a heart attack.) Some women also experience cramping, nausea, vomiting, and low-grade fever for 2 to 7 days after the procedure. This is part of what's called the postembolization syndrome.

Risks and complications. Studies have found that UAE is very safe and that complications occur in fewer than 3 percent of cases. But every medical procedure has risks. Some of the ones reported for UAE include infection of the uterus, uterine bleeding, premature menopause, persistent pain, and reaction to the x-ray imaging material. Complications may result in the need for a hysterectomy.

Unknown factors. UAE is so new that there are no studies of long-term effects, and no studies have directly compared the outcome of UAE with that of any other fibroid treatments. We don't know, for example, if the fibroids will grow back. There are questions concerning the procedure's effect on fertility, which is why it should not be recommended to women who still want to become pregnant. Perhaps the biggest concern is the unknown long-term effects of the plastic particles used to plug up the uterine arteries. They do remain behind and can make their way to other organs.

A special patient registry, sponsored by the Society of Interventional Radiology, the professional organization for interventional radiologists, is collecting information regarding the safety and effectiveness of UAE as well as its effects on fertility and quality of life over the long term in order to answer some of these questions.

Bottom line. The American College of Obstetricians and Gynecologists currently considers UAE investigational because of the possible serious complications and painful recovery. I believe it's a step beyond that and has a place among your options for treating fibroids. At this time, however, I'm not a big proponent, largely because of the lack of long-term studies.

It's understandable that physicians become enthusiastic about new procedures, which give their patients more treatment options. But I'm concerned that doctors are marketing UAE to women as their only alternative to a hysterectomy. Believe me, it's not.

Choosing a treatment that's right for you should be your personal decision, not your doctor's. And a thorough medical evaluation to determine

FIBROIDS: A VERY COMMON PROBLEM

Fibroids—also called leiomyomas—are a benign overgrowth of the layer of muscle tissue that comprises the uterus. They can range in size from a pea to a cantaloupe. Between 25 and 35 percent of women have fibroids, and for most women, they present no problems. But 10 to 20 percent of women who have them suffer severe symptoms: heavy menstrual bleeding, pelvic pain and pressure, frequent urination, and abdominal distension.

Fibroids are classified by their location within the uterus. Submucosal fibroids lie just under the endometrium, or top layer that lines the uterus, and grow into the uterine cavity; intramural fibroids grow within the uterine muscle wall; and subserosal fibroids grow on the outside wall of the uterus.

Fibroids depend on estrogen for growth, which is why they're more common in women in their forties, when hormonal changes during perimenopause result in high levels of estrogen relative to progesterone. This is also the time when they can become symptomatic. The good news is that they shrink after menopause, as long as you don't take estrogen therapy.

the location, size, and number of fibroids is the first step in determining the best course of action for long-term relief.

HOT FLASH: Losing weight is one of the best things you can do if you have fibroids. It is well-known that fat tissue produces estrogen that feeds fibroids.

Ease Worry about Hair Loss

Q: "I'm self-conscious about my hair, which has been thinning on top since I hit my forties. What can I do?"

A: *Toby Hanlon replies:* You may have female-pattern hair loss, which results in your hair's being less dense and finer. Almost half of women in their forties have it, and it's similar to the hair loss that men experience: thinning at the front of the scalp or on the top of the head. But there's no need to panic.

Vive la Différence

"The good news," says Ellen B. Milstone, M.D., clinical associate professor of dermatology at Yale University School of Medicine, "is that it's very unusual for a woman with female-pattern hair loss to have it progress to the point that she will lose hair all over her head like a man."

Yet that's her biggest fear. So Dr. Milstone reassures her patients that the gradual thinning of their hair will level off. This eases their anxiety.

Female-pattern hair loss can also happen early on (when you're in your twenties), though it's more common when women are in their forties. No matter when it occurs, it's best to check with your physician or a dermatologist to rule out other possible causes, such as an overactive or underactive thyroid (hyperthyroidism or hypothyroidism), especially if the hair loss is sudden and more diffuse at the front of the hairline or on the crown.

"A woman in her forties who complains of a gradual thinning over the past few years is more likely experiencing hair loss associated with perimenopause or the onset of menopause," explains Dr. Milstone. (Perimenopause includes the years just before menopause, when a woman begins having irregular menstrual periods and possible hot flashes, and the first year after menopause. Please see "The Menopause Timeline" on page 4.)

It's not clear just how much dwindling estrogen levels at menopause contribute to thinning hair. Dr. Milstone says that based on her experience, there may be some connection, but there's no conclusive data to support it. "There are probably multiple causes, not just estrogen loss," she speculates.

What You Can Do

Despite your fears, you're not going to lose all of your hair, and this is not a serious medical condition. But since appearance is so important, it's understandable if you're a little upset.

A recent study showed that women who experienced hair loss had feelings of powerlessness, self-consciousness, dissatisfaction with their appearance, embarrassment, frustration at not being able to style their hair the way they wanted, and concern that others would notice.

Darlene Caracappa, co-owner of Styl-Rama, a salon in King of Prussia, Pennsylvania, that specializes in hair replacement, is often the first person clients meet who can relate to their fears and concerns. "Most people tell me that their hair is their crowning glory and an important part of who they are," says Darlene. "When their hair is depleted, *they* feel depleted." Women will go to great lengths to work around their hair loss and avoid the fear and embarrassment associated with it. "They may avoid being outside and exposed to wind or rain, stop going to the gym because sweating makes the hair loss more visible, or get up at 5 A.M. to style their hair," she explains. But knowing they're not alone and that there *is* a solution is reassuring.

As for the thinning hair itself, Dr. Milstone has these suggestions.

- Don't be afraid to wash your hair. It won't lead to further hair loss. (Not washing your hair can lead to dandruff, an itchy scalp, and possible trauma from scratching.)

- Avoid brushing or teasing your hair, which can lead to some hair loss. Comb it instead.

- Try a hairstyle that layers your hair; this will help it look fuller.

- Get a perm or color your hair if you wish to give it a fuller appearance. Medically, there's no reason not to.

• Consider a hairpiece to add volume to your hair. Avoid hair weaving or any other device that can put prolonged tension on your hair or cause the hair to fracture.

What about Rogaine (minoxidil), which reportedly increases hair growth and prevents further loss? Dr. Milstone says that the 2 percent strength is minimally, if at all, effective in women, and most women don't want to put a liquid on their scalp twice a day. Besides, it does require continual use to keep the hair that has regrown.

HOT FLASH: If you're considering a hairpiece, consult with a skilled specialist to help you choose the best option.

Why You Still Need Mammograms

Q: "I keep hearing that mammograms are ineffectual, but my gynecologist still recommends them. Do you agree?"

A: *Dr. Minkin replies:* A Swedish study recently found that women who got mammograms on a regular basis reduced their risk of dying from breast cancer by 63 percent. This was encouraging news since previous landmark clinical trials showed the risk to be reduced by 30 percent.

Around the same time, the medical journal *The Lancet* published a letter in which two Danish researchers reiterated the original conclusion of a paper they published in 2000 that mammograms are "unjustified" because there is no reliable evidence that they save lives. If you're like many of my patients, you're probably frustrated, confused, and left wondering what to make of all the conflicting information.

For years, physicians, public health officials, and women's health advocates have urged women to get mammograms as a means of saving lives through early detection of breast cancer. Is this likely to change now? I'll share my perspective on this and the opinions of several breast cancer experts.

A Flawed Study

In January 2000, two Danish researchers published an analysis of seven randomized (subjects are chosen on a random basis) trials of mammography screening published in the 1980s and 1990s and concluded that it didn't save lives. (Keep in mind that this was not new research but what is called in scientific lingo "a secondary analysis of existing data.") Five of the studies from their analysis were discarded right off the bat because they were judged to be of poor quality or extremely flawed.

At the time that the analysis was published, it was discredited for being flawed in its own right. "The Danish researchers made any number of arbitrary decisions and arguable judgments about the quality of the trials," explains Robert A. Smith, Ph.D., director of cancer screening for the American Cancer Society in Atlanta. They were very critical of studies that were favorable toward mammography and very accepting of studies that showed no benefit for mammography, according to Dr. Smith. The researchers based their conclusion on two studies alone, which is "just a fraction of the existing world data," adds Dr. Smith. Many experts even wondered how the analysis got published in such a prestigious, peer-reviewed journal as *The Lancet*.

Given all the criticism, last year the Danish researchers reanalyzed their findings. To no one's surprise, in a letter they stood by their original conclusion that mammography didn't save lives. This is what made news and led to the latest controversy about mammograms' effectiveness.

What most people didn't realize, however, was that this letter contained no new research findings and was based on their original paper, which had been criticized by many in the medical and public health communities.

Check the Statistics

"If you approach the issue from a scientific perspective, it's clearly settled," says Daniel B. Kopans, M.D., professor of radiology at Harvard Medical School. Scientists have looked at mammography using the gold standard of research—randomized controlled trials—studies where randomly selected women received the treatment and were compared with women who didn't receive the treatment. They found a 25 to 30 percent statistically significant (that is, unlikely to be due to chance) mortality reduction with mammography screening. In addition, many other studies have shown that mammography found breast cancers when they were smaller and at an earlier stage, which we know translates into longer survival. "In my opinion, these data have not been refuted by the Danish researchers. They just choose not to believe them," Dr. Kopans adds.

Bert M. Petersen, M.D., director of the Family Risk Program at Beth Israel Medical Center in New York City, agrees. "Different people use the same data to make their own point. I don't think we need to continue to rehash this issue."

The death rate from breast cancer has been steadily dropping by 1 to 2 percent a year since around 1990. That's what you'd expect to see, given that mammography screening became more widespread in the United States during the mid-1980s, and breast cancer therapy became more effective.

There's no dispute about mammography's value, according to Dr. Smith. "Mammography is a matter of health policy based on a legacy of very strong scientific evidence. The recent analysis by the Danish investigators doesn't change that," he says. Women should continue to have confidence in the judgment of numerous U.S. and European groups that have reached a conclusion very different from that of the Danish researchers.

Both Dr. Kopans and Dr. Smith cite the more recent study in Sweden, which is a much more realistic measure of mammography's lifesaving potential. "Mammography won't save everyone's life, but as this study demonstrated, it provides the opportunity to reduce the death rate by as much as 63 percent—twice the benefit previously estimated," says Dr. Kopans.

Still the Best Early Detector

Realistically, no physician today will tell a woman not to have a mammogram, given that more lawsuits are brought against doctors for failure to diagnose breast cancer than for any other reason. But the truth of the matter is that mammograms are still the best way to find cancer at its earliest stage. "The tragedy, however, is that there will be women who say that mammography doesn't work, and won't get one," warns Dr. Kopans.

"Four years ago, the average size of a breast cancer detected was 2 centimeters, or about 1 inch. Now it is below 1 centimeter," says Amy Langer, executive director of the National Alliance of Breast Cancer

Organizations in New York City and a 17-year breast cancer survivor. She attributes this to early detection and the vastly improved quality of mammograms today.

Given what we know about the biology of breast cancer, when there's a smaller lesion, the chance of treating it successfully goes up. "It's the difference between fighting a war against 10,000 adversaries versus 100,000," Amy Langer adds. But the benefits of mammography aren't just about finding breast cancer. "It is never unnecessary to know that you *don't* have breast cancer," she says.

Finding breast cancer early also affects your treatment choices. This is something that tends to be ignored by studies that measure mammography's worth only in terms of death rates. "The quality of a woman's life is a big deal to me," says Dr. Petersen, "and if I can detect a tumor at an earlier stage, when it can be treated with a lumpectomy rather than mastectomy,

A KINDER, GENTLER MAMMOGRAM

If discomfort or pain is keeping you from getting regular mammograms, then here's some good news. There is now a soft foam pad, called the Woman's Touch MammoPad, that can be placed on the surface of the compression plates of the mammography machine to ease the squeeze. A study presented at the annual meeting of the Radiological Society of North America in November 2001 reported that about 70 percent of the women studied said that the pad cut their pain in half.

The special material used is "invisible" to the machine, and from initial studies, it does not appear to affect the quality of the mammogram image. Some experts, however, feel that more studies are needed to confirm this. (There is no evidence so far that the MammoPad affects the positioning of the breast during the test so that as much of the breast as possible is imaged.)

But if you or someone you know avoids mammograms because they hurt too much, then ask for the MammoPad when you schedule your appointment. About 300 mammography facilities in the United States offer it. To find one near you, call toll-free (866) 460-4141.

Most of the mammography facilities offering it are absorbing the extra cost of the MammoPad. If not, be prepared to pay extra for it: about $5.

or when a patient won't need radiation or chemotherapy, that can make a huge difference in her life."

Mammography isn't perfect: It doesn't find breast cancer 100 percent of the time. Sometimes it finds abnormalities that a biopsy later shows aren't cancer. But its limitations just mean that we have to continue looking for better ways to detect breast cancer earlier, develop treatments that can reverse it, and even find ways to prevent it. "Mammography continues to highlight the work we have yet to do," says Dr. Petersen.

The message to women and their health care providers is that the Danish study doesn't alter the fact that the preponderance of data clearly shows a benefit.

The debate about mammography may never be settled to everyone's satisfaction. In the meantime, says Amy Langer, don't forgo the opportunity to have the biggest edge against breast cancer you can by doing what is within your control. "You can't pick your genes or your parents, but you can do everything in your power to make sure you find breast cancer if it's there."

Prevention magazine recommends this schedule of mammogram screenings.

- Regular, annual mammograms starting at age 40
- Annual clinical breast examination by a trained professional
- Monthly breast self-exam

If your insurance doesn't cover a screening mammogram, call the American Cancer Society at (800) ACS-2345 (227-2345) or the Centers for Disease Control and Prevention toll-free at (888) 842-6355 for information on getting a free or low-cost mammogram.

HOT FLASH: Use your birthday as a reminder to schedule your annual mammogram.

Gas and the Hormone Connection

Q: "Now that I'm having perimenopausal symptoms, I've also started developing embarrassing gas. Is there a connection?"

A: *Dr. Minkin replies*: We know that sex-related hormones like estrogen do have an effect on gastrointestinal activity. Many women, for example, become constipated just before their periods and then have looser stools once their periods begin. This is thought to be related to changing levels of estrogen and progesterone during the menstrual cycle.

Premenopausal women also have what is known as slower gastric emptying and transit time than men, possibly due to estrogen. This means that food and liquids tend to move more slowly through their gastrointestinal tracts.

When it comes to menopause, however, there's no evidence as yet that decreasing levels of estrogen result in an increase in gas. Lin Chang, M.D., a gastroenterologist at UCLA School of Medicine, has compared complaints of bloating (typically due to gas) in premenopausal and postmenopausal women with irritable bowel syndrome. She found little difference in bloating symptoms between the two groups. "There are hormonal and age-related influences on gut function in terms of sensation and transit time," explains Dr. Chang. "But the effects of menopause on symptoms of gas and bloating have not been well-studied."

Possible Culprits

It's difficult to pin down any one reason why some women experience a "gas crisis" with menopause. Dr. Chang and her colleague, Margaret Heitkemper, Ph.D., of the University of Washington in Seattle, offer some theories.

- Since estrogen appears to slow the rate at which the stomach empties and food moves through the small intestines, the decrease in estrogen at menopause could speed up both of these, perhaps leading to more gas and bloating.

- As we age and the activity of our colons slows down, constipation increases. (It's possible that changes in parts of the nervous system that regulate bowel function are affected by aging.) More constipation could mean more gas and bloating. Slower colon transit time could also mean that less gas is expelled, resulting in bloating.

- An underlying condition—such as lactose intolerance, chronic constipation, or irritable bowel syndrome—can precipitate an increase in gas or a change in transit time, or it can lead to an enhanced perception of and sensitivity to gas.

- Women at midlife may be trying to eat a more healthful diet of fruits, vegetables, and whole grains, which could increase gas.

- What you may think is gas could be fluid retention and premenstrual bloating (both very common during perimenopause due to hormonal imbalances).

No More "Oops, Excuse Me!"

Here are suggestions from Dr. Chang and Dr. Heitkemper that should help with the gas and bloating.

- Evaluate your diet to see if you are eating more high-fiber and gas-producing foods than usual, such as beans, veggies, and fruits. Increase fiber intake gradually to avoid this common reaction.

- Check for lactose intolerance. Try eliminating all dairy products for 2 weeks. Then add them back, and see if symptoms return. If they do, eat the foods in smaller amounts, include them in meals, switch to lactose-free products, or try tablets, such as Lactaid, that help digest milk sugar. (You can probably eat yogurt with live and active cultures and experience few, if any, symptoms.)

- Try Beano, a food enzyme dietary supplement used at mealtime that may help reduce gas.

- Eliminate or reduce the amount of sugar-free foods you eat. They are sweetened with sorbitol, which can give some people gas.

- Decrease gum chewing and the use of straws, which increase the amount of air you ingest.

Persistent bloating that is not associated with your menstrual cycle should be evaluated by a physician; it could be a sign of a more serious health problem, such as ovarian cancer. If chronic constipation is a problem, or if you're experiencing symptoms of irritable bowel syndrome (recurrent or chronic abdominal discomfort, alternating constipation and diarrhea), see a physician.

While we're on the subject, don't forget that if you're over 50, you need to be screened for colon cancer. *Prevention* magazine recommends a fecal occult blood test and digital rectal exam every year, as well as either a sigmoidoscopy every 3 to 5 years or a colonoscopy every 10 years.

HOT FLASH: Give your diet (and colon) a fiber boost by trading your cornflakes for raisin bran.

"Moisturize My *What*?"

Q: "I have atrophic vaginitis. Is this an infection?"

A: *Dr. Minkin replies*: Atrophic vaginitis, or vaginal atrophy, is not an infection but a result of declining hormone levels most often seen at menopause. The delicate tissues of the vagina become thinner and drier. Low estrogen can also cause the vagina to narrow and shorten, or atrophy. These changes can lead to irritation, inflammation, and painful intercourse. Here's what you can do.

Treat the Cause

Replacing lost estrogen will treat the underlying cause of vaginal atrophy by increasing the natural moisture of the vagina as well as bloodflow, making it easier for the vagina to lubricate itself.

Oral estrogen replacement therapy will treat vaginal atrophy as well as other symptoms of menopause, such as hot flashes. But you can also just treat the problem "locally" with these forms of estrogen.

- Vaginal estrogen creams such as Estrace, Premarin, and Ogen— or the newer tablet, called Vagifem—are inserted into the vagina and absorbed directly by the vaginal tissues.

- A vaginal ring called Estring is worn in the vagina and releases a continuous dose of estrogen for 3 months.

Treat the Symptoms

If you want a hormone-free solution, try an over-the-counter personal lubricant or vaginal moisturizer. Lubricants are used during sex and coat the vagina. Examples include Astroglide and K-Y Jelly. (Orgasms naturally help lubricate the vagina by increasing blood supply.)

Vaginal moisturizers, on the other hand, act directly on vaginal tissue to replenish and maintain moisture. Their effects typically last for days, and they are most effective when used on a regular schedule. Brands include Replens, Vagisil Intimate Moisturizer, K-Y Long Lasting Vaginal Moisturizer, and Silken Secret Vaginal Moisturizer by Astroglide.

Make Peace with Your "Pot"

Q: "I have a little bubble of fat between my navel and pubic bone. It was there even when I worked out five times a week and weighed 135 pounds. Is it something I'm eating that's causing it, or is there a genetic reason for why I have this 'pooch'?"

A: *Dr. Peeke replies*: The "pooch" is an inevitable part of middle age. I have my own names for this phenomenon: It's "menopot" for women and "manopot" for men.

As we get older, especially after age 40, we accumulate more fat under the skin in the lower part of the abdomen. It's usually about 5 to 8 pounds of fat that lies above the abdominal muscle wall. The fat's not associated with any significant illness or death, but if you accumulate too much of it under the abdominal muscle wall, deep inside the tummy, that's a whole different matter. Too much fat deep inside is toxic weight, which is highly associated with increased risk of heart disease, high blood pressure, diabetes, and cancer.

You can tell the difference between the two types of fat by lying flat on your back on the floor. If your abdomen rises well above your front pelvic bones, as it would in a pregnancy, you have toxic weight. A menopot or manopot, on the other hand, will tend to flatten out and fall to the side, because the fat is external. So make peace with your pot, but get rid of any toxic weight.

RESOURCES

American Cancer Society
1599 Clifton Road NE
Atlanta, GA 30329-4251
(800) 227-2345
www.cancer.org
Comprehensive coverage of all aspects of cancer and cancer treatments.

American College of Obstetricians and Gynecologists
www.acog.org
Provides the latest updates and recommendations on hormone therapy and related issues.

American Heart Association
7272 Greenville Avenue
Dallas, TX 75231-4596
(800) 242-8721
www.americanheart.org
Provides information on risk assessment, warning signs of heart attack and stroke, and much more.

American Institute for Cancer Research
1759 R Street NW
Washington, DC 20009
(800) 843-8114
www.aicr.org
Encourages research related to diet, nutrition, and the prevention and treatment of cancer.

American Menopause Foundation (AMF)
www.americanmenopause.org
Provides support and assistance with all issues concerning menopause.

Doctors Guide to Menopause Information and Resources
www.pslgroup.com
Provides menopause-related medical news, support groups, newsgroups, and links.

A Gynecologist's Second Opinion
www.gynsecondopinion.com
Based on the book by William Parker, M.D., this Web site describes the different types of hysterectomies and discusses women's pre- and postoperative concerns. Can assist in obtaining an independent second opinion for gynecologic problems that can lead to hysterectomy.

The HERS Foundation
(Hysterectomy Educational Resources and Services)
422 Bryn Mawr Avenue
Bala Cynwyd, PA 19004
www.hersfoundation.org
Information on alternative treatments for hysterectomy, coping with a hysterectomy, counseling, etc.

Mind/Body Medical Institute
Division of Behavioral Medicine
Deaconess Hospital
One Deaconess Road
Boston, MA 02215
www.mbmi.org
Designed to help women cope with menopause and its symptoms, this program focuses on healthy behaviors that can help prevent heart disease and osteoporosis.

National Institutes of Health Women's Health Initiative
www.nih.gov/news/nf/womenshealth/5.html
This ongoing study caused the latest round of controversy on hormone therapy when it uncovered dangers in estrogen/progestin therapy (using the brand Prempro) and suspended that part of the study. Estrogen therapy without progesterone is still being studied.

National Osteoporosis Foundation
1232 22nd Street NW
Washington, DC 20037-1292
www.nof.org
Includes informative osteoporosis guides, new treatments, research findings, etc.

National Women's Health Information Center
8550 Arlington Boulevard Suite 300
Fairfax, VA 22031
(800) 994-9662
www.4women.org
Sponsored by the Office of Women's Health, U.S. Department of Health and Human Services, this site provides access to many women's health publications and organizations.

National Women's Health Resource Center
120 Albany Street Suite 820
New Brunswick, NJ 08901
(877) 986-9472
www.healthywomen.org
Provides comprehensive information on a variety of women's health topics.

North American Menopause Society
P.O. Box 94527
Cleveland, OH 44101
(800) 774-5342
www.menopause.org
Provides updates on menopause-related issues; also lists support groups, physicians, nurses, psychotherapists, and other professionals specializing in menopause in your geographic area.

Power Surge
www.power-surge.com
An Internet-only support group for women going through menopause.

Prevention magazine
www.prevention.com
Turn to *Prevention* for the latest updates on menopause research and treatments and for all women's health topics.

RECOMMENDED READING

Arnot, Bob, M.D. *The Breast Cancer Prevention Diet*. New York: Little, Brown, 1999.

Carper, Jean. *Stop Aging Now!* New York: HarperCollins Publishers, 1995.

Gillespie, Larrian. *The Menopause Diet*. Beverly Hills: Healthy Life Publications, Inc., 1999.

——. *The Menopause Diet Mini Meal Cookbook*. Beverly Hills: Healthy Life Publications, Inc., 1999.

Gittleman, Ann Louise. *Before the Change: Taking Charge of Your Perimenopause*. San Francisco: Harper San Francisco, 1999.

——. *Super Nutrition for Menopause*. Publishers' Group West, 1998.

Harrar, Sari, and Sara Altshul O'Donnell. *The Woman's Book of Healing Herbs*. Emmaus, PA: Rodale Inc., 1999.

Jones, Marcia. *Menopause for Dummies*.® New York: Hungry Minds Inc., 2002..

Leonetti, Helene B., M.D. *Menopause: A Spiritual Renaissance*. Bridger House Publications, 2002.

Lieberman, Shari, Ph.D. *Get Off the Menopause Roller Coaster.* New York: Avery Penguin Putnam, 2000.

Malesky, Gale, Mary Kittel, and the Editors of Prevention Health Books for Women. *The Hormone Connection.* Emmaus, PA: Rodale Inc., 2001.

Minkin, Mary Jane, M.D., and Carol V. Wright. *What Every Woman Needs to Know About Menopause.* New Haven, CT: Yale University Press, 1996.

Nelson, Miriam E., Ph.D. *Strong Women, Strong Bones.* New York: Perigee, 2002.

——. *Strong Women Stay Young.* Rev. ed. New York: Bantam Doubleday Dell, 2000.

——. *Strong Women Stay Slim.* New York: Bantam Doubleday Dell, 1999.

North American Menopause Society, The. *Menopause Guidebook.* Cleveland, OH: The North American Menopause Society, 2001.

Northrup, Christiane, M.D. *The Wisdom of Menopause.* New York: Bantam Books, 2001.

Smith, Kathy. *Kathy Smith's Moving Through Menopause.* New York: Warner Books, 2002.

Spilner, Maggie, ed. *Prevention's Complete Book of Walking.* Emmaus, PA: Rodale Inc., 2000.

Waterhouse, Debra. *Outsmarting the Midlife Fat Cell.* New York: Hyperion, 1999.

USING HERBS AND SUPPLEMENTS SAFELY

While herbs are generally safe and cause few, if any, side effects, you should use them responsibly. Foremost, if you are under a doctor's care for any health condition or are taking any medication, don't take any herb without your doctor knowing about it. Certain natural substances can change the way your body absorbs and processes certain medications.

Every product has the potential of causing adverse reactions. Below are cautions for the herbs mentioned in this book that may be more likely than others to cause adverse reactions in some people. Though such occurrences are rare, you should be aware of what they are and discontinue use of the herb if you experience an unusual reaction. Also, do not exceed the recommended dosages: More is *not* better.

HERB	SAFE USE GUIDELINES AND POSSIBLE SIDE EFFECTS
Alfalfa (*Medicago sativa*)	Safe
Asian ginseng (*Panax ginseng*)	May cause irritability if taken with caffeine or other stimulants. Do not take if you have high blood pressure.
Black cohosh	Do not use for more than 6 months.

HERB	SAFE USE GUIDELINES AND POSSIBLE SIDE EFFECTS
(Actea racemosa)	
Black haw *(Viburnum prunifolium)*	Do not take without medical supervision if you have a history of kidney stones as it contains oxalates, which can cause kidney stones.
Black tea *(Camellia sinensis)*	Black tea is not recommended for excessive or long-term use because it can stimulate the nervous system.
Chamomile *(Matricaria recutita)*	Very rarely can cause an allergic reaction when ingested. People allergic to closely related plants such as ragweed, asters, and chrysanthemums should drink the tea with caution.
Chasteberry (also known as vitex) *(Vitex agnus-castus)*	May counteract the effectiveness of birth control pills. Do not use during pregnancy.
Cinnamon *(Cinnamomum zeylanicum)*	Generally regarded as safe.
Cramp bark *(Viburnum opulus)*	Generally regarded as safe.
Damiana *(Turnera diffusa; T. aphrodisiaca)*	Generally regarded as safe.
Dandelion leaves *(Taraxacum officinale)*	If you have high blood pressure, see your doctor first before trying dandelion.
Dandelion root *(Taraxacum officinale)*	If you have gallbladder disease, do not use dandelion root preparations without medical approval. If you have high blood pressure, see your doctor first before trying dandelion.
Dang gui *(Angelica sinensis)*	Generally regarded as safe.
Echinacea *(Echinacea, spp.)*	Do not use if allergic to closely related plants such ragweed, asters, and chrysanthemums. Do not use if you have tuberculosis or an autoimmune condition such as lupus or multiple sclerosis because echinacea stimulates the immune system.
False unicorn root (also known as Helonias) *(Chamaelirium luteum)*	May cause nausea and vomiting in doses higher than 5 to 15 drops of tincture or ½ cup of infusion. Do not use during pregnancy.
Fenugreek *(Trigonella foenum-graecum)*	Generally regarded as safe.

HERB	SAFE USE GUIDELINES AND POSSIBLE SIDE EFFECTS
Garlic *(Allium sativum)*	Do not use supplements if you're on anticoagulants or before undergoing surgery because garlic thins the blood and may increase bleeding. Do not use if you're taking drugs to lower your blood sugar.
Ginger *(Zingiber officinale)*	May increase bile secretion, so if you have gallstones, do not use therapeutic amounts of the dried root or powder without guidance from a health care practitioner.
Green tea *(Camellia sinensis)*	Generally regarded as safe.
Guggul *(Commiphora mukul)*	Rarely, may trigger diarrhea, restlessness, apprehension, or hiccups. Do not use during pregnancy.
Helonias *(Chamaelirium luteum)*	See False unicorn.
Horsetail *(Equisetum* spp.)	Do not use the tincture if you have heart or kidney problems. May cause a thiamin deficiency. Do not take more than 2 grams per day of powdered extract or take for prolonged periods. Do not use if you're taking hypoglycemic drugs.
Lady's mantle *(Alchemilla vulgaris)*	Generally considered safe.
Licorice root *(Glycyrrhiza glabra)*	Do not use if you have diabetes, high blood pressure, liver or kidney disorders, or low potassium levels. Do not use daily for more than 4 to 6 weeks because overuse can lead to water retention, high blood pressure caused by potassium loss, or impaired heart and kidney function. Do not use during pregnancy.
Milk thistle seed *(Silybum marianum)*	Generally considered safe.
Motherwort *(Leonurus cardiaca)*	Generally considered safe. Do not use during pregnancy.
Nettle *(Urtica dioica)*	If you have allergies, your symptoms may worsen, so take only one dose a day for the first few days.
Oatstraw *(Avena sativa)*	Do not use if you have celiac disease (gluten intolerance) as it contains gluten, a grain protein.
Partridgeberry *(Mitchella repens)*	Generally considered safe.
Peppermint *(Mentha piperita)*	Generally considered safe.

HERB	SAFE USE GUIDELINES AND POSSIBLE SIDE EFFECTS
Red clover *(Trifolium pratense)*	Generally considered safe.
Rose *(Rosa* spp.)	Generally considered safe.
Sage *(Salvia officinalis)*	Used in therapeutic amounts, can increase sedative side effects of drugs. Do not use if you're hypoglycemic or undergoing anticonvulsant therapy. Generally considered safe when used as a spice.
St. John's wort *(Hypericum perforatum)*	Do not use with antidepressants or other prescription medicine without medical approval. May cause photosensitivity; avoid overexposure to direct sunlight.
Sarsaparilla *(Smilax* spp.)	May speed elimination of prescription medications thereby requiring an increase in the effective dose.
Siberian ginseng (also known as Eleuthero) *(Eleutherococcus senticosus)*	Generally considered safe.
Skullcap *(Scutellaria laterifolia)*	Generally considered safe.
True unicorn root *(Aletris farinosa)*	May cause a drug interaction with some oxytocin drugs.
Turmeric *(Curcuma domestica)*	Do not use as a home remedy if you have high stomach acid or ulcers, gallstones, or bile duct obstruction. Do not use during pregnancy.
Valerian *(Valeriana officinalis)*	Do not use with sleep-enhancing or mood-regulating medications because it may intensify their effects. May cause heart palpitations and nervousness in sensitive individuals. If such stimulant action occurs, discontinue use.
Vitex *(Vitex agnus-castus)*	See Chasteberry.
Wild yam *(Dioscorea villosa)*	Generally considered safe.
Yellow dock root *(Rumex crispus)*	If you have a history of kidney stones, do not take without medical supervision as it contains oxalates and tannins, which may adversely affect this condition.

INDEX

Boldface page references indicate illustrations. Underscored references indicate boxed text.

Photo Credits

Interior photographs on pages 90 to 97 by Hilmar

Mountain pose photograph on page 173 © Kristiane Vey/Jump

Conversion Chart

These equivalents have been slightly rounded to make measuring easier.

VOLUME MEASUREMENTS			WEIGHT MEASUREMENTS		LENGTH MEASUREMENTS	
U.S.	*Imperial*	*Metric*	*U.S.*	*Metric*	*U.S.*	*Metric*
¼ tsp	–	1 ml	1 oz	30 g	¼"	0.6 cm
½ tsp	–	2 ml	2 oz	60 g	½"	1.25 cm
1 tsp	–	5 ml	4 oz (¼ lb)	115 g	1"	2.5 cm
1 Tbsp	–	15 ml	5 oz (⅓ lb)	145 g	2"	5 cm
2 Tbsp (1 oz)	1 fl oz	30 ml	6 oz	170 g	4"	11 cm
¼ cup (2 oz)	2 fl oz	60 ml	7 oz	200 g	6"	15 cm
⅓ cup (3 oz)	3 fl oz	80 ml	8 oz (½ lb)	230 g	8"	20 cm
½ cup (4 oz)	4 fl oz	120 ml	10 oz	285 g	10"	25 cm
⅔ cup (5 oz)	5 fl oz	160 ml	12 oz (¾ lb)	340 g	12" (1')	30 cm
¾ cup (6 oz)	6 fl oz	180 ml	14 oz	400 g		
1 cup (8 oz)	8 fl oz	240 ml	16 oz (1 lb)	455 g		
			2.2 lb	1 kg		

PAN SIZES		TEMPERATURES		
U.S.	*Metric*	*Fahrenheit*	*Centigrade*	*Gas*
8" cake pan	20 × 4 cm sandwich or cake tin	140°	60°	–
9" cake pan	23 × 3.5 cm sandwich or cake tin	160°	70°	–
11" × 7" baking pan	28 × 18 cm baking tin	180°	80°	–
13" × 9" baking pan	32.5 × 23 cm baking tin	225°	105°	¼
15" × 10" baking pan	38 × 25.5 cm baking tin	250°	120°	½
	(Swiss roll tin)	275°	135°	1
1½ qt baking dish	1.5 liter baking dish	300°	150°	2
2 qt baking dish	2 liter baking dish	325°	160°	3
2 qt rectangular baking dish	30 × 19 cm baking dish	350°	180°	4
9" pie plate	22 × 4 or 23 × 4 cm pie plate	375°	190°	5
7" or 8" springform pan	18 or 20 cm springform or	400°	200°	6
	loose-bottom cake tin	425°	220°	7
9" × 5" loaf pan	23 × 13 cm or 2 lb narrow	450°	230°	8
	loaf tin or pâté tin	475°	245°	9
		500°	260°	–